Becoming a Reflective Practitioner

Becoming a Reflective Practitioner

Seventh Edition

Prof. Christopher Johns
Academy of Nursing, University of Exeter

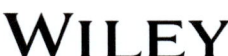

This edition first published 2025
© 2025, John Wiley & Sons Ltd

Edition History
Wiley-Blackwell (5e, 2017), 2022 John Wiley & Sons, Ltd (6e, 2022)

Registered Office(s)
John Wiley & Sons, Inc., 111 River Street, Hoboken, NJ 07030, USA
John Wiley & Sons Ltd, New Era House, 8 Oldlands Way, Bognor Regis, West Sussex, PO22 9NQ, UK
John Wiley & Sons Singapore Pte. Ltd, 134 Jurong Gateway Road, #04-307H, Singapore 600134

For details of our global editorial offices, customer services, and more information about Wiley products visit us at www.wiley.com.

The manufacturer's authorized representative according to the EU General Product Safety Regulation is Wiley-VCH GmbH, Boschstr. 12, 69469 Weinheim, Germany, e-mail: Product_Safety@wiley.com.

Wiley also publishes its books in a variety of electronic formats and by print-on-demand. Some content that appears in standard print versions of this book may not be available in other formats.

Library of Congress Cataloging-in-Publication Data

ePDF: 9781394343331
epub: 9781394343324
Paperback: 9781394343317

Cover Design: Wiley
Cover Image: © georgeclerk/Getty Images

Set in 10/12pt TeX GYRE ADVENTOR by Lumina Datamatics
Printed and bound by CPI Group (UK) Ltd, Croydon, CR0 4YY
C9781394343317_280825

CONTENTS

ABOUT THE AUTHOR

Christopher Johns

I implemented guided reflection at Burford Hospital as a doctoral study to explore its efficacy towards enabling practitioners to realise the hospital's vision of person-centred practice [1] as part of *The Burford NDU Model: Caring in Practice* [2]. A 30th anniversary edition – '*Holistic Practice in Healthcare: The Burford NDU Person-Centred Model*' was published in 2024 [3] bringing the revised Burford model to a new audience committed to realising person-centred practice as a lived reality.

Everything in this book stems from that doctoral study, the Burford model and my subsequent appointment at Luton College of Higher Education (now the University of Bedfordshire), creating the opportunity to develop guided reflection from more formal research and educational perspectives. At the university, I established reflective curriculum at post-registered undergraduate, masters and doctoral levels leading to a development of guided reflection and reflexive narrative as a distinct approach to research published by Sage as 'Reflexive narrative: self-inquiry towards self-realization and its performance' [4]. My analysis of more than 100 MSc Leadership in healthcare dissertations entitled – 'Mindful leadership: a guide for the healthcare professions' was published by Palgrave in 2016 [5]. The book showed how a collection of contextual and subjective narratives led to a deep understanding of the struggle to realise transformational leadership within transaction organisations.

In 1994, I convened the first international reflective practice conference that continued until 2015 at both national and international locations. In 2009, I experimented with a 'reflective gathering' as a more reflective type of conference with a three-day 'dialogue' held in Zakynthos.

During my time at the university, I worked as a holistic therapist at several hospices keeping a reflective journal from which I constructed an ongoing reflexive narrative spanning 12 years. The first four years were published in two books '*Being Mindful, Easing Suffering: Reflections on Palliative Care*' published by Jessica Kingsley [6] and '*Engaging Reflection in Practice: A Narrative Approach*' published by Blackwell Publishing [7]. I consider it vital that reflective guides walk the talk and live reflection in their daily practice. Dedicating one day a week to clinical practice felt vital to me, not just to write a journal but also to maintain my credibility to teach 'End of life' care from a reflective perspective.

In 2010, I was awarded a national teaching fellowship.

In 2022, I was invited to become an honorary scholar with the 'Global Academy of Holistic Nursing' (GAHN). In 2023, I joined the newly formed 'Person-centred Practice International Community of Practice CIC (PCP-ICoP)'. This is an international community of Higher Education, Health and Care Organisations and individual members interested in the global advancement of knowledge in person-centred practice. (pcp-icop.org)

In 2025, I was appointed as an honorary professor at the Academy of Nursing at the University of Exeter. I felt like the academic who came in from the cold having not been attached to an organisation for the past 10 years. The position opens the door to new possibilities to collaboratively develop reflective practices and person-centred practice.

References

1. Johns, C. (1998) *Becoming a reflective practitioner through guided reflection*. PhD thesis. The Open University, Milton Keynes.

2. Johns, C. [Ed.] (1994) *The Burford NDU Model: Caring in Practice*. Blackwell Science, Oxford.

3. Johns, C. [Ed.] (2024) *Holistic Practice in Healthcare: The Burford NDU Person-Centred Model*. Wiley Blackwell, Oxford.

4. Johns, C. (2012) *Reflexive Narrative: Self-Inquiry Toward Self-Realisation and its Performance*. Sage, Thousand Oaks.

5. Johns, C. (2016) *Mindful Leadership: A Guide for the Healthcare Professions*. Palgrave, London.

6. Johns, C. (2004) *Being Mindful, Easing Suffering*. Jessica Kingsley Publishers, London.

7. Johns, C. (2006) *Engaging Reflection in Practice: A Narrative Approach*. Blackwell Publishing, Oxford.

ACKNOWLEDGEMENTS

To all the students and practitioners I have worked with over time, especially those whose work I have drawn upon.

To all the team at Wiley who contributed to the publication of this book and who continue to support the development of reflective practice and person-centred healthcare.

To Otter.

PREFACE

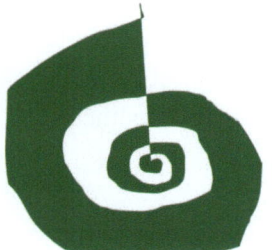

I adopted the fern as a symbol for reflective practice. It's unfurling symbolises new growth from its old roots and with its strength, resilience and enduring power.

The important thing about a book is that its ideas reach everyone.

Welcome to the seventh edition of this book. It has been nearly four years since the previous edition was published. Hardly any time and yet the world is ever changing. Writing a new edition, the canvas is already filled with words from previous editions. I approach each new edition from a reflexive perspective – how have new ideas emerged from old ones? As such, each subsequent edition is like new skin on an old animal. I have not completely discarded the old skin; its remnants can clearly be seen for the reader moving between editions, like a historian plotting the emergence of my perspective on becoming a reflective practitioner.

I ask myself – what has changed with regard to ideas about reflective practice since the previous edition? Reading through professional journals, I detect very little of significance. It is as if the dust has settled and reflective practice has 'been done'.

I imagine Plato's cave, the way the people only see what they see and cannot imagine another world. Technical rationality is the modern Plato's cave. Despite the heat of the licking flames and the hardness of the rock floor, it is a relatively comfortable place to be. I imagine the occupant's cry – 'I've found my place and I am not moving!' 'The old cliché – better the devil you know...'

This revised edition is another invitation for the reader to step outside.

Out beyond
the shadows of our thinking
a wholly different world appears;
a world of infinite possibility.

Reflective practice is being open to new possibilities. It makes clinical practice and education stimulating. Everything becomes alive. The reflective practitioner is like a new puppy, sniffing at everything, curious, questioning, turning things over, in their effort to realise their visions of practice as a lived reality. The reflective practitioner is Newton's child.

Okri [1, p. 28] writes

> 'We are like Newton's child, playing on the shore, turning over pebbles, whilst great wonders stretch out ahead of us into eternity. This is the beauty of it all. The full potential of human creativity has not yet been tapped'.

The reflective practitioner strives to reach their full potential. They open the can and play with the worms! Yet, it is so easy for the practitioner to get stuck in a rut and miss the beauty of it all. They need a guiding hand to step out of the rut and move beyond, towards realising their visions of practice. In current healthcare ideology, this vision is a person-centred or holistic practice. I use these two terms interchangeably. The vision of holistic practice and realising it through reflective practice has been the constant focus of 'Becoming a Reflective Practitioner' from its first edition in 2000.

In a practice world that becomes ever more technical and robotic with the advance of AI alongside the constant economic strain to adequately fund health and social services, the person of the patient or client and their family can easily become obscured in the organisational machinery. Through reflective practice, the persons of both the patient and the healthcare practitioner are brought into focus and attention, and with it, the possibilities of better outcomes for all involved.

Although I believe statistics are limited to demonstrate the impact of reflective practice on patient outcomes and staff morale because of the variables involved, I do offer a contribution from Ibis that suggests in 'fact' it does have positive outcomes.

They note that:

1. 70% of healthcare professionals believe that reflective practice improves patient outcomes
2. 90% of health and social care professionals believe that reflective practice improves job satisfaction

They comment –

> 'Overall, the importance of reflective practice in health and social care management cannot be overstated. It is a powerful tool that empowers professionals to grow, learn, and excel in their roles, ultimately benefiting both the individuals they serve and the organizations they work for'[i].

Encouraging words, although I do not know how Ibis arrived at these statistics. The real proof of the positive impact of reflective practice is revealed in practitioner narratives as illuminated throughout the book.

The book is a guide for students and practitioners, educators and managers, whatever their level of experience or academic achievement, to become reflective practitioners and towards realising their visions of practice as a lived reality.

I have endeavoured to write this seventh edition as previously in a reflective rather than authoritative style, illuminated through the use of journal entries and narratives. The book is not intended to be prescriptive of how to 'do reflective practice' or 'become a reflective practitioner'. What is offered are pointers along the journey to becoming both a reflective and person-centred practitioner. Indeed, I assert that one cannot be a person-centred practitioner without being a reflective practitioner, an assertion that stems from a deep conviction and considerable experience.

Structure of the Book

There are many changes from the previous edition due to giving more attention to the notion of *guiding* reflection both within clinical and educational settings, illuminated through the use of reflexive narratives. Narratives evidence the impact of guidance on enabling practitioners towards realising their visions. Their subjective and contextual nature renders them easy for readers to relate to and reflect on to inform their own practices.

The book is structured through four parts:

Part 1 sets out the basic scheme. Chapters 1–9 set out my conception of reflection, reflective practice and guided reflection. Chapter 1 offers a broad sweep on the concept of reflection, reflective practice, experience, vision, knowing in practice, the prerequisites for reflection, the reality wall and the movement of reflective learning through understanding, empowerment and transformation.

In Chapter 2, I set out the 'Six Dialogical Movements' and their assimilation within the 'Model for Structured Reflection' (MSR). Many people grasp a model of or for reflection as the essence of reflection, but that is only its technical edge. As the book illuminates, reflection is much more than that.

Chapters 3–5 apply the MSR cues in writing descriptions of experience and reflection-on-experience towards drawing tentative insights in Chapter 5. Chapter 6 is a transitional chapter between the book and 'Holistic practice in healthcare' [2] that sets out an organisational structure to develop a reflective learning culture based on the Burford NDU person-centred model notably the '9 Reflective cues' developed as a system to 'Know the person' to appreciate the pattern of a person's needs that tube the practitioner into the hospital's person-centred vision of practice. Chapter 7 considers the substance of theoretical sources to inform reflection and the development of the practitioner's knowing in practice.

Chapter 8 sets out the nature of guidance while Chapter 9 reveals the dynamic process of guidance. In Chapter 10, I apply the MSR cues to my reflection on my practice, emphasising the significance of initially working systematically working through the cues to appreciate the breadth and depth of reflection.

Chapters 11 and 12 are narratives of guiding practitioners within the clinical setting constructed through guided reflection dialogue. Both narratives extend over a period of a year. They illuminate the process of guidance and reflexive learning as the practitioners strive towards becoming leaders and realising their espoused vision of person-centred practice.

Chapter 13 is based on a leadership student's assignment to develop her leadership through establishing a clinical learning culture based on the Learning Organisation and clinical supervision.

Part 2 moves the book's narrative into formal education (Chapters 14–20). Chapter 14 offers a potential structure of the person-centred reflective curriculum. In previous editions, I termed this as just 'the reflective curriculum'. However, I want to emphasise that reflection is a means towards enabling students to realise person-centred practice, given that person-centred practice is the fundamental ideology for all healthcare curricula. It considers the necessary change process to shift towards realising the curriculum as a lived reality, considering its impact on teachers and students in shifting from a teacher-centric curriculum to a co-centric curriculum.

Chapter 15 looks at contrasting ways of teaching stroke care, one from a traditional technical rational perspective and one from a reflective perspective. It gives a flavour of difference and possibility, notably through the use of performance and cross-discipline collaboration.

Chapters 16 and 17 are exemplars of guiding first-year and third-year nursing students through guided reflection. The exemplars are grounded in real situations that I converted into group-guided reflection with nursing students. Lucy, the guide with first-year students is a lecturer practitioner, whilst Gary, the guide with third-year students is a senior lecturer. The two narratives reveal how guidance becomes less directive as students become more experienced in reflection and take more responsibility for their learning.

Chapter 18 focuses on weaving or constructing a reflexive narrative from an academic perspective using a student's assignment, 'Life begins at 40', as an exemplar.

Chapter 19 explores the creative influence of art and poetry on weaving narrative. Chapter 20 considers how reflective assignments can be meaningfully graded based on learning insights or outcomes from the reflective process rather than how the student has applied a model of reflection, using a student's assignment as an exemplar.

Part 3 comprises Chapters 21–24. These are student narratives written as educational assignments. They serve two purposes:

1. As exemplars of creative academic reflexive narratives
2. Evidence of reflective learning to bring about the practitioner's vision of person-centred practice

Part 4: The performance turn. Chapter 25 looks at narrative performance as representative of the practitioner's journey through guided reflection as illustrated through 'Jane's rap'. The performance was constructed from her narrative (Chapter 24). It has been widely performed both nationally and internationally with acclaim. The performance turn is significant considering that reflective practice *is* performance in practice. Performance is always followed by dialogue with its audience towards provoking social action – 'What can we learn from this performance and what action do we need to take as a consequence?'

Chapter 26 'wraps up' the whole book. It extols the value of maintaining a reflective journal beyond any academic programme as a natural element of being a reflective practitioner always keeping one's vision in focus. It further extols the value and validity of reflexive narratives to inform readers to draw their own insights towards becoming a reflective practitioner and realising their visions of practice, supported by practitioners' testaments.

Reference

1. Okri, B. (1997) *A Way of Being Free*. Phoenix House, London.

2. Johns C (2024) (Ed.) *Holistic Practice in Healthcare: The Burford NDU Person-centred model.* Wiley Blackwell, Oxford.

Note

i. https://www.lsib.co.uk/blog/blog.aspx?

PART 1

The Basic Scheme

CHAPTER 1

Envisaging Reflection, Reflective Practice and Guided Reflection

Reflection begins with paying attention and telling stories. So, I shall begin with a story of a conversation I overheard one morning on the train between two women:

> Sitting in the train the other day a woman hobbles on. Finds a seat to put her leg up. She says to her mate 'They just don't care anymore. She didn't look properly at my foot. She wasn't interested. Told me it was probably a corn. Wasn't listening to me. Told her the pain was in me 'eel. In the end she said 'Your 10 minutes are up got to see someone else'. Her mate rolls her eyes 'Bloody awful ain't it, chiropody on the NHS'.

The woman's comments reflect her dissatisfaction with her care. You might accept her word that the chiropodist wasn't listening to her and ponder the reason for that. Had the chiropodist's practice become so time routine requiring little thought and engagement with the patient? Was the woman just a task to do? The bottom line is that every professional, no matter what discipline, must take responsibility for ensuring effective person-centred practice. This requires practitioners not only to be reflective after the event but also, more significantly, to reflect within practice, to have a finger on the pulse of practice. To be a reflective practitioner.

Experience

Listening to the above conversation was an experience. Life and practice are made up of a continuous stream of experiences. Most are taken for granted, reflecting the way things are. Yet experience is a rich learning opportunity when paid attention to.

O'Donohue [1, p. 26] writes

> 'Everything that happens to you has the potential to deepen you. This potential is actuated through reflection as a self-inquiry into experience to find meaning, gain insight and prompt action that will deepen you'.

Practitioners live practice through a succession of experiences. Most of these experiences are taken for granted as normal. They do not disturb the practitioner's smooth flow of practice. However, sometimes something disturbs the practitioner, leading to a breakdown of its smooth running. The practitioner feels uncertain or anxious about what is happening. The experience becomes conscious and leaves a trace in the mind. It is these types of experiences that most often trigger reflection. However, as the practitioner becomes increasingly reflective, then all experiences become available for reflection, challenging and opening up one's normal practice to scrutiny in light of realising one's vision. Experience is made manifest through our stories of everyday practice.

Reflection

My interest in reflection was triggered by Margaret Clarke's paper 'Action and reflection: practice and theory of nursing [2]. It turns upside down the relationship between theory and practice. Learning through reflection on experience is practice-based, informed as appropriate by theory, rather than theory-based to apply to practice. For a practice discipline such as nursing, it made absolute sense.

The words *reflection* and *reflective practice* are often used glibly in everyday discourse as if reflection is simply a normal way of thinking about something that has happened and that requires little skill or guidance. Smyth [3, p. 285] writes

> 'Reflection can mean all things to all people ... it is used as a kind of umbrella or canopy term to signify something that is good or desirable ... everybody has his or her own (usually undisclosed) interpretation of what reflection means, and this interpretation is used as the basis for trumpeting the virtues of reflection in a way that makes it sound as virtuous as motherhood'.

Smyth's words are both salutary and provocative. They remind us to be careful about grasping reflection in any casual or authoritative way. The Compact Oxford English Dictionary [4, p. 86] defines 'reflect' as:

- throwback heat, light, sound without absorbing it
- [of a mirror or shiny surface] show an image of
- represent in a realistic or appropriate way
- bring about a good or bad impression of someone or something [on]
- think deeply or carefully about

Hence, reflection can be viewed as a mirror to see images or impressions of self *thrown back* in context of the particular situation. It is thinking deeply about the way the practitioner has responded and reasons for that response in light of what they were trying to achieve. It is *self-judgmental* – did I act in accordance with my vision? It is *wake up call* because so much of practice is non-reflective, merely a matter of habit and automatic response.

Edward Bear

An image of reflection can be discerned in the story of Edward bear and Christopher Robin [Milne 5, p. 1]

> 'Here is Edward bear, coming down stairs now, bump, bump, bump on the back of his head behind Christopher Robin. It is, as far as he knows, the only way of coming downstairs, but sometimes he feels there really is another way, if only he could stop bumping for a moment and think about it. And then he feels that perhaps there isn't'.

Reflection is creating the space to 'stop bumping' to think about what is happening, why it is happening and ways it might change for the better, and yet recognising that both finding a better way and affecting change may be difficult because we are locked into patterns of behaviour and relationships, including our relationship with the Christopher Robins of this world.

Perhaps, it is easier to conform and take pain killers for the sore head! Perhaps, we need an altogether different Christopher Robin to show us the way.

The reflective practitioner is someone who lives reflection as a mindful way of being within everyday practice where every action is focused on living one's vision of practice. The gateway to becoming a reflective practitioner is through reflection on everyday experiences.

Defining Reflection

I describe reflection as –

> 'Being mindful of self, either within or after an experience, as if a mirror in which the practitioner can view and focus self within the context of a particular experience, in order to reveal, understand, and be empowered to resolve contradiction between their envisaged their vision of practice and actual practice as revealed through reflection. In this process, the practitioner gains insight to develop their knowing in practice towards realising their vision of practice as a lived reality'.

Pinar [6, p. 184] picks up the idea of reflection as a mirror

> 'We are not mere smudges on the mirror. Our life histories are not liabilities to be exorcised but are the very precondition for knowing. It is our individual and collective stories in which present projects are situated, and it is the awareness of *these stories* which is the lamp illumining the dark spots, the rough edges'.

Reflection opens up *these stories* as a learning space. The learning space is resolving contradictions. Senge [7, p. 142] terms contradiction as 'creative tension' – the tension between our vision (where we want to be) and our current reality (where we actually are as recalled through reflection). Our recall may be smudged due to our subjective perspective on their experience. Guidance will help the practitioner to clean the reflective mirror to see reality more clearly (Chapters 8 and 9).

Activity

Next time you are at work, look into the self-mirror and ask yourself:

- 'Why am I responding as I am?'
- 'Am I responding in tune with my vision of practice?'
- 'Am I being effective?'
- 'Could I respond in different, perhaps more effective ways?'

These are reflective questions any serious practitioner would naturally ask self as they go about their practice that open the doorway to self-inquiry. As a consequence, do you become more sensitive to your practice? You are stepping along the reflective journey.

Vision

At the core of reflection is holding a vision of practice. It sets up contradiction and creative tension. Vision is the practice rudder to steer practice in a certain direction. It gives meaning and purpose to practice. It shapes one's attitude. It energises practice.

A vision is ideally developed with colleagues so that everybody pulls in the same direction. However, holding a personal vision is essential to contributing to a shared vision. As Senge writes [7, p. 231]

'If people don't have their own vision all they can do is 'sign up' for someone else's. The result is compliance, never commitment'.

In reality, practitioners are often at a lost to say what their vision is as if practice is concerned with 'what I do' rather than 'what I believe'. As such, vision is a rare thing beyond such taken for granted rhetoric of 'individualised care' or 'person-centred practice'. Indeed, practitioners may scoff at the need to have a vision or take offence that someone might suggest what their vision should state or that somehow they are deficient or incompetent in some way.

An inquiry into a vision of practice would expect to be professionally informed. The Royal College of Nursing UK[i] define nursing as –

'Registered nurses use evidence-based knowledge, professional and clinical judgment to assess, plan implement and evaluate high quality *person-centred* nursing care. Compassionate leadership is central to the provision and co-ordination of nursing care. They have high levels of autonomy within nursing and multi professional teams'.

The RCN represents professional nursing in the UK and, as such, it is reasonable to accept this definition as the primary focus for practice. This position is supported by the Nursing and Midwifery Council, the regulatory nursing body in the UK who state[ii] –

'Kindness and respect mean different things to different people. That's why it matters to be *person-centred*. Being *person-centred* means thinking about what makes each person unique, and doing everything you can to put their needs first'

These statements clearly point towards person-centred practice as being nursing's vision. Yet many practitioners do not explicitly hold a vision or merely pay lip service to an ideal such as person-centred practice but have never inquired into its nature. It is easy for any practitioner to believe that they are person-centred. Indeed, it would be difficult to admit they were not. Yet if practitioners were to be observed, the contradictions between a vision of person-centred practice and its reality would be evident. Thus, learning through reflection is learning to become a person-centred practitioner whatever that means as something lived. It is complex when viewed against the bigger picture of society. Issues such as gender, culture, diversity, race, climate change, politics, refugees, poverty, ageing population and health all impact on everyday clinical practice and education. As Rolling Thunder [8, p. 7] writes

Mankind's strength and ultimate survival depend not upon an ability to manipulate and control but upon an ability to harmonize with nature as an integral part of the system with life'.

From a person-centred perspective practitioners strive to harmonize with persons in relationship. Just as practitioners strive to grow through reflection so practitioners strive to enable persons to grow through their health-illness experience.

Mandy[iii] reflects on having a vision for practice

'In one reflective practice workshop Chris shared his experience of constructing the Burford model vision. This was a sharp wake up call. I recalled that the department had its own philosophy but if I was challenged as to its contents I would have failed miserably. Once back in the department, I eventually found the operational policy buried away in a filing cabinet. Included in its contents is the department's philosophy of care; however, it did not state who had devised it and when. I asked one of my colleagues who had worked in the department for many years as to the origin and author of the philosophy she looked at me blankly and said "I am sorry, I did not know we had one duck".

In my next management supervision, I raised this issue with my manager who also was ignorant of these facts but thought it might have been based upon the acute services philosophy. I compared the department's philosophy with one of the acute inpatient wards, only to discover that it was exactly the same. Johns [9] draws attention to the difficulties caused by having an imported philosophy imposed on a practice: it denies articulation of the practitioner's own beliefs and values and is easily forgotten. What then is the point in having a generic philosophy devised by someone else, locked away in a filing cabinet? Non-whatsoever. Reflecting upon this, I established that the team believes that we provide a high standard of individualised care for patients within the department. However, we lack evidence to validate this. By not having a philosophy of care constructed on our collective beliefs and objectives of our practice, how do we know where we are going and the rational for the journey?

Running in Place

We can only know person-centred practice as something lived. Beck describes this as 'running in place' [10, p. 123] –

> 'Suppose we want to realize how a marathon runner feels: if we run two blocks, or two miles, or five miles, we will know something about running those distances, but we won't know anything about running a marathon. We can recite theories about marathon running, we can describe tables about the physiology of marathon runners, we can pile up endless information about marathon running but that doesn't mean we know what it is. We can only know when we are the one doing it. We can only know our lives when we experience them directly, instead of dreaming about how they might be if we did this or have that. This we can call running in place, being present as we are, right here and right now'.

Life is paid attention to through reflection. Through reflection, practitioners learn quite quickly they are not running in place. Indeed, they have not given that much thought, locked into non-reflective modes of practice.

Take the example of caring. Frank [11, p. 13] writes –

> 'Caring is one of those activities that people know only when they are involved in it. From within, and only from within, caring makes sense. To try and explain care leads to the circularity expressed in statements such as "caring for this person requires doing this, and I do this because I care for this person". Philosophy teaches that, for some activities, there is only practice'.

It follows that if we accept Frank's position, we can only know caring from within caring. Caring cannot be known as a technical or abstract thing. The practitioner knows self as caring only within the moment. It can be scrutinised and developed through reflection.

Reflective practice *is* person-centred/holistic practice[iv]

- Learning is embedded in practice; thus, learning is practice. There is no division between them. Every moment is a learning experience for both practitioners and persons.
- Learning is grounded in the practitioner's whole experience and then seeks to understand the significance and relationship of issues within the whole that mirrors the person-centred practitioner's approach to persons.
- Learning acknowledges that the practitioner is ultimately self-determining and responsible for her or his own practice in context with their practice environment that mirrors the person-centred practitioner's approach to persons.
- Learning seeks to facilitate the individual practitioners' growth to reach their full practice potential that mirrors the person-centred practitioner's approach to persons.

Knowing in Practice

The fact is, practitioners cannot easily control their experiences. They just happen to confront the practitioner moment by moment.

Salzberg notes [12, p. 76]

> 'No matter how much we want it to otherwise, the truth is that we are not in control of the unfolding of our experience. We can affect and influence and impact what happens, but we can't wake up in the morning and decide what we will encounter and feel and be confronted by during the day'.

The practitioner responds to situations with their knowing in practice. Schön [13, p. 22] terms this knowing as 'professional artistry'. Artistry captures how this knowing is expressed through performance. Knowing in practice is always tentative. It is never certain. Every situation needs to be approached from a position of 'not-knowing' and thus inquired into and interpreted for its meaning and response simply because it has never been experienced before. If knowing is perceived as certain, it closes down possibility.

As Wheatley and Kellner-Rogers [14, p. 69] write

> 'The future cannot be determined. It can only be experienced as it is occurring. Life doesn't know what it will be until it notices what it has just become'.

Knowing in practice is a *reflexive knowing*. Every reflected-on experience results in tentative insights or understanding that informs future experiences [15] within a deepening hermeneutic spiral of understanding (see Chapter 2). Reflexivity is 'looking back' through experiences to discern the pattern of deepening their knowing in practice towards realizing their vision of practice and expanding their horizon of knowing. As Gadamer writes [16, p. 183]

> 'Our own horizon is constantly in the process of formation, not least through our encounters with the past'.

Schön [13] notes that everyday practice is tacit, complex and indeterminate that defies technical solutions to its problems. He notes (p. 49)

> 'When we go about the spontaneous, intuitive performance of the actions of everyday life, we show ourselves to be knowledgeable in a special way. Often, we cannot say what it is that we know. When we try to describe it, we find ourselves at a loss. Or, we produce descriptions that are obviously inappropriate. Our knowing is ordinarily tacit, implicit in the patterns of action and in our feel for the stuff with which we are dealing. It seems right to say that our knowing is in our action'.

Reflection enables the practitioners to lift this tacit knowing to the mind's surface to explore in the context of the particular experience. Tacit knowing is like a wave flowing just beneath conscious thought, yet it is accessible and obliquely articulated through reflection, where it can be scrutinised and developed.

Knowing in practice, because of its tacit nature, is intuitive and contextual. The reflective practitioner has a sense of knowing what to do. King and Appleton [17] and Cioffi [18] both note that reflection accesses, values and develops intuitive processes. Technical rational knowledge has been claimed as necessary for nursing's disciplinary knowledge base because it can be observed and verified [19]. Historically, professions such as nursing have accepted the superiority of technical rationality over tacit or intuitive knowing [13]. Yet, a technical rational mentality inevitably leads to stereotyping, fitting the patient to the theory rather than using the theory to inform the situation, thus reducing the patient/client to some object and the practitioner to the status of a technician carrying out a prescription irrespective of the person's humanness. A technical rational approach gives dominance to theory and objective facts rather than subjective opinions and feelings. Indeed, feelings may be denigrated as unprofessional and stories as mere anecdotes with little learning potential. From this perspective, reflective practice is likely to be adapted to fit this dominant culture rather than see the potential for reflection to transform both educational and organisational culture. Hence, a radical shift of mind is necessary to accommodate reflective practice. Yet, people get locked into a paradigmatic view of knowledge and become intolerant of other claims because such claims fail the technical ratio- nality injunction as to what counts as truth [20] (I pick this idea up in Chapter 26).

Since the Briggs Report [21] emphasised that nursing should be a research-based profes- sion, nursing has endeavoured to respond to this challenge. However, the general under- standing of what 'research based' means, has followed an empirical pathway reflecting a dominant agenda to explain and predict practice. This agenda has been pursued by nurse academics seeking academic recognition that nursing is a valid science within the University settings. Whilst abstract knowledge has an important role in informing practice, it certainly cannot predict and control, at least not without reducing the patient and nurses to the status of objects to be manipulated like pawns in a chess game. The consequence of this position in nursing has been the repression of other forms of knowing that has perpetuated the oppres- sion of nurses of their clinical nursing knowledge [22]. Has it improved in the past 30 years? I see no evidence to support that.

☐   Tick the box 'I am not a robot'.

Developing a Reflective Attitude

Learning through reflection requires a 'reflective attitude'. Fay [23] identified certain qual- ities of mind that he considered pre-requisite to reflection: commitment, curiosity and intel- ligence. These are significant to counter more negative qualities of mind associated with defensiveness, habit, resistance and ignorance.

Commitment

Commitment is energy that sparks life. Yet, for many practitioners, commitment for their practice has become numbed or blunted through working in non-challenging, non-supportive and generally stressful environments, where work satisfaction is making it through the work with minimal hassle. These practitioners are unlikely to appreciate reflection. They turn their heads away from the reflective mirror because the reflected images are not positive. They do not want to face themselves and accept responsibility for their practice. Things wither and die without commitment. When those things are people, then the significance of commitment is only too apparent. Commitment is fuelled by vision, which helps them face up to difficult situations simply because realising their vision matters to them. The small child is ambivalent about learning to walk; he stumbles and falls, he hurts himself. It is a painful process. Yet, the satisfaction of developing his potential far outweighs the bumps and bruises [24].

Curiosity

Curiosity is self-inquiry, questioning who I am and what I do. It is the opening up of possi- bility. As Gadamer [16, p. 266] writes –

> 'The opening up and keeping open of possibilities is only possible because we find ourselves deeply interested in that which makes the question possible in the first place. To truly question something is to interrogate something from the threat of our existence, from the centre of our being'.

Curiosity is fundamental to the creative life and yet many practitioners are locked into habitual patterns of practice that are taken for granted as normal. They get stuck in a non-reflective habitual groove going through the motions.

Through reflection, the practitioner becomes innately curious in taking nothing for granted and exploring new ways of being and responding towards realising one's vision. Curiosity moves the practitioner away from an uncritical, pre-reflective state of being, where aspects of practice were not questioned but simply taken for granted [25].

Curiosity is turning over pebbles, wondering what lies on the other side, while open to the possibilities of viewing the same thing from different perspectives. Curiosity helps us pay attention as if each new experience is to be explored for its meaning and response. As Loori [26, p. 74] writes –

> 'When we truly pay attention, we see each object or situation for the first time- and it always seems fresh and new, no matter how many times we've encountered it before. We break free of our habitual ways of seeing'.

Intelligence

Intelligence opens the practitioner to new ideas in contrast with being ignorant, where new ideas are viewed as a threat and dismissed. Intelligence is about being a thinking person questioning the very basis for practice. Intelligence is tuning into one's intuition and a deeper awareness of self rather than a reliance on abstract knowledge.

Krishnamurti writes [27, p. 89]

> 'There is an intelligent revolt [against environment] which is not reaction but comes with self-knowledge through the awareness of one's own thought and feeling. It is only when we face experience that we keep intelligence highly awakened; and intelligence highly awakened is intuition, which is the only true guide in life'.

The practitioner may lack these qualities of mind. However, these qualities of mind are naturally nurtured through reflection, especially with guidance.

Spectrum of Reflective Practices

Reflective practices as a spectrum (Figure 1.1) characterised by three developing themes:

- From 'doing' reflection towards 'being' reflective
- From a technical rational to a professional artistry knowing
- An increasing criticality

'Doing' reflection reflects a technical-rational approach, whereby reflection is viewed as a tool or device. 'Being' reflective reflects an ontological approach rooted in 'who I am' rather than 'what I do'. Bulman, Lathlean and Gobbi [28], in their investigation of student and teacher perspectives on reflective practice, revealed that a focus on being rather than doing was significant. The ontological approach acknowledges that the way we think about and do things must involve who we are to think about things in the first place. An increased criticality reflects a shift from reflection to critical reflection whereby the assumptions that underpin practice are understood, challenged and worked towards shifting towards realising one's desired vision.

Reflection-on-Experience

When people refer to reflection, they usually refer to reflection-on-experience. Indeed, most theories of reflection are based on this idea of looking back on an experience after the event with learning intent towards anticipating future experiences.

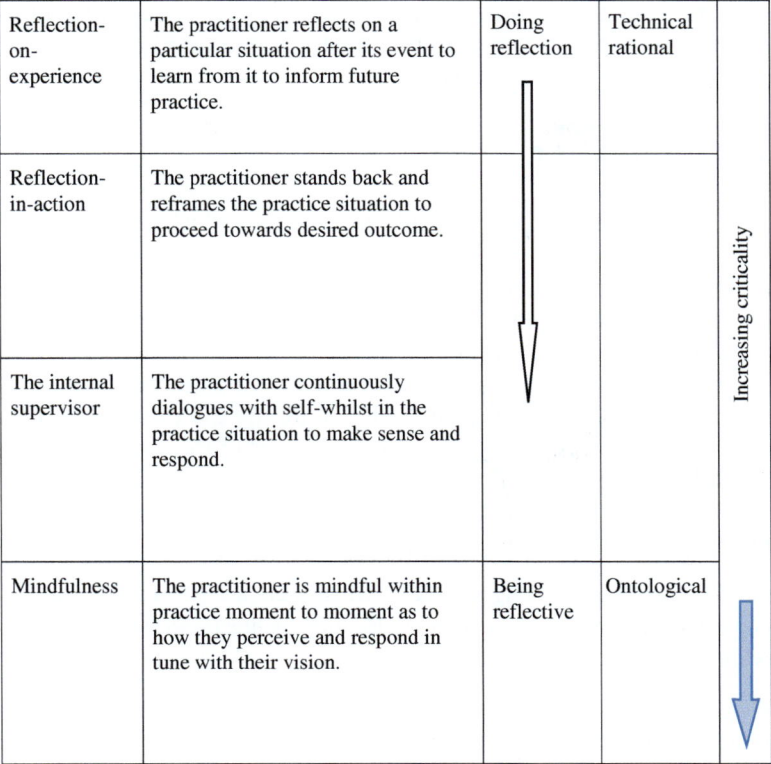

Reflection-on-experience	The practitioner reflects on a particular situation after its event to learn from it to inform future practice.	Doing reflection	Technical rational	
Reflection-in-action	The practitioner stands back and reframes the practice situation to proceed towards desired outcome.			
The internal supervisor	The practitioner continuously dialogues with self-whilst in the practice situation to make sense and respond.			
Mindfulness	The practitioner is mindful within practice moment to moment as to how they perceive and respond in tune with their vision.	Being reflective	Ontological	

FIGURE 1.1   Spectrum of reflective practices.

Reflection-in-Action

Schön [13, 29] distinguished reflection-*on-action* with reflection-*in-action* as a way of thinking about a situation whilst engaged within it, to reframe it as necessary to overcome some obstruction. The practitioner can naturally adjust to minor interruptions within the smooth flow of experience because the body has embodied knowing. However, the practitioner is sometimes faced with situations that require the practitioner to stop and reframe the situation to proceed. This requires a shift in thinking and contemplating new ways of responding. As such, it is problem solving yet recognising that old ways of thinking are inadequate. Reflection is the practitioner's unique encounter and conversation with a situation through which, as Schon [29, p. 163] puts it, 'he shapes it and makes himself part of it'.

Schön [13] drew on exemplars from music and architecture, situations of engagement with inanimate forms. His example of counselling is taken from the classroom not from clinical practice. The classroom is a much easier place to freeze and reframe situations in contrast with clinical practice grounded within the unfolding human encounter. It is easy to misunderstand reflection-in-action as merely thinking about something whilst doing it.

Schön [29] responded to the idea that reflection interferes with action. He acknowledges the difficulty of 'being in the firing line' when the practitioner must respond quickly and intuitively. However, I make a distinction between cognitive thinking and embodied thinking based on the body's tacit knowing. Hence, the quick intuitive response is an example of embodied thinking – the body knows how to respond. Subsequent reflection on the experience, as with all reflection on experience, feeds tacit knowing and the intuitive response even if the practitioner does not recognise it as such. As Schon concluded [29, p. 281], 'there is nothing in reflection, then, which leads necessarily to paralysis of action'.

Perhaps when reflection has not been embodied, as for novice reflective practitioners, an attempt to reflect-in-action can seem to interfere with action as if cognitive thinking gets in the way of intuitive thinking and response.

The Internal Supervisor

Casement [30] coined the expression the 'internal supervisor' as a continuous dialogue the practitioner has with themselves in response to the unfolding situation – 'what is going on here', 'how am I responding' and so on. The practitioner if also mindful of intent – 'what am I trying to achieve?' It is a more dynamic form of reflection-in-action. Reflection opens the practitioner's awareness to what they know, mindful of the assumptions they make and ideas they have. This awareness or openness to the unknown 'leaves more room for the patient to contribute to any subsequent knowing; and what is jointly discovered has a freshness that belongs to both. More than this, it may be a significant part of the process of therapeutic gain is achieved through the patient coming to know that the practitioner can learn from him or her' [30, p. 26].

Casement notes [30, p. 9] that Reflection counters

'a tendency to experience a feeling of déjà vu when there are elements of similarity between a current clinical situation and others before it, leading the practitioner to a false sense of recognition or a closing down of understanding'.

Thus, when a practitioner thinks they know, they close down other possibilities. The reflective practitioner is aware of the tension between their knowing and not-knowing yet runs with a tacit sense of not-knowing, knowing they can learn through subsequent reflection.

Mindfulness

In the previous editions of this book, I referred to mindfulness as reflection-within-the-moment. I prefer mindfulness because it is a constant state of being rather than just within the moment. The practitioner is mindful of the way they perceive and respond to practice in tune with their vision of practice. Reflection is the gateway to mindfulness.

Goldstein [31, p. 89] notes

'Mindfulness is the quality of mind that notices what is present without judgment, without interference. It is like a mirror that clearly reflects what comes before it'.

Mindfulness is a heightened state of awareness. It is being aware moment by moment of things and the world around us, of our body, our feelings and thoughts and ourselves in relationship with others. Wheatley and Keller-Rogers [14, p. 26] write –

'The more present and aware we are as individuals and as organisations, the more choices we create. As awareness increases, we can engage with more possibilities. We are no longer held prisoner by habits, unexamined thoughts, or information we effuse to look at'.

Miller offers a vivid description of being mindful of the world around him [32, p. 27]

'Nothing was too petty to escape my attention, seeing the everyday things in this new light I was transfixed. The moment you give close attention to anything, even a blade of grass, it becomes mysterious, awesome, indescribably magnified world in itself'.

Miller's words reflect how mindfulness leads to a much greater attention of practice to the extent that all practice is no longer routine but alive and awesome. McIlvanney [33, p. 250] offers a compelling perspective of mindfulness –

'While mind seeks to vet our behaviour, the mind itself must always be on probation and must give itself up constantly to have its own behaviour vetted'.

Each of these above quotes reflects the essence of mindfulness as the ability to stand outside self to see self. Yet, as McIlvanney notes [33], mindfulness is not the mind but the mind's awareness of itself. Rather than jumping to action in response to thoughts and feelings, the mindful mind says to the practitioner – 'hang on a moment, note how you are feeling and how are you interpreting this situation. Take a breath and ask yourself how is this man feeling and thinking to make you frustrated and angry', 'how best do I respond?' Mindful mind creates a clearing in the emotional midst and cognitive reaction to see oneself in the situation clearly for what you are trying to achieve within the particular situation. It is the state of poise whereby the practitioner is vigilant against unskilful actions and negative emotions, such as anger, arrogance, resentment, hatred, envy and greed [34] that might negatively influence the practitioner's response. In Buddhism, this quality of mind is *apramada* or non-heedlessness. I refer to it as 'as the ever watchful guardian at the gate of the senses'.

Being mindful may sound exhaustive, as the idea of 'normal practice' or 'the taken for granted' is no longer tenable. Yet mindful practice is creative, energising and satisfying. It is accrued through reflective experience in a subtle manner.

Self-inquiry as Research

Reflection is self-inquiry towards self-realisation, however, that might be expressed presented as a reflexive narrative that plots the journey of becoming. When guided, reflection has been utilised as a formal research process at every academic level [35]. In constructing 'Reflexive narrative' as a construct, I have been influenced by a bricolage of various philosophical and theoretical ideas that give depth to its nature (Figure 1.2).

Kincheloe, McClaren and Steinberg [36, p. 168] note that –

'Bricolage in a contemporary sense, is understood to involve the process of employing these methodological processes as they are needed in the unfolding context of the research situation enabling the researcher to move beyond the blinders of particular disciplines and peer through a conceptual window to a new world of research and knowledge production'.

These methodological ideas served to inform and deepen my understanding of reflexive narrative and the process of guided reflection towards its construction. Many of these influencing factors have already been touched upon in the above exploration of reflection and are apparent throughout the book.

Critical Social Theory

Critical social theory asserts that change is not rational but resisted by factors to maintain the status quo. Thus, reflection is an inquiry into these factors deeply embedded in the practice

Narrative inquiry and literary theory	Reflective and guided reflection theory	Non-western thought
Critical social science	Reflexive narrative as a journey of self-inquiry towards self-realisation.	Hermeneutics
Feminist slant	Auto-ethnography and performance	Chaos theory

FIGURE 1.2 Reflexive narrative bricolage.

culture. Without emphasising this criticality, reflection is likely to be superficial, focusing on problem solving. It will tend to avoid challenging underlying assumptions that govern the way the practitioner thinks and responds to situations. Brookfield poses the question – what makes reflection critical? He writes [37, p. 8]

> 'To put it briefly, reflection becomes critical when it has distinctive purposes. The first is to understand how considerations of power undergird, frame and distort educational processes and interactions. The second is to question assumptions and practices that seem to make our lives easier but actually work against our long-term interests'.

Narrative Inquiry

Chase notes [38, p. 421], drawing on narrative theorists, defines narrative as

> 'A distinct form of discourse; as meaning making through the shaping or ordering of experience, a way of understanding one's own and others' actions, of organising events and objects into a meaningful whole, of connecting and seeing the consequences of actions and events over time'.

Chase explores the diverse forms narrative inquiry can take, notably through revealing experience as storytelling and how the experience is contextualised from within one's environment leading to an analysis of the impact of environment on experience.

Feminist Slant

A feminist slant acknowledges that learning and practice must break through the glass ceiling of patriarchy. Thus, guided reflection is explicitly concerned with liberating practitioners to fulfil their vision against the grain of patriarchy that has dominated bureaucratic organisations, such as the NHS in the UK, where women need to think and act like a man to be successful.

It explicitly acknowledges the significance of intuition, imagination, emotions and creativity, all regarded as right brain activity that has been largely neglected in technical rational curriculum and practice.[v]

Hermeneutics

Hermeneutics is the study of interpretation of text. It is the root of learning through experience to draw out and co-create insights to reflexively inform and deepens one's knowing in practice within the hermeneutic spiral of deepening understanding (see Chapter 2).

Auto-ethnography and Self-inquiry

Auto-ethnography and self-inquiry are very similar ideas. In her book 'The ethnographic I' [39], a doctoral student asks Carolyn Ellis – 'Auto-ethnography? What is that? Ellis replies "I start with my personal life and pay attention to my physical feelings, thoughts and emotions. I use what I call 'systematic sociological introspection' and 'emotional recall' to try and understand an experience I've lived through. Then I write my experience as a story. By exploring a particular life, I hope to understand a way of life, as Reed-Danahay [40] says' [38, p. xvii].

Auto-ethnography is self-inquiry yet without its reflexivity. Neither is it vision oriented. It is communicated ideally through performance.

Chaos Theory

Learning through reflection is 'chaos' by focusing on the wholeness of the situation governed by the quest to realise a vision of practice. Hence, reflection is standing back and seeing the pattern of things within wholeness. Vision is the strange attractor around which practice is organised. As Wheatley [41, p. 119/120] notes –

> 'It is chaos's great destructive energy that dissolves the past and gives us the gift of a new future. It releases us from the imprisoning patterns of the past by offering us its wild ride into newness. Only chaos creates the abyss in which we can recreate ourselves. The shape of chaos materialises from information feeding back on itself and changing in the process'.

Thus, guided reflection is this abyss. The feeding back on itself is reflexivity. The journey of self-inquiry and self-transformation is evidenced through the reflexive narratives offered in the book.

I must emphasize that the bricolage only serves to inform my construction of reflexive narrative whereby practice *is an unfolding reflexive narrative*. The bricolage is not prescriptive. My appreciation of it is tentative due to its deep philosophical nature and the inevitable partiality of my interpretation, as I engage with these influences in deepening my understanding of reflexive narrative.

Self-inquiry is a unique ontological experience. It is learnt 'by running in place' [10] informed as appropriately by ideas. As Mishler [42, p. 422] notes:

> 'Skilled research is a craft, and like any craft, it is learnt by apprenticeship to competent researchers, by hands-on experience, and by continual practice. It seems remarkable, if we stop to think about it, that research competence is assumed to be gained by learning abstract rules of scientific procedure. Why should working knowledge be learned anymore easily, or through other ways, than the competence required for playing the violin or blowing glass, or throwing pots?'

A Brief Review of Reflective Theories

Imagine the practitioner's cry – 'tell me what reflection is so I can do it!' However, it is not as simple as that. It is more complex than simply applying a technique, although on the surface, it might seem that a prescription is just what is required. Indeed, many practitioners and educators may misguidedly view it as such. If so, reflection becomes a task to be done rather than something meaningful and transformative.

Besides Schön's [13, 29] work (as discussed), the following reflective theorists complement my understanding of reflection:

- Boyd and Fales [43]
- Boud, Keogh and Walker [44]
- Gibbs [45]
- Mezirow [46]

It is not my intention to review these theories in any depth. The reader is directed to the primary sources to explore these theorists more deeply if inclined and to explore more recent ideas.

It is important to note that any model of reflection should be viewed through a sceptical lens. Rather like the skilled craftsman, the practitioner will choose the tool that is most helpful. Models are not prescriptions for reflection. They must always be viewed as heuristic, as a means to an end. In a technical rational society, reflective models are likely to be grasped as authoritative. The risk, from this perspective, is that practitioners will fit their experience to the model of reflection rather than use the model creatively to guide them to gain insight. It is easy to get wrapped up in the technology of reflection, especially in a learning culture dominated by technical rationality.

Boyd and Fales (43)

These Authors Define Reflection

> 'As the process of creating and clarifying the meaning of experience (present or past) in terms of self (self in relation to self and self in relation to the world). The outcome of the process is changed conceptual perspective. The experience that is explored and examined to create meaning focuses around or embodies a concern of central importance to the self'. [43, p. 101]

From their research with counsellors, they extrapolate reflection through six components (p. 106):

1. A sense of inner discomfort;
2. Identification or clarification of the concern;
3. Openness to new information from internal and external sources, with ability to observe and take in from a variety of perspectives, and a setting aside of an immediate need for closure;
4. Resolution, expressed as 'integration', 'coming together', 'acceptance of reality' and 'creative synthesis';
5. Establishing a continuity of self with past, present and future;
6. Deciding whether to act on the outcome of the reflective process.

In relation to stage 6, they note

> 'The new insight or changed perspective is analyzed in terms of its operational feasibility involving the practitioner's sense of rightness, values and potential acceptance by others'. [43, p. 112]

Boyd and Fales offer little practical guidance on how to explore experience. I generally agree that reflection is triggered by 'inner discomfort' for practitioners when first engaging reflection. However, as the practitioner becomes more mindful, then all experience, not just 'inner discomfort' becomes available for reflection. I equate the idea of changed conceptual perspective as synonymous with insight to inform future experiences.

Boud, Keogh and Walker (44)

These authors they describe reflection as –

> 'Reflection, in the context of learning, is a generic term fort those intellectual and affective activities in which individual engage to explore their experiences in order to lead to new understandings and appreciations. It may take place in isolation or in association with others'. [44, p. 19]

They posit reflection as moving through three key stages:

- returning to experience
- attending to feelings
  - utilising positive feelings
  - removing obstructing feelings

- re-evaluating experience
  - re-examining experience in the light of the learner's intent
  - associating new knowledge with that which is already possessed
  - integrating this new knowledge into the learner's conceptual framework
  - appropriation of this knowledge into the learner's repertoire of behaviour

Appropriation is akin to gaining insight; that the practitioner is changed through the reflective process, that when faced with a similar situation they will respond differently. This differs from Boyd and Fales's approach, in that the practitioner makes a choice whether to respond differently in light of learning. Boyd and Fales [43, p. 112] write – 'The need to test one's self-changes [insights] against the mirror of others is an essential component of all growth'.

These words emphasise that all individual learning must be set within its context.

As with Boyd and Fales, they give little practical guidance on how to 'return to experience'.

Gibbs (45)

Gibbs offers a practical reflexive circle moving through six stages suggesting that each stage is important to inform the next stage ultimately resulting in an action plan for responding in future similar situations.

1. Description [of the situation],
2. feelings [what were you thinking and feeling],
3. evaluation [what was good and bad about the experience]',
4. analysis [what sense can you make of the situation],
5. conclusion [what else could you have done],
6. action plan [if it arose again what would you do].

Gibbs' approach shared the broad outline of the Model for Structured reflection yet without its detail.

Mezirow (46)

Mezirow viewed reflection as a process leading to emancipatory action. He posited a depth of reflection through seven levels of reflectivity spanning from consciousness, the way we might think about something, to critical consciousness, where we pay attention and scrutinise our thinking processes. Thinking is inherently problematic. Hence, our thinking is a focus for reflection. Hence, I need to think differently to perceive the situation differently, and in doing so, to unearth those assumptions that govern thinking. If reflection is viewed merely as a problem solving, and we used the same thinking to solve the problem that caused the problem, then we wouldn't get very far. Our solutions would quickly break down. Mezirow [46, p. 6] conceptualised the outcome of reflection as *perspective transformation* –

> 'The process of becoming critically aware of how and why the structure of psycho-cultural assumptions has come to constrain the way we see ourselves and our relationships, reconstituting this structure to permit a more inclusive and discriminating integration of experience and acting upon these new understandings'.

Mezirow's focus on understanding assumptions takes reflection into what is generally regarded as a 'critical' domain. The focus on emancipatory action is to rewrite one's own and collective assumptions to govern a more satisfactory state of affairs however that might be framed. Not easy stuff for the humble practitioner to grasp as Smith [47, p. 212] acknowledges –

> 'Despite widespread and long standing commitment to the notion of critical reflection across the health and social care professions, it can be difficult to assimilate into teaching because the language is complex, and the same terminology is used in different ways in different contexts so carries different nuances'.

Balancing the Winds

The above theories all stem from a western rational cognitive tradition reflected in the words, ideas and language used. As such, they fit easily into a technical rational mindset. An appreciation of Buddhism and Native American lore gave me wider, more esoteric, perspectives [48].

To become a reflective practitioner is to develop mindfulness and wisdom beyond rational thinking as explored earlier in this chapter. Reflection is a way to connect with all things, gain respect, inner strength and to realize one's vision as reflected in the idea of *bimadisiwin*. Blackwolf and Jones [49, p. 47] write –

> 'Bimadisiwin is a conscious decision to become. It is time to think about what you want to be. The dance cannot be danced until you envision the dance, rehearse its movements and understand your part. It is demanding for every step needs an effort in becoming one with the vision. It takes discipline, hard work and time. It is freeing, for its frees the spirit. It releases you to become as you believe you must'.

Put another way, Bimadisiwin is reflection. It is a ritual dance of becoming. Listen to the drum!

Believe in the vision of you
   Practice the vision
      Become the vision

Blackwolf and Gina Jones's book 'Earth Dance Drum' is an invaluable book on reflection [49]. In striving to become the vision the practitioner prepares for war, the war from outside and the war within the mind. Reflection becomes the practitioner's metaphoric war shield to defend against and transform the forces that obstruct realising one's vision. As a guide, I use an art workshop to invite practitioners to draw and decorate their warshield with colour and meaningful words such awareness, belief, courage and strength to remind the practitioner 'I am a warrior fighting to realise my vision!' One profound Native American word to put on the warshield is 'Namaji' which is respect, honour, dignity and pride. As Blackwolf notes 'we wear Namaji for all to see'. It raises such questions as 'how do you show respect for your self?', 'How do you wear your dignity?', 'What are you proud of?' and 'How do you extend Namaji to others?' [49, p. 12]

Making a warshield spurs the imagination that has a profound empowering impact.

Barriers to Rational Change (Facing the Reality Wall)

Rationally, the practitioner can decide to be a person-centred practitioner. I assume that all practitioners are concerned with realising desirable practice yet, for one reason or another, such realisation is difficult, either for reasons embodied within themselves or embedded in the work environment.

Embodiment	- the way people have been socialized to think, feel and respond to the world in a normative and pre-reflective way.
Tradition	- a pre-reflective state reflected in the assumptions and habitual practices that people hold about the way things should be.
Authority and power	- the way normal relationships are constructed and maintained through authority's use of power.

FIGURE 1.3 Barriers to rational change (Fay 23).

However, practice is not rational. The self has embodied a certain way of being that is continuously reinforced through everyday practice. Through exposing contradiction, the practitioner strives to understand its causes and explore what must be done to resolve it.

Pinar [6, p. 177] notes

'It is only when practitioners truly understand themselves and the conditions of their practice, can they begin to realistically change and respond differently. To understand, the reflective practitioner creeps underneath habitual explanations of his actions, outside his regularized statements of his objectives'.

The practitioner must question – 'what barriers constrain me from responding in tune with my vision?' These barriers may not be easy to recognize and shift because they form the fabric of everyday practice and are largely taken for granted. I term this the reality wall.

Fay [23] identified the three barriers of tradition, authority and embodiment (Figure 1.3) that govern the fabric of our social world. Fay [23, p. 75] writes from a critical social science perspective that gives reflection its critical nomenclature –

'The goal of a critical social science is not only to facilitate methodical self-reflection necessary to produce rational clarity, but to dissolve those *barriers* which prevent people from living in accordance with their genuine will. Put in another way, its aim is to help people not only to be transparent to themselves but also to cease being mere objects in the world, passive victims dominated by forces external to them'.

Embodiment

Practitioners have embodied a way of being and doing in practice that governs their behaviour in ways that may not be compatible with their vision of practice. Because one's behaviour is normal; it is not usually scrutinised for its appropriateness although the practitioner may often have disquiet that things could be different. Through understanding the nature of contradiction, the practitioner becomes cognizant of their embodied practice as the first step to disembody old ways of being necessary to embody a new way of being. The process of stripping away the old may create considerable dissonance as old ways of being compete with new ways of being. Newman [50, p. 13] commented that

'To view the world from a different perspective requires a paradigm shift that incorporates the old paradigm and transforms it'.

In reality, it may feel like taking two steps forward and one step back.

One embodied barrier is the practitioner's embodiment of subordination whereby their practice is controlled by others resulting in a lack of autonomy to respond in tune with their vision [Roberts, 51]. It is pertinent to note that Roberts wrote her paper more than 30 years ago and yet, in my experience of guiding practitioners, this embodied subordination continues to haunt them.

Tradition

Tradition is reflected in the norms that govern organisation and practice. It has been determined over time perhaps shifting slightly to accommodate new ideas and directives. It constitutes 'normal practice' – 'the way things are done around here' and is largely taken for granted. Practice is contextual set within the particular organisational setting. Dawson [52, p. 25] notes –

> 'Context refers to the grand societal narratives, those clusters of beliefs and cultural norms that give shape and meaning to the human cultures within which we live'.

When tradition is dissected through reflection, its underlying assumptions and associated prejudices can be revealed. Bohm [53, p. 69] writes-

> 'Normally, we don't see that our assumptions are affecting the nature of our observations. But the assumptions affect the way we see things, the way we experience them, and consequently the things we want to do. In a way we are looking through our assumptions; the assumptions could be said to be an observer in a sense'.

Responding in more desirable ways will almost certainly disturb normal practice. As such, it is likely to be resisted by those with an investment in maintaining normal practice and the status quo. You might say 'I believe in treating patients with dignity and compassion' and believe your practice reflects that. However, on reflection you may acknowledge that your responses lack these qualities leading to uncaring behaviours what Jameton [54] and Corey and Goren [55] have labelled the 'dark side of nursing'. So next morning you set out to remedy this in your own practice and get criticised by other staff for getting 'to involved with your patients' or 'there's work to be done'. The pressure is immediately put on you to conform to normal practice. You feel the creative tension and the difficulty in resolving it. As such, the practitioner conforms to 'fit-in' to be recognised as a 'good team-player' but, in doing so, compromises their values of how practice should be, resulting in cognitive dissonance. Such compromise creates stress, as if living a lie, reflecting how normal culture can be toxic.

Authority and Power

One aspect of tradition is the way authority works through power. Power is embodied through socialisation processes and reinforced through everyday authoritative patterns of relating. Hence it is normal and largely unchallenged.

Force is the negative aspect of power used to ensure people conform to certain ways of behaviour endemic within transactional organisations such as the NHS whereby people are subordinate to authority transmitted down through its hierarchy where power is invested in positional roles. Positional power is laced with a coercive threat of sanction [56] to constrain the practitioner from acting 'out of line'. This works at every level of the organisation. Hence those who exert power over others at one level have power exerted on themselves from a higher level all the way from the 'top down' within a bureaucratic pyramidal structure characterised by an endemic anxiety that results in the need to control [57]. Control demands subordination where practitioners are viewed as fundamentally irresponsible (see embodiment above). Subordinates get told what to do. Play the game, do as you are told, keep your head down to avoid sanction, and then one day you too will gain authority with power over others. In such a transactional culture creativity is stifled and visions perish. Fear of sanction is a powerful deterrent for being different. It suppresses practitioners from voicing their opinions and asserting autonomy. Yet how comfortable are people in their illusions of truth? Is it better to conform than rock the boat? Is it better to sacrifice the ideal for a quiet life and patronage of more powerful others? Better keep your head down than have it shot off above the parapet for daring to speak up?

Power is also invested in professional roles. Doctors often perceive themselves as superior to nurses and other healthcare professionals, coining such expressions that nurses were the 'doctor's handmaiden', although now muted with the fear of sexist behaviour and misogyny.

However, nursing as a largely female workforce has been oppressed by patriarchal attitudes that has rendered it docile and politically passive, and thus limits its ability to fulfil its therapeutic potential. If so, then realising desirable practice would require an overthrow of oppressive political and cultural systems. The link between oppression and patriarchy is obvious, considering the way nursing has been viewed as women's work, and the suppression of women's voices in 'knowing their place' within the patriarchal order of things. Images of 'behind the screens' where women conceal their work, themselves, and their significance [58] and images of emotional labour being no more than women's natural work, therefore unskilled and unvalued within the heroic stance of medicine [59] are powerful signs of this oppression.

Those in authority have vested interests to maintain the status quo, to keep people 'in their place' rather than 'in-place', where they need to be in tune with realizing their vision. Hence being in place becomes a contested arena.

Mayeroff [60, p. 68] notes –

> 'I am in-place because of the way I relate to others. And place must be continually renewed and reaffirmed; it is not assured once and for all, for it is our response to the need of others to grow which gives us place'.

Nurses are taught to 'know their place' within the order of things. It is traditional for dominant professions such as medicine to reinforce subordinate behaviour in other health care professions, such as nursing [61]. In other words doctors are always motivated to maintain the status quo and resist rivalry for power. Nurses rationalise their compliance with medical domination because of the need to be valued. Chapman [62] suggested that doctors reinforce nurses' subordination through humiliation techniques that become a normative pattern of relating. Hence it becomes difficult for nurses to claim autonomy to move into the right place to practice desirably, kept in place by both managers and doctors. It is also the same with students and teachers. Even in Universities, teachers traditionally set the agenda and control the classroom. Students learn to be 'good' otherwise sanctions will ensue. Of course, some students like practitioners rebel against stifling authority. They are labelled 'trouble makers'. They often quit rather than lead unsatisfactory lives.

Empowerment

Through reflection, the barriers to rational change can be understood. They lie thick within any experience. It is obvious that to bring about *realisation of vision*, these barriers need to be understood and practitioners skilful and empowered to overcome them. However, acting on understanding may be difficult. Yet, when practitioners are committed to realizing their vision of practice, then they are likely to become restless knowing that there is a more satisfactory way to practice. No easy task. It can be painful and frustrating and consequently the practitioner may feel it's not worth tackling. As Smyth [63, p. 40] notes –

> 'Most of us, unless we feel uncomfortable, shaken, or forced to look at ourselves, are unlikely to change. It is far easier to accept our current conditions and adopt the least line of resistance'.

Lieberman [64] (cited by Day [65, p. 88]) notes –

> 'Working in bureaucratic settings has taught everyone to be compliant, to be rule governed, not to ask questions, seek alternatives or deal with competing values'.

Reflection intends to un-conceal these barriers. Greene [66, p. 58] writes –

'Concealment does not simply mean hiding; it means dissembling, presenting something as other than it is. To "unconceal" is to create clearings, spaces in the midst of things where decisions can be made. It is to break through the masked and the falsified, to reach toward what is also half-hidden or concealed. When a woman, when any human being, tries to tell the truth and act on it, there is no predicting what will happen. The "not yet" is always to a degree concealed. When one chooses to act on one's freedom, there are no guarantees'.

Empowerment is enhanced when practitioners are committed to and take responsibility for their practice, have strong values, and understand why things are as they are. It requires an assertive and political voice that is heard and listened to within the corridors of power. Yet so many nurses' voices are silent or suppressed for fear of sanction. Such practitioners are not so much lost for words but have no words to say [67]. Perhaps you can remember being silenced, not so much by others but by yourself. Practitioners often say- 'I wish I had said something but ...'

I know that so many practitioners feel that they have little control over the circumstances of their practice working in transactional organisations, often leading to a feeling of resignation or a victim of the system mentality [57]. In such worlds practitioners often feel like objects or bits within systems that impose control over their lives and stifle their professional aspirations. The transactional world is resistant to change. Then reflection can be reduced to like swimming in the shallow end of a deep swimming pool, literally splashing about with surface issues rather than tackling the deeper political and systems issues necessary to realise one's vision. However, that is not to say that tackling surface issues is not important, as indeed is developing reflective skills, and understanding of the deeper issues even if they are not amenable to change on an individual level. The need for collective reflection and action becomes vital for organisational change. If practitioners are to realise desirable practice with integrity they need to take such action. Yet is that possible against the transactional machine that will crush them? Becoming empowered will certainly need a guiding hand.

Reflection as Agentic Action

One way to view empowerment is in terms of realizing and sustaining agency. Agentic people are clear on what they want to accomplish, understand how intended actions will contribute to their accomplishments, and are confident that they can complete the intended actions and attain their goals. The core ingredients of personal agency are self-determination; self-legislation; meaningfulness; purposefulness; confidence; active-striving; playfulness; and responsibility [68].

In contrast, the practitioner may perceive themselves as a victim, feeling powerless to take action towards realising their vision of practice [69]. To view self as a victim is to experience a loss of personhood and to project the blame for this loss onto others rather than taking responsibility for self. Victimic people depict their lives out of control, shaped by events beyond their influence. Others' actions determine practice outcomes, and the accomplishment or failure to achieve life goals depend on factors they are unable to change. Bruner [70, p. 41] notes that persons construct a victimic self by –

'Reference to memories of how they responded to the agency of somebody else who had the power to impose his or her will upon them, directly or indirectly by controlling the circumstances in which they are compelled to live'.

Bruner's notes that the construction of life plots is always in relation to others. Victimic selves are oriented towards avoiding negative possibilities than to actualizing positive possibilities. Clearly, a victimic self is a contradiction with realising a vision of person-centred practice. Cochran and Laub [68] considered the shift from a victimic to agentic identity consisted of two correlative movements: the progressive construction of a new agentic life story, and the destruction of and detachment from the victimic life story. The victimic life story does not simply fade away, it must be actively confronted. This confrontation can be viewed as moving through four phases within guided reflection:

Phase 1

This phase is dominated by the practitioner's sense of entrapment or incompleteness, being controlled and helpless to change that – described as being 'trapped in a world in which most of what makes practice worthwhile is gone, and threatened by the possibility that this bleak existence might extend indefinitely' [68, p. 90]. Realising their vision of practice seems a hopeless task.

Phase 2

Practitioners become involved in activities that will assist in regaining an agentic life. Through reflection on experience they can formulate new ways of responding in tune with their vision of practice that is worthwhile and attainable. The practitioner begins to take ownership of their practice and can see that their efforts make a difference and effect outcomes. They monitor their progress and success through subsequent reflection on experiences in achieving progressively more person-centred practice. Experience of success in achieving their vision is crucial to validate the practitioner's capacity to make a difference and fuel their optimism for a better future and produce a sense of freedom and control.

Phase 3

Practitioners engage in activities more closely related to realising their vision in more self-directed ways in progressive independence from guidance. Cochran and Laub [68] describe this as actually playing the game, whereas phase 2 was practising the game. In other words, responding in tune with one's vision has become increasingly embodied. The person becomes aware that the remaining major barriers to a fuller, more agentic life, resides as much in their own beliefs and attitudes, as in factors outside self.

Phase 4

Practitioners experience a liberating sense of realising their vision. As Cochran and Laub [68, p. 94] note – 'Now one lives with a sense of life being on course, full, open to possibilities, unrestricted'. The person has achieved a sense of wholeness that is no longer threatened by former recollections. They have become the author of their own life and taken control of their practice.

An Encouraging Note

Learning through reflection is moving through three phases of understanding, empowerment and transformation set against a background of realizing a vision of practice. At each phase insights can be gleaned. Reflection creates stories of resistance and possibility; chipping away at resistance by confronting and shifting those barriers of resistance and opening up possibility. Nothing can be more meaningful for the serious practitioner intent on realizing desirable and effective care.

Reading about critical reflection and its implications may feel daunting to many readers. Just the language can feel intimidating. Yet think again about vision. What does it mean to you? Are you motivated to shifting barriers to realize it? Perhaps this stems back to your motivation to be a health care practitioner, to remember what that was before it was knocked out of you by the harsh realities of everyday practice and training.

Fay writes [23, p. 29] –

> 'It is highly unlikely that practitioner will change unless the level of discontent they are experiencing is really quite high; otherwise, what might be called the 'natural resistance' to fundamental change will act as a counterweight to the desire for change, and will induce these people to accommodate themselves to the discontent they are suffering'.

In other words, faced with daunting reality, you may prefer to rationalize your discontent and turn your back on reflection at least in any deep and meaningful sense. Better to swim along the surface of practice rather than dive deep within its murky depths. Understanding barriers is one thing. As I discuss in Chapters 8 and 9, guidance is vital to enable practitioners to become empowered to act on their insights. It requires communities of practitioners to work collectively to act on insights and change things. Perhaps even more it requires organisational shift towards transformational cultures and leadership that actively facilitates reflection rather than resist it as a threat to its status quo as evident in transactional organisations that seek a docile and subordinate workforce. Yet the individual can make a mark. As Carson [71, p. 139] writes –

> 'When you change the way an individual thinks of himself, you change the way he lives in his community and thereby you change the community in some way to a greater or lesser extent'.

The reflective practitioner actively works towards influencing and changing the practice environment. If practitioners truly wish to truly live their visions of practice, then they must become political in working towards establishing the conditions of practice where that is possible.

References

1. O'Donohue, J. (1997) *Anam Cara*. Bantam Press, London.
2. Clarke, M. (1986) Action and reflection: practice and theory in nursing. *Journal of Advanced Nursing* 11, 3–11.
3. Smyth, J. (1992) Teachers' work and the politics of reflection. *American Educational Research Journal* 29, 267–300.
4. Compact Oxford English Dictionary (third edition) (2005) C. Soanes, S. Hawker [Ed]. Oxford University Press, Oxford.
5. Milne, A. A. (1988) *Winnie-the-Pooh*. Dutton's children's Books, New York.
6. Pinar, W. (1981) 'Whole, bright, deep with understanding': issues in qualitative research and autobiographical method. *Journal of Curriculum Studies* 13(3), 173–188.
7. Senge, P. (1990) *The Fifth Discipline: the Art and Practice of the Learning Organization*. Century Business, London.
8. Boyd, D. (1976) *Rolling Thunder*. Delta, London.
9. Johns, C. (2013) *Becoming a Reflective Practitioner* (fourth edition). Wiley-Blackwell, Oxford.
10. Beck, C. Y. (1989) *Everyday Zen*. Thorsons, London.
11. Frank, A. (2002) Relations of caring: demoralization and remoralization in the clinic. *International Journal of Human Caring* 6(2), 13–19.
12. Salzberg, S. (2002) *Faith: Trusting your own Deepest Experience*. Riverhead Books, New York.
13. Schön, D. (1987) *Educating the Reflective Practitioner*. Jossey-Bass, San Francisco.
14. Wheatley, M., Kellner-Rogers, M. (1996) *A Simpler Way*. Berrett-Koehler Publishers, San Francisco.

15. Dewey, J. (1933) *How we Think*. J. C. Heath, Boston.

16. Gadamer, H-. G. (1960) Truth and method. G. Barden, J Cumming [Eds.] Seabury Press, New York.

17. King, L., Appleton, J. (1997) Intuition: a critical review of the research and rhetoric. *Journal of Advanced Nursing* 26, 194–202.

18. Cioffi, J. (1997) Heuristics, servants to intuition, in clinical decision making. *Journal of Advanced Nursing* 26, 203–208.

19. Kikuchi, J. (1992) Nursing questions that science cannot answer. In J. Kikuchi, H. Simmons [Eds.] *Philosophic Inquiry in Nursing* Sage, Newberry Park.

20. Wilber, K. (1997) *The Eye of Spirit: an Integral Vision for a World gone Slightly Made*. Shambhala, Boston.

21. Department of Health & Social Security (1972) *Report of the Committee on Nursing* [Chairperson, Professor Asa Briggs] HMSO, London.

22. Street, A. (1992) *Inside Nursing: A Critical Ethnography of Clinical Nursing*. State University of New York Press, Albany.

23. Fay, B. (1987) *Critical Social Science*. Polity Press, Cambridge.

24. Rogers, C. (1969) *Freedom to Learn: A View of What Education might Be*. Merrill, Columbus, OH.

25. Cox, H., Hickson, P., Taylor, B. (1991) Exploring reflection: knowing and constructing practice. In G. Gray, R. Pratt [Eds.] *Towards a Discipline of Nursing*. Churchill Livingstone, Melbourne. 373–389.

26. Loori, J. (2005) *The Zen of Creativity: Cultivating your Artistic Life*. Ballantine Books, New York.

27. Kishnamurti, J. (1996) *Total Freedom*. Harper, San Francisco.

28. Bulman, C., Lathlean, J., Gobbi, M. (2012) The concept of reflection in nursing: qualitative findings on student and teacher perspectives. *Nurse Education Today* 32, e8–e13.

29. Schön, D. (1983) *The Reflective Practitioner*. Avebury, Aldershot.

30. Casement, P. (1985) *On Learning from the Patient*. Routledge, London.

31. Goldstein, J. (2002) *One Dharma*. Rider, London.

32. Miller, H. (1964) *Henry Miller on Writing*. New Directions Books, New York.

33. McIlvanney, W. (1996) *The Kiln. A Sceptre Paperbook*. Hodder and Stoughton, London.

34. Sangharakshita. (1998) *Know your Mind*. Windhorse, Birmingham.

35. Johns, C. (2021) *Reflexive Narrative: self-Inquiry towards Self-Realisation and its Performance*. Sage, Thousand Oaks.

36. Kincheloe, J. L., McClaren, P., Steinberg, S. R. (2011) Rethinking critical pedagogy and qualitative research. In D. K. Denzin, Y. S. Lincoln [Eds.] *The Sage Handbook of Qualitative Research* (third edition). Sage, Thousand Oaks, 163–177.

37. Brookfield, S. (1995) *Becoming a Critically Reflective Teacher*. Jossey-Bass, San Francisco.

38. Chase, S. E. (2011) Narrative inquiry: still a field in the making. In N. K. Denzin., LY. V. Lincoln [Eds.] *The Sage book of Qualitative Research* (fourth edition). Thousand Oaks, 421–434.

39. Ellis, C. (2004) *The Ethnographic I: a Methodological Novel about Autoethnography*. AltaMira Press, Walnut Creek.

40. Reed-Danahay, D. (1997) *Auto/Ethnography: Rewriting Self and the Social*. Berg, Oxford.

41. Wheatley, M. J. (1999) *Leadership and the New Science*. Berrett-Koehler, San Francisco.

42. Mishler, E. (1990) Validation in inquiry-based research: the role of exemplars in narrative studies. *Harvard Educational Review* 60, 415–442.

43. Boyd, E., Fales, A. (1983) Reflective learning: key to learning from experience. *Journal of Humanistic Psychology* 23(2), 99–117.

44. Boud, D., Keogh, R., Walker, D. (1985) Promoting reflection in learning: a model. In D. Boud, R. Keogh, R. D. Walker [Eds.] *Reflection: Turning Experience into Learning*. Kogan Page, London, 18–40.

45. Gibbs, G. (1988) *Learning by doing: a Guide to Teaching and Learning Methods*. Further Education Unit, Oxford Polytechnic.

46. Mezirow, J. (1981) A critical theory of adult learning and education. *Adult Education* 32(1), 3–24.

47. Smith, E. (2011) Teaching critical reflection. *Teaching in Higher Education* 16(2), 211–223.

48. Johns, C. (2005) Balancing the winds. *Reflective Practice* 5(3), 67–84.

49. Blackwolf, C., Jones, G. (1996) *Earth Dance Drum*. Commune-E-Key, Salt Lake City.

50. Newman, M. (1994) *Health as Expanded Consciousness* (second edition). National league for Nursing Press, New York.

51. Roberts, S. (1993) Oppressed group behaviour: implications for nursing. *Advances in Nursing Science* 5(4), 21–30.

52. Dawson, J. (2015) We need new stories. Resergence and Ecologist Issue 289 March/April, p25–29.

53. Bohm, D. (1996) In L. Nichol [Ed.] *On Dialogue*. Routledge, London.

54. Jameton, A. (1992) Nursing ethics and the moral situation of the nurse. In E. Friedman [Ed.] *Choices*

and Conflict. American Hospital Publishing, Chicago, 101–109.

55. Corey, M. C., Goren, S. (1998) The dark side of nursing: impact of stigmatizing responses on patients. *Scholarly Inquiry for Nursing Practice* 12(2), 110–121.

56. French, J., Raven, B. (1968) The bases of social power. In D. Cartwright, A. Zander [Eds.] *Group Dynamics*. Row Peterson, Evanston, IL, 150–67.

57. Johns, C. (2016) *Mindful Leadership: a guide for the Health Care Professions*. Palgrave, London.

58. Lawler, J. (1991) *Behind the Scenes: Nursing, Somology and the Problems of the Body*. Churchill Livingstone, Melbourne.

59. James, N. (1989) Emotional labour: skill and work in the social regulation of feelings. *Sociological Review* 37(1), 15–42.

60. Mayeroff, M. (1971) *On Caring*. Harper Perennial, New York.

61. Oakley, A. (1984) The importance of being a nurse. *Nursing Times* 83(50), 24–27.

62. Chapman, G. (1983) Ritual and rational action in hospitals. *Journal of Advanced Nursing* 8, 13–20.

63. Smyth, W. J. (1987) *A Rationale for Teachers' Critical Pedagogy*. Deakin University Press, Melbourne.

64. Lieberman, A. (1989) *Staff Development in Culture Building, Curriculum and Teaching: the next 50 Years*. Teachers' College Press, Columbia University, New York.

65. Day, C. (1993) Reflection; a necessary but not sufficient condition for professional development. *British Educational Research Journal* 8, 83–93.

66. Greene, M. (1988) *The Dialectic of Freedom*. Teachers College Press, Columbia University, New York.

67. Belenky, M. F., Clinchy, B. M., Goldberger, N. R., Tarule, J. M. (1986) *Women's ways of Knowing: the Development of Self, Voice, and Mind*. Basic Books, New York.

68. Cochran, L., Laub, L. (1994) *Becoming an Agent: Patterns and Dynamics for Shaping your Life*. State University of New York Press, Albany.

69. Polkingthorne, D. (1996) Transformative narratives: from victimic to agentic life plots. *The American Journal of Occupational Therapy* 50(4), 299–305.

70. Bruner, J. (1994) The remembered self. In U. Neisser, R. Fivush [Eds.] *The Remembering Self: Construction and Accuracy in the Self Narrative*. Cambridge University Press, New York.

71. Carson, J. (2008) *Spider Speculations: a Physics and Biophysics of Storytelling*. Theatre Communications Group, New York.

Notes

i. https://www.rcn.org.uk/Professional-Development/Definition-and-principles-of-nursing.

ii. https://www.nmc.org.uk/standards/code/code-in-action/person-centred.

iii. Mandy was a MSc leadership in healthcare student (see Chapter 14).

iv. I use the terms 'person-centred practice and holistic practice interchangeably as essentially meaning the same thing.

v. As with so many aspects of the book's text, googling concepts reveals a wealth of information. For example, https://www.verywellmind.com/left-brain-vs-right-brain-2795005.

CHAPTER 2

The Six Dialogical Movements Set Within the Model for Structured Reflection

The Six Dialogical Movements

Learning through reflection can be conceived as moving through the 'Six Dialogical Movements' set within the hermeneutic spiral of deepening one's knowing in practice (Figure 2.1).

The first movement is the practitioner paying attention to a particular experience and writing a descriptive account or story text of that experience. The second movement is standing back from and engaging with the story text prompted by a series of reflective cues as set out in the reflective phase of the model for structured reflection (Figure 2.2) to penetrate the breadth and depth of the experience in order to draw tentative insights towards realising a vision of practice.

The third movement is to dialogue with relevant sources of information to deepen and develop insights. The fourth movement is to dialogue with a guide to further deepen and co-construct insights. The third and fourth dialogical movements are interwoven. The fifth movement is to represent insights into reflexive narrative form. The sixth movement is to dialogue the narrative text with an audience (usually through performance) towards social action.

The Hermeneutic Spiral

Hermeneutics is the interpretation of text [1] through reflection on the practitioner's experience (text) resulting in understanding and insights that inform and deepen the practitioner's 'knowing in practice' to inform future experiences.

Imagine throwing a stone into a pool. It makes a splash and sends out ripples over the whole surface of the pool. The pool represents the whole of one's existing pool of knowing in practice that is the background against which each new experience is explored. The stone is the experience drawn attention to by the splash. The ripples are the insights gained through reflection that provide new understanding to deepen the whole pool's knowing in practice. These insights emerge from the existing pool of knowledge. Thus, there is always movement between the whole and its significant parts drawn out from the reflection and subsequently fed back into the 'whole' within an ever-expanding spiral of understanding towards realising one's vision, which is always to be achieved [2].

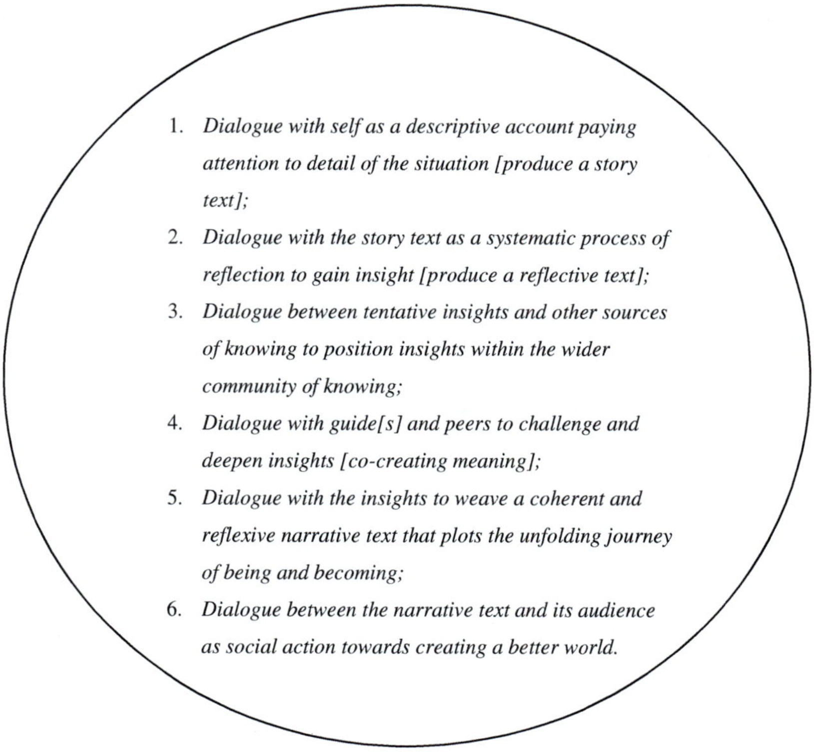

1. *Dialogue with self as a descriptive account paying attention to detail of the situation [produce a story text];*
2. *Dialogue with the story text as a systematic process of reflection to gain insight [produce a reflective text];*
3. *Dialogue between tentative insights and other sources of knowing to position insights within the wider community of knowing;*
4. *Dialogue with guide[s] and peers to challenge and deepen insights [co-creating meaning];*
5. *Dialogue with the insights to weave a coherent and reflexive narrative text that plots the unfolding journey of being and becoming;*
6. *Dialogue between the narrative text and its audience as social action towards creating a better world.*

FIGURE 2.1 The Six Dialogical Movements of reflective learning within the hermeneutic spiral.

Wilber [3, p. 1] alludes to the hermeneutic spiral –

'We move from part to whole and back again, and in that dance of comprehension, in that amazing circle of understanding, we come alive to meaning, to value, and to vision: the very circle of understanding guides our way, weaving together the pieces, healing the fractures, lighting the way ahead – this extraordinary movement from part to whole and back again, with healing the hallmark, of each and every step, and grace the tender reward'.

Wilber's words have poetic resonance. Reflection is coming alive to meaning. Vision is the light ahead. Resolving contradictions is healing the fractures. Moving towards realising one's vision is a movement towards finding grace.

Hermeneutics is not primarily seeking understanding of the movement. It is the movement or flow of experience. In finding meaning, the practitioner comes closer to be who they seek to become. One finds oneself through reflection. As Weinsheimer [2, p. 71] writes –

'It is an event of being that occurs. But this event changes who she is in such a way that she becomes not something different but rather herself'.

As such, reflection is always lived, a way of being in the world rather than an intellectual technique. Reflection is always moving beyond one's own horizon through understanding. Again Weinsheimer [2, p. 182]

'It is possible to become more aware of our historical situation, the situation in which understanding takes place. Having such awareness does not mean that once the situation has become more fully conscious, we can step outside of it, anymore than seeing our own shadow means we can outrun it. Rather our shadow moves along with us. The situation of understanding can also be called our horizon. It marks the limit of everything that can be seen from a particular point of view, but the idea of horizon also implies that we can see beyond our immediate standpoint'.

In other words, there is a world of possibility beyond our existing horizon of understanding, a world pointed at by a vision we seek to become through the dialogue.

Dialogue

Each learning movement is dialogical. Bohm notes that dialogue stems from the Greek word *dia-logos* – 'meaning flowing among and through us, out of which may emerge some new understanding' [4, p. 6].

Isaacs [5, p. 25] describes dialogue as –

> 'A discipline of collective thinking and inquiry, a process for transforming the quality of conversation and, in particular, the thinking that lies beneath it … a movement towards creating a field of genuine meeting and inquiry where people can allow a *free flow of meaning* and vigorous exploration of the collective background of their thought, their personal pre-dispositions, the nature of their shared attention, and the rigid features of their individual and collective assumptions. As people learn to perceive, inquire into, and allow transformation of the nature and shape of these fields, and the patterns of individual thinking and acting that inform them, they may discover entirely new levels of insight and forge substantive and, at times, dramatic changes in behaviour. As this happens, whole new possibilities for coordinated action develop'.

Six Rules of Dialogue

Bohm [4] discerned six 'rules' of dialogue:

1. Commitment to work with others towards consensus for realising a collective vision of practice.
2. Awareness and suspension of one's own assumptions and prejudices in order to participate with an open mind.
3. Proprioception of thinking – becoming aware of one's thoughts at any time – 'This is how I am thinking'. It is mindfulness in action.
4. Open to possibility and free from attachment to ideas that governed previous ways of viewing practice.
5. Listening with engagement and respect to what others are saying.
6. Those involved having a mutual appreciation of dialogical rules.

Dialogue is a deliberate form of communication. This may be difficult to achieve when normal forms of talk or communication have been non-dialogical. It needs to be cultivated.

As Issacs notes [5, p. 24] –

> 'Most forms of organizational conversation, particularly around tough, complex, or challenging issues lapse into debate (the root of which means "to beat down"). In debate, one side wins and another loses; both parties maintain their certainties, and both suppress deeper inquiry. Debate reflects patterns of power relationships and rivalry, were people jostle for control typified by people lining up to get their point across and win the argument. Very little genuine listening takes. People partially listen to what they want to hear, seeking feedback to reinforce their position rather than be open to new possibility through dialogue'.

Bohm's ideas on dialogue were strongly influenced by Krishnamurti's belief that dialogue could penetrate and transform the way people thought about issues, enabling new ways of seeing and responding to issues that could uproot old ways of thought, and in doing so liberate the mind from traditions and habits. In Krishamurtis's words [6, p. 93] –

To inquire and learn is the function of the mind. By learning I do not mean the mere cultivation of memory or the accumulation of knowledge, but the capacity to think clearly without illusion.

As such, the foremost intention of dialogue is the process of dialogue itself rather than its results. This requires careful listening that requires an awareness and suspension of personal ambition, dominant perspectives, values, defensiveness and weight of tradition. Yet, listening is a rare quality in the patterns of talk that dominate practice and education. Do we listen to what we want to hear, or distort what we hear to fit into our own scheme, to confirm our own assumptions?

Given the powerful influence of tradition on how people respond to the world, the dialogical intent is to surface and understand the way the practitioner's prejudices and assumptions create contradiction with what is desirable and work to shift these prejudices and assumptions so they are no longer contradictory.

Bohm [4] notes how thought is infiltrated with these notions. As such, dialogue requires people to be critically conscious of their own thinking, so it does not corrupt the effort to find true meaning. Bohm terms this proprioception of thought in much the same way the body is aware of itself in space. This does not mean the listener has to agree with what is being said, but to understand what is being said without a sense of judgment to allow the dialogue to flow. The aim of dialogue is to understand and explore divergent perspectives and the assumptions that support such perspectives moving towards consensus and harmony. Bohm notes [4, p. 4] –

> 'It is clear that if we are to live in harmony with ourselves and with nature, we need to be able to communicate freely in a creative movement in which no one permanently holds to or otherwise defends his own ideas'.

Thus, to dialogue, participants must be ready to drop old ideas and intentions towards making something in common or 'co-creating meaning'.

As Gadamer [1, p. 263] writes –

> 'If understanding always meaning coming to an understanding, then it always involves two— and two different—participants. The ideal is not that one party should understand the other but rather they should reach an understanding between them. This "between" is the true locus of hermeneutics'.

To dialogue, people must not only know and suspend their assumptions and opinions but also be aware of the thinking that gave rise to these assumptions in the first place. Where do they arise from, and how tenacious do we cling to them? Why do we cling to them? Within the dialogical process, there is a shift from problem-solving towards acknowledging and resolving paradox that requires thinking about the way people think about things. If we use the same thinking that caused the problem to try and solve the problem, we fail. Hence, we need to change the way we think to view the problem differently. As Bohm [4, p. 25] writes –

> 'We could say that practically all the problems of the human race are due to the fact that thought is not proprioceptive. Thought is constantly creating problems that way and then trying to solve them. But as it tries to solve them it makes it worse because it doesn't notice that it's creating them, and the more it thinks, the more problems it creates—because it's not proprioceptive of what it's doing'.

Only then can people transform their perspectives to see things differently. Finally, dialogue requires that those involved in dialogue have a mutual appreciation of dialogue and ensure when in dialogue with others that the dialogical rules are both known and nurtured.

The Model for Structured Reflection (MSR)

Throughout the book, I advocate that practitioners use the Model for Structured Reflection to reflect on their experiences although, as noted in Chapter 1, other approaches to reflection have been constructed. The MSR was designed to enable practitioners to access the depth and breadth of experience necessary to reflect, gain and deepen insights to develop the necessary knowing in practice to realise their visions of practice as a lived reality.

The first version of the MSR was constructed in 1991 through analysing the pattern of recorded dialogue in guided reflection, framed within Strauss and Corbin's grounded theory paradigm model [7]. Since then, the MSR has evolved through reflection on its efficacy as evidenced through subsequent editions of 'Becoming a Reflective Practitioner'. The 'Six dialogical movements' are now merged within the successive phases of the MSR.

Figure 2.2 sets out the 19th edition of the MSR structured through six phases;

---

1. *Preparatory phase:*
   Bringing the mind home or clearing the head of distractions to bring oneself fully available to reflect

2. *Descriptive phase:* Write a description of the experience

3. *Reflective phase cues*
   - What is significant to reflect on?
   - Why did I respond as I did?
   - Did I respond in tune with my vision?
   - Did I respond effectively in terms of consequences?
   - Did my feelings and attitudes influence me?
   - Did past experiences influence me?
   - Did I respond ethically and morally?
   - Did other factors influence me?

4. *Anticipatory phase*
   - Given a similar situation, how could I respond more effectively, for the best and in tune with my vision?
   - What might be the consequences of responding differently?
   - Am I able to respond as I envisage?
     Consider:
   - Am I skilful and knowledgeable to respond differently?
   - Do I have the authority respond differently?
   - Do I have the right attitude?
   - Am I poised to respond differently?

5. *What tentative insights do I draw from this experience?*

6. *Informing insights phase*
   - How has theory informed and deepened my insights and knowing in practice?
   - How has guidance deepened my insights? (If in guided reflection)

7. *Wrap up*
   'How do I now feel about the experience?'
   Summarising the actions I intend to take in a reflective journal (to pick up reflexively in subsequent reflections)

8. *Representative phase*
   Communicating my experience(s) and insights to an audience

---

FIGURE 2.2 Model for structured reflection (19th edition).
Source: Christopher Johns/19th edition – June 2024.

1. Preparatory phase
    The preparatory phase of bringing the mind home is simply bringing the mind present to the moment, clearing away distracting thoughts. It is achieved through using the breath (see Chapter 8 for a more detailed exploration through guidance).
2. Descriptive phase
    The descriptive phase is writing a descriptive account of an experience, what I term as 'story text'. This is explored in Chapter 3.
3. Reflective phase
    The reflective phase explores the breadth and depth of the particular experience guided by a series of cues towards drawing tentative insights explored in Chapter 4.
4. Anticipatory phase
    The anticipatory phase considers how the practitioner might respond differently in tune with their vision of practice in future experiences and factors that might constrain them.
5. Insightful phase
    Throughout the reflective process, the practitioner pays constant attention to drawing tentative insights as explored in Chapter 5.
6. Deepening insights phase
    The deepening insights phase is developed through dialogue with sources of information and guidance (Chapters 7– 9).
7. Wrap up phase
    Wrap up as two functions. Firstly, the practitioner to ask themselves – 'How am I now feeling?' This is significant considering that most reflected-on experiences will have a strong affective negative component. Dealing with residual feelings is one reason why guidance is so beneficial (see Chapters 8 and 9).
    Secondly, recording insights gained and consequential actions to take in the practitioner's journal (see Chapter 8).
8. Representative phase
    The representative phase is communicating one's experience and insights to an audience. This may be written as an educational assignment, a publication or as a performance (see Chapter 18).

References

1. Gadamer, H-.G. (1975) *Truth and Method*. Seabury Press, New York.

2. Weinsheimer, J. C. (1985) *Gadamer's Hermeneutics: A Reading of Truth and Method*. Yale University Press.

3. Wilber, K. (1988) *The Eye of Spirit: An Integral Vision of a World Gone Slightly Mad*. Shambhala, Boston.

4. Bohm, D. (1996) *On Dialogue* L. Nichol [Ed.]. Routledge, London.

5. Issacs, W. (1993) *Taking Flight: Dialogue, Collective Thinking, and Organizational Learning*. Centre for Organizational learning's Dialogue project. MIT, Boston.

6. Krishnamurti, J. (1996) *Total Freedom*. Harper, San Francisco.

7. Johns, C. (1998) *Becoming A Reflective Practitioner Through Guided Reflection*. PhD thesis. The Open University, Milton Keynes.

CHAPTER 3

Writing Self: The First Dialogical Movement

'Writing my journal was finding my voice'

(Clare)[i]

Reflection begins with writing an account of a particular experience to create a 'story text' in a journal. Writing self is the raw data of experience. The more detailed the description the more text to reflect on. Through writing self the practitioner learns to pay attention, to become aware of self in context of their environment.

Journal Entry 3.1

Many of the students do not keep a reflective journal. Why? They are not used to keeping a journal. Between sessions they get caught up in their everyday work worlds that distract them. Lucy says she does reflect, but only in her head. I challenge her to write it down; that something deeper happens when we write it down. She agrees she is more attentive to the experience when writing. Other students agree that they must be disciplined to set aside time to write and reflect. They admit they are not used to keeping a journal and that they get caught up in their everyday work worlds.

   Coleman and Willis [1, p. 910] note from their research –

> 'In summary students were in agreement that the writing down of experiences helped them learn more from them, with models of reflection helping to scaffold the process'.

Journal Entry 3.2

Priest and Johns [2, p. 200] write – 'I commenced a journal to help me track my emerging leadership style. Its white pages, however, remained blank for a few weeks. I didn't want to spoil its pages with dull and uninspiring entries. I sought some scandalous event to analyse or an argument to reveal my leadership style, but little came to fruition. My mind kept returning to a sketch by Tony Hancock who excitedly bought a diary and his first entry began with 'I had eggs for breakfast today'. I made a conscious decision to write uninhibitedly, for it seemed the only way to unblock my retained self. I found it hard not to filter my thoughts because of guilt, self-righteousness and a fear of fraudulent existence. To let the words and emotions flow onto the page, I just wrote, even if it made no sense, I just wrote.

Even if it made me feel stupid, I just wrote. Even if I felt vulnerable, I just wrote. I wrote it as if no one was watching. Because the truth is, when the mud settled down and the clouds cleared away, everything became a little clearer each day, I just wrote'.

These words capture the essence of writing self-*just write*. What is written is the raw data of one's practice, the raw data for reflection. However, practitioners may struggle to write as if they hit a mental block. Perhaps telling stories is more spontaneous, whilst writing is more considered, more cognitive and more self-conscious as if an internal censor is at work trying to fit the description into learnt ways of writing that may inhibit expression and stifle the imagination. Some people will always struggle to write despite advice to just let the words spontaneously flow.

Writing is taking ownership of one's experience. It enables the practitioner to pay attention to and become aware of their practice, the first step to becoming a reflective practitioner and realising one's vision. I cannot emphasise enough the significance of paying attention in becoming a reflective practitioner. It is an awakening and inquiry into self.

Tufnell and Crickmay [3, p. 63] note how –

'Writing gives us time to absorb the feel of what has just happened. While movement is ephemeral, quickly vanishing from our memory, written language remains, giving us a means of dwelling upon and finding significance in what has just occurred'.

The practitioner writes to recall their experience through rich description, paying attention to detail and drawing on the senses. It is 'replaying the situation in the mind's eye' [4, p. 27]. Recalling the experience is subjective, viewed from the practitioner's particular perspective. It is best written from the perspective of 'I' rather than in the third person that depersonalises the experience as if turning self into an object. It is 'I' in relationship with others.

Gully [5, p. 151] writes –

'The process of journaling is by far the most significant act in my practice, for it records the process of my evolving as a human being and connects me with the other in my nursing relationship; it is the journey from the "I" to the "we"'.

Writing a journal is the search for meaning of one's vision as something lived and understanding why things are as they are.

As one student noted [6, p. 94].

'Having my diary is like having my own personal textbook, a reference to my own practice and no one else's. I can look back and add further thoughts days after the event. I have been able to identify learning domains, recurring issues and tie them together and begin to make sense of them'.

Writing exposes the self and opens a world of possibilities.

As Manjusvara [7, p. 10] writes –

'The practice of writing takes us to the heart of ourselves and makes it palpable how alive with possibilities we really are'.

Manjusvara's words suggest that writing wakes the self up to our human potential, a self that might have become deadened to the world for whatever reason, where potential has shrunk to virtual nothing. Writing is cathartic, enabling the discharge of strong feelings, feelings that will later be explored through reflection.

One student wrote [6, p. 92]

'This patient was blind with anger. I used a cathartic response that acknowledged this anger. It enabled the patient, whilst still angry to exclaim "I'm angry because ...!" Reflection has helped me reflect on confronting people with their anger. Writing my reflective diary has also helped me – normally I would absorb all that anger – although professionally you know you shouldn't carry it around with you alongside my own feelings. – writing about it helped me discharge some of it – I felt better about it after I had written about it'.

Writing spontaneously lifts unconscious matters to the surface.
As Ferruci [8, p. 41] writes –

'Writing can be much more powerful that we may think at first. We should not be surprised that unconscious material surfaces so readily in our writing'.

Keeping a Reflective Journal

I carry a small notebook for making notes that I can later reflect on. These notes are reminders me about the situation or noting dialogue that I might not quite remember later. These notes can then be worked up on the computer [my digital reflective journal]. I write in the present tense to better capture the moment. I let the words come as a spontaneous flow in rich description, paying attention to as much detail as possible, pursuing signs, running off on tangents.
As Wheatley [9, p. 143] writes –

'We paint a portrait of the whole, surfacing as much detail as possible'.

Recalling the moment, paying attention to the look on the person's face, a word said, a tear shed, a feeling, a harsh word spoken, uncertainty, the dance of the trees outside the window. These things may seem insignificant on the surface of things but they all add up.

Writing is perhaps best done as a letting go into imagination rather than a rigid attempt to remember every fine detail. In this way, images and ideas emerge. Tufnell and Crickmay note [3, p. 63] that writing –

'May be fluent, or clumsy, abundant of brief, poetic or plain. We have to assume it will be the necessary expression for this moment'.

These words offer helpful advice to the practitioner not to be over concerned about what or how they write. The practitioner should feel free to write in any linguistic form such as poetry or draw images in whatever way best suits them. Remember – you are writing yourself for yourself. It is honouring self, warts and all. It should never be a chore.

Journal Entry 3.3

One evening I wrote in my journal after a shift at the hospice where I work as a voluntary therapist –

Indigo lies on her bed. Her arm tucked up behind her head, her eyes are closed. She makes little movements of her waxed lips. Shifts of her pelvis as if trying to get comfortable, little furrows of pain between her eyes. Her swollen abdomen incongruent with her emaciated body. The staff tell me they struggle to keep on top of her pain. The diamorphine dose has reached 160 mg. via the syringe driver. I listen to its regular pulse infuse its cargo into Indigo's tired veins. For a moment technology holds the gaze and then I see Indigo again against a backdrop of flowers with white and yellow heads that adorn the bedside. A friend from church sits with her. The quiet waiting room. The aroma-stone has gone. I find it in the clinical room 'in soak'. I feel the conflict stir within me, mindful of the merry-go-round of careless action. A care assistant says it went dry, adding 'They have not had time to replenish it'. The conflict rises inside like a malevolent energy. I would like to say 'It is not a question of time it is a question of attention'. But mindful of the critical parent rising within me, I refrain. Bottle up the anger. Not good!

This description simply says what happened. What you write should not be written to suit others although there are some useful tips to help the writer.

1. Pay attention to everything that seems to impinge upon the experience no matter how tangential it is. Do not discard anything. It may emerge as significant.
2. Write as spontaneously as possible. To facilitate spontaneous expression, I assert *'write without taking the pen of the paper'*. Spontaneity is a helpful instruction because it encourages the writer not to over think the description but let it flow as if it is the body writing rather than the mind. When we lift the pen, we pause, and think and get stuck.
    Manjusvara [7, p. 37] notes –

    > 'As the hand begins to overtake the brain it is amazing how often there emerges a coherent statement of what I had previously been struggling to say'.

3. Draw on all your senses. What did things look like, smell like, sound like, even taste like, what did I sense? Paying attention to detail- the colour of the walls, what noises permeated the situation? What time of day? Such things may seem immaterial at the time of writing but on reflection may gain significance. The more detail the better.
4. Prepare yourself to pay attention to your experiences and write your journal by finding a quite space free from distraction.
5. Give free rein to your imagination. Writing should be approached with a playful and creative spirit. IT is YOU! In writing, you are writing yourself, your body, nurturing your precious and unique self. In writing you change yourself on a subliminal level. As Ferruci [8, p. 42] says 'It is like cutting a new pathway in a jungle'.
6. Capture 'talk' that took place during the experience using actual words as recalled. It leads to recall of the moment and better description.
7. Ask yourselves questions – 'I wondered what she was thinking?' These will highlight points that can be picked up later on reflection. You do not have to answer the questions in the description.
8. Considering the points above, it doesn't matter what you write and if you just write just a few words to jolt the memory at a later time to pick up on reflection.

Journal Entry 3.4

In the reflection workshop, the practitioners write furiously for the allotted 20 minutes. Afterwards, many say they were surprised by what they have written. They note how their writing went off on tangents to the extent that some of them did not write about what they had intended to or hadn't yet come to the specific point. They all seemed to enjoy this creative form of writing even though it some of them say it first seemed alien and difficult to start. Revealing the storied self. Putting together the pieces of self, of life itself. It is a creative and restorative act.

Tufnell and Crickmay [3, p. 41] note how

> 'Creating is a way of listening and of trying to speak more personally from within the various worlds we inhabit. It is a way of discovering our own stories, refreshing and reawakening our language and giving form to the way we feel'.

I advocate people write about the experience soon after it happens. My own edict is to write within 24 hours of the experience. Although I have no hard evidence to support this.

However, practitioners' feedback that this is useful advice. Of course, I don't always achieve this edict. Sometimes a week or even a month goes past and I haven't written about the experience for whatever reason. I can still recall it clearly and yet I wonder if my recall has become more distorted through time. It might suit some people to write at a later time when the immediacy of the experience has settled. Writing too soon after a situation may not be enough time for the emotional mud to settle and for things to become clearer.

Sylvia Plath [10, p. 147] writes in one letter to her mother

> 'The thing about writing is not to talk, but to do it; no matter how bad or even mediocre it is, the process and production is the thing, not the sitting and theorizing about how one should write ideally, or how one could write if one really wanted to or had the time'.

Plath's words are a reminder about not getting caught up in technique.

Journal Entry 3.5

One student asks – 'How do I write?'
I respond – 'Just do it. Let if come and flow as naturally as water flowing in a stream'.
'Give me a clue' the student asks.
'Were you at work yesterday? I respond
'Yes'
'Think of one patient you nursed?'
'Well a couple of days ago I thought about one patient who was sad'
'Ok so now write a story about that'.

He wrote – 'Mr Smith is 46. He sits in his chair by the bed. He seems sad. I am frustrated that I do not have enough time to spend with him and the moments I have made time I 'm not sure how to help him which makes me want to stay away from him. So I feel caught in a dilemma'.

Later I ask 'How was that?'
'It has opened a real work of cans to reflect on'.

Triggers

When practitioners commence writing, they are more likely to focus on situations that for whatever reason have caused anxiety and become lodged in the mind accompanied by uncomfortable feelings, such as anger, guilt, sadness, frustration and resentment [11]. These emotions create a sense of drama in the mind. It may be triggered by what the practitioner has written before, as if what is written is a continuation of previous experiences. This is likely as the practitioner becomes more experienced in reflection and begins to see patterns emerging through reflection. In other words, writing becomes more reflective than simply descriptive over time.

The student mentioned in *Journal entry 6* was at a loss to know what to write about. It was his anxiety at not knowing how to respond to a sad man that caught his attention. It follows that the practitioner may *naturally* reflect either consciously or subconsciously to defend against this anxiety. They may distort, rationalise, project or even deny the situation that caused these feelings. Chodron [12, p. 12] helps us view negative feelings more positively as an opportunity for learning and growth. She writes –

> 'Generally speaking, we regard discomfort in any form as bad news. But for practitioners or spiritual warriors – people who have a certain hunger to know what is true – feelings like disappointment, irritation, resentment, anger, jealousy and fear, instead of being bad news, are actually

very clear moments that teach us where it is that we're holding back. They teach us to perk up and lean in when we feel we'd rather collapse and back away. They're like messengers that show us with terrifying clarity, exactly where we're stuck. This very moment is the perfect teacher and, lucky for us, it's with us wherever we are'.

Chodron advocates practitioners face up to their anxiety to see anxiety as an opportunity for learning.

In a similar vein Paramananda [13, p. 58] writes –

'Whenever we begin to feel frustrated in what we are doing, we should slow down and pay closer attention to it. Frustration takes us away from ourselves; we become alienated from our experience. When we feel this beginning to happen we need to pay more attention to our experience'.

Some practitioners may find writing helps them face up to and work through their feelings, but others may find it difficult and require guidance. Writing about experience may stir up uncomfortable feelings. As Jade noted –

'I haven't written about it in my diary – I suppose I was trying to avoid it the issue – you churn it all up again writing the notes' [14, p. 92].

Gray and Forsstrom [15, p. 360] write –

'The process of "Journaling" may sound simple and easy to execute, but at times it was extremely difficult. Mostly the incidents recorded were identified because there was an affective component. This may be related to feelings of personal inadequacy to cope with the demands of the situation. Alone, it was emotionally painful to journal events that were largely self-critical'.

Perhaps this is a strong reason why many practitioners want to steer clear of reflection or merely pay lip service to it. They don't want to go there because it is uncomfortable to look at oneself in a critical way. It may challenge one's self-image of being a caring and effective practitioner.

A consequence of only paying attention and writing about negative stuff is that the practitioner may get into a pattern of negative thinking about self and practice. They may despair about oneself, the organisation and colleagues. Not much fun. However, it is significant to experience our anger, our sorrow, our failure and our apprehension; for these feelings are all our teachers when practitioners do not try and defend against them. Then, learning is not possible. That's not hard to understand, just hard to do [16].

Useful advice to practitioners is to balance writing about positive experiences so as to give oneself positive feedback. However, it is less likely practitioners will pay attention to positive experiences because they are often taken for granted, especially for the novice reflective practitioner. I know through auditing the experiences practitioners share in guided reflection a shift from solely reflecting on negative experiences to affirming experiences as they become more experienced with reflection and have learnt to pay attention to all experience as they begin to live reflection in their everyday practice.

In my action research study of working with an NHS Trust to implement clinical supervision [14], Holly [one of the participants] noted in response to the question, 'Was keeping a diary helpful?'

'Yes, but I wish I had managed to do so on a daily basis. When I reflected in the group on experiences I had previously written down I feel we were able to get much further than when I talked about something off the top of my head'.

In the same study, Lisa noted

'I feel a reflective diary would be very helpful although I was not able to keep a diary which I put down to time constraints. I feel it would useful as the experiences that I wrote out in preparation for supervision encouraged me to reflect further'.

Tapping the Tacit

Writing may be difficult for practitioners because much of their knowing is tacit and not easily explainable [17]. In other words, practitioners may struggle to write what they know.

Schon [17, p. 49] writes –

> 'When we go about the spontaneous intuitive performance of the actions of everyday life, we show ourselves to be knowledgeable in a certain way. Often we cannot say what it is we know. When we try to describe it we find ourselves at loss, or we produce descriptions that are obviously inappropriate. Our knowing is ordinarily tacit, implicit in our action and in our feel for the stuff with which we are dealing. It seems to right to say that our knowing is in our doing'.

However, I would argue that no description is obviously inappropriate. Writing is what it is. The practitioner need not be concerned with tapping tacit knowledge. Through subsequent reflection and guidance tacit knowing will naturally bubble to the surface. Writing is only the first step.

As Holly [18, p. 71] writes –

> 'It [keeping a reflective journal] makes possible new ways of theorizing, reflecting on and coming to know one's self. Capturing certain words while the action is fresh, the author is often provoked to question why ... writing taps tacit knowledge; it brings into awareness that which we sense but could not explain'.

Summarising the benefits of keeping a reflective journal:

1. Writing enables the practitioner to relive the experience, lifting it into consciousness and significance.
2. Writing is cathartic and healing given that most experiences are triggered by emotional disturbance.
3. Writing is paying attention to one's practice leading the practitioner to become increasing self-aware and perceptive within practice.
4. Writing prepares the practitioner for revealing their experiences within guided reflection. This leads to a more productive use of guided reflection time.
5. Writing is energetic and stimulating curiosity and commitment to the one's practice.
6. Writing enables the practitioner to take responsibility for their practice and development.
7. Writing gives the practitioner 'a voice', enabling the expression of feelings, thoughts and opinions.

Susan Brooks' [19] reflects on the benefits of keeping her reflective journal

> 'Having never attempted to keep a reflective journal before, the journey ahead seemed a little daunting as evidenced by the first recorded entry – "Today I start my journal. What shall I write? I'm really worried about this whole thing – will I get time to do it – will I want to do it – will I do it right? If I'm honest in it will it matter if others read it? Reflective practice – what is it really? I think I know but I don't think I've ever really done it properly. I feel so uncertain about everything at the moment and a bit scared and threatened. I don't feel I know anything about myself really and I suppose I just do what I do to fit in. I need to get over this and get on with it – pull yourself together Sue – you know you can do it'".

This first journal entry reveals my initial uncomfortable reactions to the prospect of journal writing. I had doubts about my capacity to write, felt threatened by having to face myself on paper, questioned my ability to manage my internal censors that may inhibit complete honesty and held the naïve assumption that there is a correct way to keep a journal – all classic reactions to journaling [20]. My initial fears were quickly dispelled as the value of my journal soon became evident. After a while, it became a powerful emancipatory tool in giving my innermost thoughts voice. I was the only person with access to the journal and, possibly because of this, it became a very cathartic experience to write. As the process continued, I soon recognised that I did not need to confront all the chaos of my personal or professional life at any one time and became more discriminatory about the events that I considered worthy of deeper reflection and subsequent action [20]. The journal became, in a sense, my autobiography, containing both positive and less than positive experiences – a non-hagiographic record of my daily life. My journal had, after just a few months on the course, become a silent but very powerful and challenging teacher – perhaps more persuasive and influential than any human embodiment that I had met. The following entry signifies just how my attitude had changed since that first entry at the start of the course. 'I read of a teacher today who got very excited about writing his journal. He wrote that he felt especially good about writing for himself instead of someone else. His written thoughts were entirely his own regardless of lack of style, format or academic expression. He had never written like this before and felt that he was really communicating with and understanding himself'. That's just how I feel now and I wish I had started writing like this ages ago. To be unrestricted by structural rigour, academic expectations and the approval of others is so liberating!'

From the practical aspect, a double entry technique was used with the factual account (data collection) of the experience written on the left of the page and the reflective thought (the analysis) on the right [21]. Both the ordinary and extraordinary events of every day practice were included to prevent selective inattention, particularly to the seemingly mundane, where habitual routine practice is thought most likely to occur [22]. I considered myself to be the primary research tool here. If the journal was to accurately and consistently record my own experiential world I needed to maintain a strong sense of commitment to the task and demonstrate the skills necessary to the reflective cycle – self-awareness, description, critical analysis, synthesis and evaluation [23]. Keeping a journal enabled me to enter into a dialogue between my objective and subjective self and it transformed my feeling self into a spectator and analyst of my own personal professional drama [20]. Street [20] writes that journaling provides the reflector with a process for meta-theorising, that is thinking about the processes of thinking. This significantly developed not only my skills of reflection but also my skills as a learner in general, moving me away from my previously held attitude that knowledge (and not necessarily enhanced learning skills) was the goal to be achieved'.

Susan extols the virtue of keeping her journal. Note her technique of dividing the page. And yet, at the beginning she felt daunted. It is a serious matter for the practitioner to enter into reflective practice. It requires commitment and responsibility reflecting why practitioners might struggle to keep a reflective journal. They are tired at the end of the day, they want to switch off, they don't see the value, they do not have the discipline, they don't find it meaningful, they lack technique or they don't see the point. Perhaps writing needs the stimulus of a specific purpose, such as an educational course, clinical supervision or demand to keep a professional portfolio. Put another way, practitioners might need to do something with their writing, a means towards an end rather than just an end in itself. I found this true for myself as I wrote and reflected on my experiences with the intention of constructing a reflexive narrative or performance, or using my stories for teaching, and analysing the learning process as an educational and research approach. As Susan comments, some practitioners will find writing story easy whilst others struggle as if some mind censor constrains the writing potential. If you have never written about self before it may feel strange, even threatening. The reflective mirror is not always kind, especially if we write about things, we find difficult for whatever reason. Then, we may subconsciously distort our recall and create false impressions of ourselves. Hence, writing is courageous. It requires effort, honesty and perseverance.

The Therapeutic Benefit of Writing

Writing a story of experience is healing [24]. Without doubt, healthcare work is stressful, embracing suffering on a daily basis and working under conditions that do not necessarily facilitate caring work. As such, it seems imperative that practitioners have a mode for expressing and sharing their feelings.

The subtitle of Rachel Remen's [25] book *Kitchen Table Wisdom* is 'stories that heal'. She claims that in telling our stories, we connect with something vital in us, something healing. She writes [25, p. 70] –

> 'Whatever we have denied may stop us and dam the creative flow of our lives ... avoiding pain, we may linger in the vicinity of our wounds ... without reclaiming that which we have denied, we cannot know our wholeness or have our healing'.

The reclaiming is in telling or writing the story. Writing is the creative flow of our lives. If we do this consistently, then it washes away traumatic debris before it can accumulate into a dam. Then, we have a crisis. Jourard [26] argues that self-disclosure of upsetting experiences serves as a basic human motive. As such, people naturally discuss daily and significant experiences with others. Talking through a trauma with others can strengthen social bonds, provide coping information and emotional support and hasten an understanding of the event; the inability to talk with others can be unhealthy.

In reviewing the therapeutic benefit of telling and writing experience, the work of Pennebaker's [27] (1990) book title – 'Opening up the healing power of confiding in others' tells his overall message – the idea of story as 'opening up'. And in opening up, letting go of the tension within. Pennebaker [28, p. 213] writes –

> 'When given the opportunity, people readily divulge their deepest and darkest secrets. Even though people report they have lived with these thoughts and feelings virtually every day, most note that they have actively held back from telling others about these fundamental parts of themselves. Over the past several years, my colleagues and I have learned that confronting traumatic experiences can have meaningful physiological and psychological benefit. Conversely, not confiding significant experiences is associated with increased disease rates, ruminations and other difficulties'.

Pennebaker and his various colleagues [29, 30] demonstrated the therapeutic benefit of therapeutic journaling in well-being, notably the benefit of connecting strong feelings to past traumatic events. Smyth et al.'s [31] review of the literature suggested that emotional expression has a salutary health effect, whereas emotional inhibition has a detrimental health effect. Smyth et al. cite Pennebaker et al.'s [30, p. 865] claim that

> 'Written emotional expression leads to a transduction of the traumatic experience into a linguistic structure that promotes assimilation and understanding of the event, and reduces negative affect associated with thoughts of the event'.

Smyth et al. [31] reviewed 10 studies that demonstrated significant superior health outcomes in health participants; psychological well-being, physiological functioning, general functioning and reported health outcomes, but not for health behaviours. They noted that these studies demonstrated that short-term distress was increased but is thought to be related to long-term improvement, indicating a need to support or guide practitioners in writing about their emotional experiences.

Pennebaker et al. [29, p. 536] write

> 'The present experiment, as well as others that we have conducted, found that writing about transition to college resulted in more negative moods and poorer psychological adjustment by the end of the first semester. Our experiment may have effectively stripped the normal

defences away from the experimental subjects. With lowered defences, our subjects were forced to deal with many of their basic conflicts and fears about leaving home, changing roles, entering college'.

Indications from this study suggest that writing my initially have had a detrimental effect that learnt defensive mechanisms had protected them from. In the follow-up questionnaires, the overwhelming majority of the subjects wrote that the value of the experimental condition derived from their achieving a better understanding of their own thoughts, behaviours and moods, suggesting the subjects had developed healthier defence mechanisms to cope with reality shock.

Ann Saunders [32] writes

'My journal has been a comfort, friend and critic enabling me to view situations from a variant slant. It has made me stand still and enabled me to select issues from the unending data that Wheatley [33] describes as being barely noticeable in the fast pace of our lives. I hesitated to write honestly and openly towards self. Street [20] likened this to the recognition of an "internal censor," which regulates emotions, feelings and failings which flags them up to myself and others to criticize. The internal censor however is also open to questioning through self, being honest and in recognizing the need for truth. This is the practitioner's responsibility and one I did not take to lightly. As one continues to journal and the benefits become apparent, the unfolding moments are unveiled in greater depth and insight. Sometimes I surprise myself with my writing. Writing transcends the rational mind, and as we write we stumble upon and discover images, metaphors, analogies and symbols that sharpen perception, hold meaning and "open ourselves into intuition of which our rational side is barely conscious"' [7, p. 12].

Writing self is just a question of doing it. Do it your own style, whatever works best for you. So –

1. Think of the last time you were at work. Now think about one particular situation. It needn't be dramatic. It can simply be something mundane or ordinary, perhaps something you wouldn't normally give a second thought.
2. First relax and bring your mind home. Now write a description of this situation for 15–20 minutes. Do not to take your pen off the paper. Do not stop and think about the why's of the situation. Just let the pen or keyboard flow spontaneously, in rich graphic description, paying attention to detail, drawing on all your senses. Capture actual dialogue spoken. Just write.
3. After you finish writing, pause, and stand back. Read what you have written with an open and curious mind. Ask yourself – 'what is significant in what I have written?' Responding to this question you enter the reflective spiral.

Moving into Reflective Mode

Whilst writing, the practitioner may pause and dialogue with what they have written to dig deeper into their description of the experience and moving into a reflective mode whereby writing self merges into reflection. In Chapter 4, I consider how the Model for Structured Reflection can scaffold the reflective process.

References

1. Coleman, D., Willis, D. S. (2015) Reflective writing; the student nurse's perspective on reflective writing and poetry writing. *Nurse Education Today* 35(7), 906–911.

2. Priest, J.-M., Johns, C. (2010) More than eggs for breakfast. In C. Johns [Ed.] *Guided Reflection: A Narrative Approach to Advancing Professional Practice* (second edition). Wiley-Blackwell, Oxford, 195–214.

3. Tufnell, M., Crickmay, C. (2004) *A Widening Field: Journeys in Body and Imagination.* Dance Books, Alton.

4. Boud, D., Keogh, R., Walker, D. (1985) Promoting reflection in learning: a model. In D. Boud, R. Keogh, D. Walker [Eds.] *Reflection: Turning Experience into Learning.* Kogan Page, London.

5. Gully, E. (2005) Creating sacred space: a journey to the soul. In C. Johns, D. Freshwater [Eds.] *Transforming Nursing through Reflective Practice* (second edition). Blackwell Publishing, Oxford.

6. Johns, C. (1997) Reflective practice and clinical supervision. Part 1: The Reflective Turn. *European Nurse* 2(2), 87–97.

7. Manjusvara. (2005) *Writing your Way.* Windhorse, Birmingham.

8. Ferruci, P. (1982) *What we may be.* St. Martin's Press, New York.

9. Wheatley, M. J. (1999) *Leadership and the New Science: Discovering Order in a Chaotic World.* Berrett-Koehler, San Francisco.

10. Plath, S. (1975) *Letters Home.* Harper & Row, New York.

11. Boyd, E., Fales, A. (1983) Reflective learning: key to learning from experience. *Journal of Humanistic Psychology* 23(2), 99–117.

12. Chodron, P. (2000) *When Things Fall Apart.* Shambhala, Boston.

13. Paramananda. (2001) *A Deeper Beauty: Buddhist Reflections on Everyday Life.* Windhorse, Birmingham.

14. Johns, C. (1997) *Implementing Clinical Supervision [guided reflection] within an NHS Trust: Study 1.* Unpublished Report. Centre for Reflective Practice, Institute for Health Services Research, University of Luton, Bedfordshire.

15. Gray, G., Forsstrom, S. (1991) Generating theory from practice: the reflective technique. In G. Gray, R. Pratt [Eds.] *Towards A Discipline of Nursing.* Churchill Livingstone, Melbourne, 355–372.

16. Beck, C. Y. (1989) *Everyday Zen.* Thorsons, London.

17. Schön, D. (1983) *The Reflective Practitioner.* Avebury, Aldershot.

18. Holly, M. L. (1989) Reflective writing and the spirit of inquiry. *Cambridge Journal of Education* 19(1), 71–80.

19. Brooks, S. (2004) '*Becoming A Transformational Leader*'. Unpublished Masters in Leadership dissertation. University of Bedfordshire, Bedford.

20. Street, A. (1995) *Nursing Replay.* Churchill Livingstone, Melbourne.

21. Moon, J. (2002) *Reflection in Learning and Professional Development: Theory and Practice.* Routledge, London.

22. Heath, H., Freshwater, D. (2000) Clinical supervision as an emancipatory process avoiding inappropriate intent. *Journal of Advanced Nursing* 32, 1298–1306.

23. Atkins, S., Murphy, K. (1993) Reflective practice. *Nursing Standard* 9(45), 31–37.

24. De Salvo, L. (1999) *Writing as a Way of Healing: How Telling our Stories Transforms our Lives.* The Women's Press, London.

25. Remen, R. (1996) *Kitchen Table Wisdom.* Riverhead Books, New York.

26. Jourard, S. (1971) *The Transparent Self.* Van Nostrand, Newark.

27. Pennebaker, J. (1990) *Opening Up: The Healing Power of Confiding in others.* Morrow, New York.

28. Pennebaker, J. (1989) Confession, inhibition and disease. *Advances in Experimental Social Psychology* 22, 211–244.

29. Pennebaker, J., Colder, M., Sharp, L. (1990) Accelerating the coping process. *Journal of Personality and Social Psychology* 58, 528–537.

30. Pennebaker, J., Mayne, T., Francis, M. (1997) Linguistic predictors of adaptive bereavement. *Journal of Personality and Social Psychology* 7, 863–871.

31. Smyth, J., Stone, A., Hurewitz, A., Kaell, A. (1999) Effects of writing about stressful experiences on symptom reduction in patients with asthma or rheumatoid arthritis. *Journal of the American Medical Association* 281, 1304–1309.

32. Saunders, A. (2006) *Transforming Self Through Transformational Leadership.* Unpublished MSc Leadership in Healthcare, University of Bedfordshire, Bedford.

33. Wheatley, M. (1999) *Leadership and the New Science.* Berrett-Koehler, San Francisco.

Note

i. Clare's narrative 'Life begins at 40' is shown in Chapter 18.

CHAPTER 4

Engaging the Reflective Spiral: The Second Dialogical Movement

In Chapter 3, I explored *writing self* as the first Dialogical Movement. Having written a description of an experience, the practitioner stands back from the descriptive text to view it more objectively and move into the second dialogical movement to reflect on the experience guided by the Model for Structured Reflection (MSR (Figure 2.2)).

The MSR cues guide the practitioner to penetrate the breadth and depth of experience towards gaining insight. Thus, the practitioner always keeps in mind – 'what insights can I draw'. As Caitlin noted (cited from Chapter 12)

> 'Using the MSR cues was very helpful to open up aspects of the experience. The cues made sense and were easy to use'.

The novice reflective practitioner will benefit from systematically applying the cues until they become second nature and used more intuitively. Then, the descriptive and reflection phases will tend to merge to the point, whereby the practitioner is using the cues in writing their descriptions.

Using the cues will naturally shape the practitioner's awareness and perception of practice, nurturing the development of reflection within practice.

Janet Graham noted (1, p. 91–92)

> 'I personally feel that I would have been lost without the model for structured reflection that I used for my journal keeping. I fear this would have remained at the descriptive level. Describing events but not knowing what to do with the description is almost like sitting in a car without wheels forever stuck on the starting line of reflection without the ability to move down the road to being a more effective practitioner'.

The Reflective Cues

The cues can be viewed are markers along a reflective spiral from significance – 'what lies on the surface of the experience' to drawing insights – 'what lies deeper within the practitioner'.

'What Is Significant to Reflect on?'

What is significant is usually obvious from what triggered the practitioner's attention to the particular experience. It gives reflection its initial focus. However, in writing description other significant issues emerge as if one thing leads to another, unravelling the complexity of everyday practice.

'Why Did I Respond as I Did?'

Having surfaced what might be significant, the practitioner inquires into how they responded within the situation in context of what they were trying to achieve. In doing so, they explore the reasoning behind their actions. This may be complex as many decisions are often made reactively or intuitively.

It became evident through guiding practitioners that they tend to respond based on three criteria:

- Responses they have used before;
- Responses that have worked before;
- Responses they are comfortable using.

What was not evident was practitioners responding towards realising a vision. This reflects how doing tasks in contrast with realising a vision was generally governing practice.

The practitioner can review how they responded through the 'cycle of clinical judgment'. This comprises four movements: assessment, judgement, response and evaluation (Figure 4.1). 'How did I appreciate or assess the situation?' asks the practitioner to reflect on how they perceived the situation. The most obvious issues are whether they knew the person adequately in terms of 'Who is this person?' leading to an appreciation of the person's health-illness experience.

Based on reflection of assessment, the practitioner can then reflect on their rationale for the decisions they made in terms of what they were trying to achieve, and consequently on the actions they took and whether these actions were effective in light of outcomes for both the person(s) involved in the experience and for themselves.

To ask the question – 'Was I effective?' requires the practitioner to have a grasp of what effectiveness would look like. Some situations can be observed or measured, for

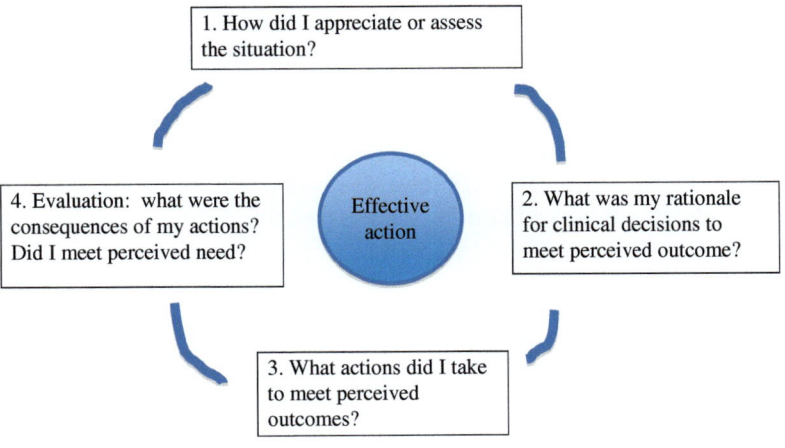

FIGURE 4.1 Cycle of clinical judgement.

example, wound healing. Other situations less so, such as giving advice whereby judging effectiveness is subjective and best perceived from the patient's perspective.

'Did I Respond in Tune with My Vision?'

This cue lifts the practitioner's vision or lack of vision into scrutiny – 'Did I act in tune with my vision?' or 'What is my vision?' It challenges the practitioner to consider what their vision is and what it means as something lived beyond the words used to express it. It sets up the basic contradiction as the core element of learning through reflection.

'Did I Respond Effectively in Terms of Consequences?'

Actions have consequences. This cue prompts the practitioner to reflect on the consequences of their actions linked to effectiveness. On the surface, consequences may be quite obvious. Others will be less so. Imagine throwing a pebble into a pond. The splash is the immediate consequence and the ripples spreading out are further, longer-term consequences that are less easy to perceive and may only be revealed over time.

Considering the consequences of one's actions facilitates the development of foresight – the ability to weigh up the likely consequences of actions as part of the decision-making process. Whilst foresight can be informed by previous experience and theory, it is predominantly intuitive, for how can consequences be known given the uncertainty of the human experience? Aristotle [2] termed this ability 'phronesis' or practical wisdom as being mindful of the best way to respond within a particular situation considering its ethical consequences.

'Did My Feelings and Attitudes Influence Me?'

Feelings and attitudes influence decision-making [3]. They need to be understood and shifted, especially if they are not conducive towards realising the practitioner's vision of practice. Feelings and emotions most often trigger reflection, notably negative feelings, such as a sense of failure, frustration, distress, anger and fear of authority with its threat of sanction for doing the wrong thing. They create an emotional tension within the practitioner. Senge [4] argues that we need to release emotional tension before we can focus on creative tension, as if emotions smudge the mirror and distort rational thought. Boud, Keogh and Walker [5] also suggest that we need to remove obstructive feelings as part of the reflective process. As noted in Chapter 3, writing about feelings helps to dispel emotional tension.

By paying attention to their feelings, the practitioner works towards developing the poise to know and manage their emotional self [6]. Hence, knowing what made the practitioner frustrated, angry or fearful, they can work towards resolving these strong emotions and associated feelings. Understanding is a balm for the worried mind simply because it brings some element of control.

As practitioners reflect, they can begin to accept their feelings and emotions as something they can learn through rather than something to defend against. It is not easy learning as feelings are often deeply embodied. Through reflection negative feelings are chipped away.

As Rosenberg [7, p. 145] notes –

'Little by little, we're not so enslaved to things'.

Beck [8, p. 42/3] recognises the discomfort reflection on feelings may incur but its benefit in long run –

> 'For a time our life may feel worse than before, as what we have concealed becomes clear. But even as this occurs, we have a sense of growing sanity and understanding, of basic satisfaction. To continue practice through severe difficulties we must have patience, persistence and courage ... we learn in our guts not just in our brains'.

Ramos [9] writes of an 'emotional impasse', where practitioners resist engagement with persons to avoid responding to patients' emotional or psychological needs. Because negative feelings and fears are uncomfortable, practitioners are likely to reflect to defend themselves against negative feelings, drawing on defence mechanisms, such as rationalisation, sublimation and projection [10], rather than face up to them. However, negative feelings drain the practitioner's energy. How often have you heard the practitioner's cry 'I'm drained!'

Feelings reflect deeper underlying attitudes and assumptions the practitioner may hold about the world but which they may not be aware of. As Cox notes [11, p. 100] –

> 'The therapist's attitudes colour the atmosphere of therapeutic space. He is never as neutral as he thinks'.

Assumptions govern the way people perceive and respond to their practice. They reflect 'who we are' as people, learnt through socialisations processes stemming from childhood, education and professional 'training' and reinforced daily through systems, ways of relating and habitual practice. Thus, they clearly influence clinical judgment. Yet, the practitioner may ask – 'Are my assumptions compatible with realising my vision of practice?' For example, Jane (Chapter 24) had assumed deliberate self-harm patients in Accident and Emergency department were 'time wasters', an attitude not conducive to her vision of person-centred practice. Once she realised this contradiction, she was able to explore it and shift it over time in guided reflection.

Negative attitudes lead to such phenomena as the 'difficult patient', the 'interfering relative' and racism. For example, issues surrounding racism continue to surface [12, 13], perhaps more so in light of the 'Black lives matter' movement[i] and the global response to George Floyd's death by a policeman in the USA on 25 May 2020 demanding justice and equality. As Puzan [12, p. 194] writes –

> 'There is so much familiarity in talking about the alleged racial differences of non-white people in public discourse and so little familiarity in talking about those racial properties attached to being white, that the concept of whiteness (or a recognition of racial formation) has little resonance within nursing. While issues related to cultural difference are not ignored, they rarely include the difference specifically engendered by "whiteness", which is structured to avoid and deflect interrogation or critical reflection'.

Puzan's words challenge all health care practitioners, health organisations and health systems about the right attitude to hold towards all people irrespective of race to ensure cultural safety and health equity. A commonly used definition of cultural safety is that of Williams [14, p. 213] who defines cultural safety as –

> 'An environment that is spiritually, socially and emotionally safe, as well as physically safe for people; where there is no assault challenge or denial of their identity, of who they are and what they need'.[ii]

From a health care perspective, *Cultural safety* is the effective nursing practice of a person or family from another culture that is determined by that person or family. An unsafe cultural practice is defined as 'an action, which demeans the cultural identity of a particular person or family' [15, p. 9].

The practitioner may reflect superficially to avoid going deeper that might reveal deeper psyche factors or emotional scars that may be better left alone [16]. It is these deeper reaches of the mind where old stuff lies buried, stuff that is fundamental to the assumptions we hold, the feelings we express, that govern our practice. If we are to gain insight, then it is necessary to access and shake up these assumptions. If not, then we may merely scratch at the surface of our experience without meaning. However, it may seem better to reflect superficially rather than get out of our depth. It depends on how significant such feelings are perceived and the help of guidance.

'Did Past Experiences Influence Me?'

Practitioners often get into a groove or rut of habitual practice, whereby their response is a repetition of their previous responses, especially when they consider previous responses had been effective (at least in their view) and which they felt confident and comfortable in applying. Habitual responses are non-reflective as if the practitioner is on 'auto-pilot'. Whilst past experiences may seem similar, they are not the same. Every experience is unique from a perspective of person-centred practice. The person as a patient is not an object to do things to. Previous experiences obviously do inform (lessons from the past) but should not dictate the practitioner's response.

Blackwolf and Jones [17, p. 78] write –

> 'If we don't stay connected and remember the lessons from the past, are we not doomed to repeat them?'

Reflection is connection. Through reflection, we learn the lessons of the past to inform future practice as a continuous unfolding narrative.

Clandinin and Connelly write [18, p. 29] –

> 'When we see an event, we think of it not as a thing happening at that moment but as an expression of something happening over time. Any event, or thing, a past, a present as it happens to us, and an implied future'.

By connecting their reflection on experience with past experiences, the practitioner can begin to discern any pattern to their responses and reflect whether such patterns need shifting towards future experiences and realising their vision of practice as a lived reality.

They can begin to climb out of the rut of normal practice to see each encounter creatively as unique.

'Did I Respond Ethically and Morally?'

Another influencing factor is responding ethically and morally. These are related concepts. Ethics are external rules or principles, whereas morals are personal beliefs and values. This cue guides the practitioner to reflect on their ethical response to reveal any dilemma about acting ethically or morally. Often personal morals may conflict with ethics. 'Ethical mapping' offers the practitioner a framework to reflect on such dilemmas (Figure 4.2) set against appreciation of ethical principles and the perspectives of those people involved in the experience to understand the most ethical response.

The first step is to frame the dilemma – 'How do we respond for the best in this particular situation?' It is broader than a simple choice between two alternatives.

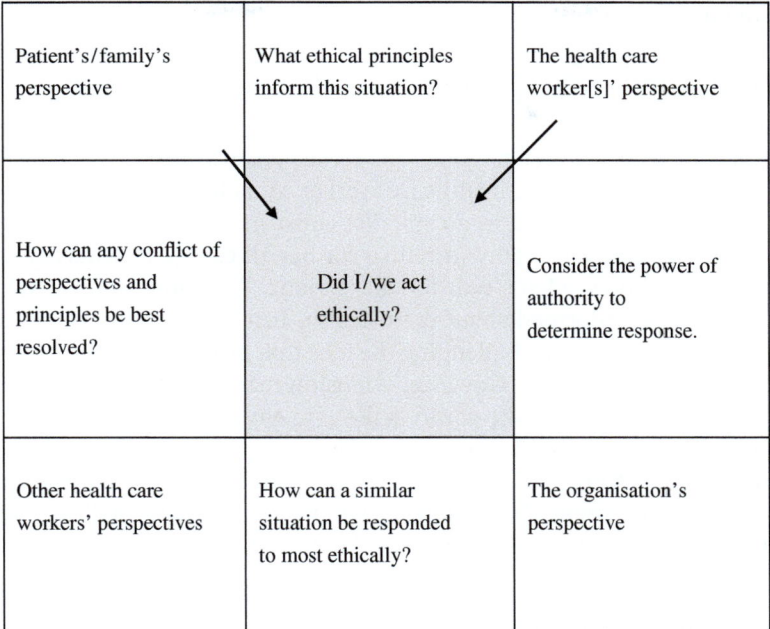

Patient's/family's perspective	What ethical principles inform this situation?	The health care worker[s]' perspective
How can any conflict of perspectives and principles be best resolved?	Did I/we act ethically?	Consider the power of authority to determine response.
Other health care workers' perspectives	How can a similar situation be responded to most ethically?	The organisation's perspective

FIGURE 4.2 Ethical mapping (adapted from Johns [21]).

Different Perspectives

The second step is to consider the perspectives of those involved within the particular experience. Every experience involves a web of different people: patients, relatives and diverse professionals set within an organisational background. Each person will have a perspective on the particular situation. These perspectives are often contradictory, in that people may see the situation differently. Hence, it is necessary for the practitioner to inquire into these different perspectives beyond her or his own perspective and partial view.

Inquiry into other perspectives is termed empathic inquiry.[iii] It is the path to connect with the other and opens a gate to tune into the other's wavelength and talk about issues towards consensus. Imaging the other's perspective requires stepping back and taking an objective stance free from one's own personal perspective. It is akin to putting yourself in the other person's shoes to consider their perspective on the situation. It expands the practitioner's view of the situation, challenging the practitioner's own partial perspective to give a bigger picture of the situation. It sets up the potential for resolving any ethical dilemma and conflict over what is the most consensual way to respond within practice itself.

Ethical Principles

The third step is to consider ethical principles. Ethics is acting for the best or good. Yet how is the 'ethical' known? Guidance is offered by a code of professional ethics that set out the way a practitioner should always treat the patient with dignity and respect.

There are a number of ethical principles that the practitioner needs to appreciate: autonomy, benevolence, non-malevolence, utilitarianism, justice, equality and confidentiality set against the background of professional integrity and duty.

However, these are only principles to guide rather than determine the practitioner's ethical response. Deciding how to act for the good always needs to be interpreted within each moment [19, 20].

Autonomy

Autonomy is the person's right to be self-determining. Seedhouse [22] views autonomy as the highest ethical principle. In respecting a person's autonomy, the practitioner works with the person, as possible, to make the best decisions about the person's health care. This is in contrast with professional autonomy for the healthcare worker to make such decisions. Professional autonomy was universally accepted in a capitalist construction of health care whereby the patient gave up his rights to autonomy in return for health care [23], whereby practitioners perceive themselves to know what's best for the patient. This situation is now very different. People are now more informed about their health. Just 'Google' any health condition to reveal an overload of information, challenging the idea that professional knowledge is beyond the public's general understanding. However, a tension may exist between professional and patient autonomy that challenges who controls the care environment.

For whatever reason, patients may be passive. Perhaps it is easier for the patient to say to the health professional – 'you know best'. If the practitioner accepts the patient's passivity, then they must act in the person's best interests, what is termed 'paternalism'. Benjamin and Curtis [24] set out three criteria to legitimate such action;

- Harm – would the patient come to some harm if I hadn't act for them?
- Autonomy – is the patient able to act for themselves?
- Ratification – would the patient at a later time thank me for my actions?

These criteria offer a focus for reflection on respecting the person's autonomy.

Benevolence and Non-malevolence

Beneficence and non-malevolence are enshrined within the Hippocratic oath that doctors should do good [beneficence] and not do harm, [non-malevolence]. This is the governing principle underlying all ethical action. It often involves an element of risk when outcomes are unpredictable. The professional's role is to explain the risks in enabling the patient to decide on what action to take.

Utilitarianism

Utilitarianism is based on the principle of 'the greatest good' whereby the needs of the individual may be in tension with the needs of society as a whole usually due to finite resources, such as time and money. Hence, the health care practitioner is always concerned with managing resources to the best effect. It involves establishing priorities and pitching the need of the individual against the needs of many.

This inevitably creates tension with the person's autonomy. It becomes an issue of justice and goodness. Gilligan [25] argues that women and men have different criteria to judge 'moral goodness'. Men tend towards a view that the highest moral claim is justice based on the utilitarian ethic, whereas women tend towards a view that the highest moral claim is caring and responsibility based on respecting the person's autonomy. Gilligan [25] suggests that within a patriarchal culture, the masculine ethic is deemed a higher level of ethical development, whereby the needs of society as a whole are morally greater than the needs of the individuals within that society. This position is supported by Kant's categorical principle of doing your duty even if it acts against what you would like to do.[iv]

The reader will appreciate the way this tension is played out in everyday life, reflected in the media, about the way decisions are made about health care – what is funded and what is not, as supported by the National Institute of Clinical Excellence. As such, the person's right to make decisions about their health care is constrained by resources available as determined by others with greater authority. Hence, the practitioner will reflect on how utilitarianism affects the ability to give patient-centred care, raising issues about the number of staff available, how priorities are made, how much time can be spent with one patient, what equipment is available and staff development. It behoves the practitioner to become political to assert necessary resources to create an environment where their vision can be realised. Compromise between giving the best care and resources to give the best care is frustrating and, as such, a constant focus for reflection.

Confidentiality

Confidentiality is enshrined in the Data Protection Act (1998)[v] to protect information about a patient being disclosed to others without the patient's permission. This may create a dilemma for the practitioner's care for relatives who are anxious for information that the patient doesn't want disclosed or is unable to give permission because of their condition.

The Ethical Demand

Practitioners have a duty of care, what Logstrup [26, p. 18] terms the 'ethical demand'.
He states

> 'By our very attitude to one another we help to shape one another's world. By our attitude to the other person we help to determine the scope and the hue of his or her world; we make it large and small, bright or drab, rich or dull, threatening or secure. We help to shape his or her world, not by theories and views but *by our very attitude* to him or her. Herein lies the unarticulated and one might say anonymous demand that we take care of the life which trust has placed into our hands'.

Logstrup's words are a powerful challenge to the practitioner – 'Do you hold such an attitude?' 'If not, why not?' His words reflect the dynamic impact the practitioner can have on the person's well-being. It returns the practitioner back to 'Did my feelings and attitudes influence me?'

'Do as You Would be Done by'[vi]

The biblical idea of 'do as you would be done by' is a subjective, and often emotional response, rather than a rational response. It runs the risk of imposing your own values into the situation. For example, viewing an elderly patient as if she was my mother. The problem with this principle is that the patient is not your mother and that imposing such a position may be misguided because of identification and emotional entanglement.

The fourth step is to consider any difference between ethical principles and perspectives towards resolving any conflict between them to determine the best ethical response.

Authority to Act

The fifth step is to consider who has the authority to determine the ethical response. In reality, decisions are not necessarily made in terms of what's best for the patient or family but in terms of professional interest and dominance implicit within normal patterns of relating between professionals. Hence, to act for the best, the practitioner may need to challenge the authority of others by championing the most ethical response in context of person-centred practice. Thus, vision is itself an ethical principle to respond accordingly. The use of ethical mapping in guided reflection is illustrated in Chapter 16.

Following the ethical map trail

1. Frame the dilemma – did /I we act for the best?
2. Consider different perspectives commencing with the practitioner's own perspective:
3. Consider which ethical principles apply in terms of the best decision;
4. Consider what conflict exists between perspectives / values and how these might be resolved.
5. Consider who has authority to determine response?

Loxley [27] identified some questions that are useful to inform the question of authority:

- Who defines the problem?
- Whose terms are used?
- Who controls the domain or territory?
- Who decides on what resources are needed and how they are allocated?
- Who holds whom accountable?
- Who prescribes the activity of others?
- Who can influence policy makers?

'Did Other Factors Influence Me?'

The normality and exigencies of everyday practice are influential in determining the practitioner's response within the particular situation. As I noted in Chapter 1, issues of embodiment, tradition and authority are powerful determinants of normal practice. Normality is a reflection of tradition and is very influential determining 'the way things get done around here'.

Going against normality is likely to be resisted by others entrenched and comfortable in normal ways of working. As a consequence, the practitioner may feel it better 'to fit in' and 'do as your told' rather than 'rock the boat' with its incipient threat of sanction.

Reflection challenges the practitioner to challenge the rationale behind 'do as your told' to voice their own thoughts opinion and risk 'rocking the boat'.

In challenging the rationale, the practitioner's response will certainly be influenced by learnt theory, especially received knowledge that prescribes what the practitioner should do under the presenting circumstances. Indeed, learning 'facts' is the foundation of a technical rational curriculum (see Chapter 14). Reflection exposes any prescribed influencing theory to scrutiny for its appropriateness to inform, theory that previously may have been received as authoritative. Other influencing factors may include issues, such as motivation, morale, stress that affect commitment and resources such as time and staffing.

Anticipatory Reflection

The cue 'Given a similar situation, how could I respond more effectively, for the best and in tune with my vision?' opens the creative space to generate alternative responses to plant seeds of possibility in the practitioner's mind [28]. Generating options is both a cognitive search for logical alternatives and drawing on our imagination of how things could be for responding differently Michael Moorcock says 'Our imagination is our greatest gift. It gives us moral sensibility' [29, p. 102], whereby sensibility is being able to appreciate and respond to complex emotional or aesthetic influences, things that you sense rather than analyse logically.[vii]

Considering alternative responses is an invitation to throw open the shutters of the mind to see the experience laterally, for the practitioner to get out of their normal frame of reference to challenge their habitual ways of perceiving and responding to practice. It is like opening different windows in the mind to see similar things from new perspectives, to reframe the familiar.

As O'Donohue [30, p. 163–4] writes –

> 'Through these different windows, you can see new vistas of possibility, presence and creativity. Complacency, habit and blindness often prevent you from feeling your life. So much depends on the frame of vision – the window through which we look'.

In generating alternatives, the practitioner keeps their vision in mind, inquiring into what their vision really means as something lived rather than words. In weighing up alternatives, the practitioner considers the potential short- and long-term consequence of each option. It may not be easy for the practitioner to see beyond their existing horizon of knowing necessary to generate alternatives. Sometimes the rut of habitual practice is very deep and difficult to climb out of, one reason why guidance is beneficial to see beyond the practitioner's existing horizons of knowing (see Chapters 8 and 9).

'Am I Able to Respond as Envisaged?'

Having envisaged the 'best' alternative, the practitioner must then weigh up whether they are able to respond accordingly due to constraining influences – what I term 'the reality wall'. In previous MSR versions, I posited 'the influences grid' that pointed the practitioner towards potential constraining factors. These potential factors were interpreted from practitioners' experiences revealed in guided reflection sessions (see Figure 4.3) some of which the practitioner may have been previously identified through reflecting on the MSR cue 'what other factors influenced my response'.

In constructing the sixth edition of this book, I converted these influencing factors into four cues:

- Am I skilful and knowledgeable to respond differently?
- Do I have the right attitude?
- Do I have the authority to respond differently?
- Am I poised to respond differently?

These cues offer a more dynamic approach for the practitioner to consider whether they are able to respond as envisaged. They incorporate the barriers to rational change identified by Fay [31] of authority, embodiment and tradition as (see Chapter 1).

Expectations of myself to respond as envisaged.	Factors that constrain me:
	• Expectations from others how I should respond (issues of authority, tradition) with ensuing fear of conflict and sanction • Self embodiment of 'normal practice' (issue of embodiment) • Existing and contrary assumptions and attitudes • Lack of skill and knowledge • Conflicting ethical concern – issues of control, time and priorities

FIGURE 4.3 Potential constraining factors to taking envisaged action (adapted from Johns [32, p. 38]).

'Am I Skilful and Knowledgeable to Respond Differently?'

The practitioner will need to reflect on their skill base as to whether they are skilful to respond as envisaged. The mind set of 'I know what I need to do but can I do it?' This is where guidance is very beneficial to explore and act on this question. Knowing whether their skills were effective cannot be known until reflected on in subsequent experiences – 'the proof is in the pudding' so to speak, meaning the value, quality or truth of something must be judged based on direct experience with it.[viii] The cue opens the door for the practitioner to expand their repertoire of skills and ways of knowing as necessary to realise their vision of practice.

'Do I Have the Right Attitude and Assumptions?'

To respond differently, the practitioner may need to review their attitudes and assumptions as previously explored in the MSR cue – 'Did my feelings and attitudes influence me?' To respond differently, for example, in light of realising person-centred practice, the practitioner must adopt assumptions to support that. This may take some time, especially when 'normal' ways of working are fundamentally different, for example, a functional approach to practice, especially when 'normal practice' is constantly reinforced by other practitioners. Research [33–35] suggests that practitioners are less likely to relate to people who are different from them for whatever reason epitomised by the phrase 'the unpopular patient'. Such people as patients are labelled 'time wasters' (see Chapter 24), 'difficult', 'ungrateful', a nuisance and the like. Labelling reflects a culture where the patient is expected to fit into the practitioner's expectations of the 'good patient' to lighten the caring burden.

So, consider the shift of practitioner assumptions to support person-centred practice [36]. Some examples include the following:

- Shifting for doing to, for or at patients to working with persons in relationship.
- Patients are unique persons with complex 'holistic' needs.
- All care is based on 'knowing the person' and understanding the meanings the person gives to his current health-illness experience.
- Each caring encounter has never been experienced before.
- Working with persons and their families involves myself in relationship whereby 'Who I am' is my primary therapy, requiring a shift from 'professional detachment' to 'professional involvement'.
- Practice is carried out within a therapeutic team where colleagues are available to support each other.
- There is no such thing as an 'unpopular patient' only a suffering human being in need of care.

'Do I Have the Autonomy and Authority to Respond Differently?'

Within the authority matrix, practitioners may feel they do not have either the autonomy or authority as an individual practitioner to respond as envisaged. Practitioners work in transactional organisations structured through a hierarchy of authority transmitted from the top down. As I noted above, authority is a powerful influence on the practitioner's response.

However, the practitioner can claim autonomy for responding differently. This may not be an issue working with individual patients until it impinges on the interests of colleagues who may resist variance from 'normal practice'. As such, changing practice is best done collectively through dialogue. However, the conditions for dialogue need to exist or be established whereby the voices of all practitioners are heard and respected, working collectively towards realising its vision.

To claim autonomy to choose how best to respond, practitioners need an assertive voice. This can be developed using 'the assertive action ladder' (Figure 4.4), a step by step climb to becoming assertive.

Step 1 stems from acknowledging contradiction between practice and vision; a sense that something is not right. Step 2 gives this sense of not being right moral and ethical substance. Step 3 – 'authority to assert self' is a belief that one has the authority to assert their voice because I have a responsibility to the person. It stems from step 2, whereby if I don't assert myself, the patient's care will be compromised. Step 4 'arms' this voice with *good argument* so that the practitioner's voice cannot easily be dismissed. Step 5 is calculating the best moment to assert self for the greatest effect. It may be best in private at a quiet moment, or in public with an audience (see Chapter 11 for an example).

Step 6 is 'just do it!' It is taking the leap, shedding fear of any ensuing conflict or sanction.

Step 7 is using effective communication skills through which to assert self, what is termed communicative competence –

> 'The ability to achieve communicative goals in a socially appropriate manner. It is organized and goal-oriented, i.e., it includes the ability to select and apply skills that are appropriate and effective in the respective context. It includes verbal and non-verbal behaviour'.[ix]

Step 8 is to keep self and the other person in adult-adult mode vital for dialogue. It is being poised – knowing and managing one's emotional self in order to be fully present to the moment.[x] This step is based on transactional analysis [37]. The practitioner is mindful of not

10	Treading the fine line between pushing and yielding
9	Playing the power game
8	Staying in adult mode
7	Being communicatively skilful
6	'Just do it!' [JDI]
5	Creating the optimum conditions to assert self
4	Making a good argument
3	Authority to assert self
2	Ethically right to assert self
1	Feeing the need to assert self

FIGURE 4.4 The assertiveness action ladder.

being flipping into parent or child mode in the face of the other's response. It is essentially taking responsibility for one's actions and not being intimidated.

Step 9 is to force the issue by reminding others of their unsatisfactory response yet remaining in adult mode. Being assertive is likely to challenge normal power relationships with other colleagues especially those perceived to hold power over you with threats of sanction if you step out of line and forget your place within the system. It is moving self and other from a competitive to collaborate mode of conflict management to see the situation being asserted from a personal to a professional issue [38].

Step 10 is yielding when the issue cannot be forced further. Yielding is a strength not a weakness. It is an awareness that pushing an issue may have negative consequences. Better to live and fight another day. Retreat with dignity, with one's integrity intact.

Blackwolf and Gina Jones note [39, p. 281] –

> 'Yielding is not passive. It is being sensitive to energy flows and extending wisdom. Allow the winds of change to flow through you rather than against you. Be flexible with what is happening today. Yield to the circumstance, yet rooted with who you are'.

Assertiveness is an essential skill for the practitioner to develop to take envisaged action and be available to the persons. Nothing gets changed if practitioners are fearful of consequences. All steps are easier to climb with a collective voice. The reflective practitioner, mindful of potential resistance, can rally the support of colleagues, thus raising collective consciousness and a collective voice that is harder to resist if others are of a similar mind. Raising the stakes of the power game.

(Utilising the ladder in guided reflection is illustrated in Figure 4.4).

'Am I Poised to Respond Differently?'

Reflection is often triggered by strong feelings and emotions that, if unresolved, impact on the practitioner's ability to respond as envisaged. I have previously noted the significance of poise in asserting oneself and this difficulty especially with people perceived as having authority over the practitioner. Thus, to respond differently requires that practitioners develop the necessary poise to know and manage one's emotional self in whatever situation they find themselves.

Person-centred practice, by its very nature, involves the practitioner into a human–human relationship with persons. On a clinical level, this may often result in vulnerability to the person's suffering. Menzies-Lyth [10] wrote of the need for practitioners to develop professional detachment as a defence against the vulnerability and anxiety associated with caring. However, this defence no longer holds up. However, from a person-centred perspective, it now requires practitioners to develop professional involvement and the poise as a defence against vulnerability. Practitioners often wear metaphoric suits of armour to protect themselves from the anxiety and emotions of caring and the suffering of others. As Jade, one of the primary nurses at Burford Hospital said 'I don't come to work dressed in protective armour' [40].

Dewey [41, p. 30] observed –

> 'Unconscious fears also drive us into purely defensive attitudes that operate like coats of armour – not only to shut out new conceptions but even to prevent us from making new observations'.

Dewey believed that anxiety limited the practitioner's ability to learn through experience. The professional is closed to protect self rather than open to possibility. 'Armour' is akin to professional detachment. Logstrup noted the radicality of the ethical demand [26, p. 44] –

> 'The demand asks me to take care of the other person's life not only when it strengthens me but also when it is very unpleasant because it intrudes disturbingly into my own existence'.

Coming to an understanding of one's vulnerability begins a journey to unlearn existing defence mechanisms and learn the necessary poise for person-centred practice. In my experience, there is little organisational sensitivity to the profound nature of caring work and its impact on practitioners. Both James [42] and Bolton [43] refer to this as 'emotional labour', that emotional work is natural women's work, and therefore is unskilled, doesn't need to be taught, and is not valued, when emotional work is the greatest gift nurses can offer patients. Taylor [44, p. 1042] noted a theme within the literature of how nurses have been dispossessed 'of their essential humanness as human beings and as people, by emphasising their professional roles and responsibilities'. Taylor draws attention to the fact that nurses are human too and, as such, are vulnerable to the same issues that face their patients and families. The lack of recognition of humanness in nursing through a focus on roles and responsibilities has led practitioners to strive to be something they were clearly struggling to cope with. Consequently, they risk becoming alienated from themselves in their efforts to cope with and live with the contradictions in their lives. Jourard [45] noted that such striving damages 'the self' and reinforces the need to cope in a vicious downward spiral of self-destruction towards burnout and a state of anomie.

The Problem of Stress

Poise is a sense of feeling good about oneself. This can be seriously impaired by unresolved stress with consequences for the practitioner's health and morale. The reality of today's NHS is that nurse shortages are reportedly reaching crisis point [46] bed occupancy is constantly 'red alert'. In such an environment, Wall et al. [47] note that NHS staff suffer considerably more stress than any other workforce with 28% recording levels above the symptom threshold. Wind the clock forward. BBC News reports that NHS Foundation Trusts need to resubmit their financial plans. Only essential posts should be filled. The news asks what impact on patient care. What impact on staff morale and stress. Perusing my local newspaper (West Briton- Thursday 12 March 2015) I read that staff morale at Royal Cornwall Healthcare Trust is low.

The Royal College of Nursing Report (April 2024)[xi]

> 'NHS England data shows that for nursing staff, the proportion of sick days attributed to stress, anxiety, depression and other psychological illnesses increased from 21.0% in 2022 to 24.3% in 2023. A chronic workforce crisis is driving the pressure on staff. Thirty-four thousand nursing posts are unfilled across the NHS in England, leading to consistently understaffed shifts. The College is calling upon NHS leaders and the government to stop normalising poor mental health amongst staff and bring forward[xii] an action plan to tackle dangerous levels of stress and anxiety, including measures to boost recruitment into the nursing profession and ease the pressure on staff'.

I have made the point that writing and reflection is healing. Yet reflection can bring awareness of the practitioner's frustration but leave them stewing in their own juices. It is not healthy. It drains the practitioner's energy. Stress accumulates if not released. Imagine your body is like a *water butt* – slowly filling with stress. As it fills the practitioner becomes more tired and more intolerant but contains it, using up valuable energy for persons' care. There comes that moment when the practitioner unable to contain stress anymore feels they are drowning. Then one of two things happens. Either you blow up inside and have a breakdown or else you snap and 'blow your top'. You rage at events or people [20, 48, 49].

Pike [48, p. 351] writes –

> 'Moral outrage ensues when the nurse's attempts to operationalize a choice is thwarted by constraints. The outrage intensifies when these constraints not only block action, but also force a course of action that violates the nurse's moral tenets'.

This outrage is evident in practitioner's shared experiences. However, the water butt does have a drainage tap. Through reflection, the practitioner can learn to monitor their stress and open the tap to drain the stress by converting it (negative energy) into positive energy to take the appropriate action to resolve the sources of stress just as the gardener draws water from the water butt to water the flowers and nourish their growth. However, the tap might be blocked, requiring help to unblock it. If stress accumulates, then the risk of burnout looms large on the horizon. Burnout is a descent into a black hole when the caring self has been scrapped away on the uncaring sharp edges of systems. Cherniss [50, p. 5] describes burnout as a process in which 'the professional's attitudes and behaviours change in negative ways in response to job strain'. Maslach [51, p. 6] suggested that the major negative change in those experiencing burnout in people-centred work was 'the loss of concern for the client and a tendency to treat clients in a detached, mechanical fashion'. McNeeley [52] observed that when practitioners felt they had lost the intrinsic satisfaction of caring, they became focused on the conditions of work, for example, off-duty rosters and workload issues, characteristic of bureaucratic models of organisation. McNeeley [52] believes that bureaucratic conditions are antithetical to human service work and strongly advocated that such organisations needed to move to collegial ways of working with staff to offset the risks of burnout. Put another way, a shift from transactional management to transformative leadership.

And yet burnout can be a healing space, where the practitioner can recover/discover themselves. It may be dark, lonely and painful but it can still be a necessary healing space. Such healing is a journey to discover rather than recover, because recovery suggests returning to what she was before, only for the hurting to start all over again.

Benner and Wrubel [53] believe that the answer to stress and burn-out is to reconnect to caring rather than the development of personal detachment as advocated by Menzies-Lyth [10] as previously noted. Caring is a reciprocal relationship. If nurses and other health care practitioners are expected to care, then they need to work in caring environments. If the practitioner is suffering it is likely that other colleagues also suffer, sapping their energy and limiting their availability to be with patents. And yet often, practitioners seem to need to cope, to not expose their vulnerability as if it is a weakness not to cope or admit to strain. They would prefer a collusive silence. To care, we need ways to penetrate the silence to support each other and create a therapeutic team, whereby its members are actively and genuinely available to support each other. Then suits of armour can be discarded.

Consider the following questions –

- Are people stressed or worse, burnt-out?
- Are adequate support systems in place?
- If so – why do you think that is?
- Do you see seeking help as a strength rather than weakness?
- Do you explore your anxiety as a learning opportunity?
- Are you truly available to support your colleagues?

Practitioner may well sacrifice integrity to manage their anxiety and stress and thus view the reflective project as an overt threat to their security or rather their insecurity. In my experience, very little practitioner education focuses on the development of poise.

Tools such as the feeling fluffy-feeling drained scale can help practitioners reflect on stress factors and working to reduce them. (The scale is illustrated in Chapter 17 guiding third-year nursing students within a guided reflection session).

The cue – 'Am I able to respond as envisaged' has the potential to guide the practitioner into deep self-inquiry, reinforcing the fact that reflection without guidance can be difficult. Experience is a story to share.

Summary

Through writing and reflection, the practitioner learns to pay attention to their everyday experiences. In doing so, their practice becomes more alive and meaningful. They become increasingly mindful of self within practice, no longer taking things for granted as normal. Practitioners become more curious, more questioning. The gate is open to becoming a reflective practitioner as someone who *lives* reflection in his or her everyday practice. Besides enabling practitioners to explore reflection, the MSR facilitates the development of clinical skills as learning from the cues spills over into everyday practice. The MSR cues draw the practitioner to frame tentative insights (Chapter 5) and subsequently, to deepen their insights through dialogue with sources of information and guidance (Chapters 7–9). The final phase of the MSR 'Wrap up' is also a focus of Chapter 9. An application of the MSR is set out in Chapter 10.

References

1. Johns, C. (1997) Reflective practice and clinical supervision- part 1: the reflective turn. *European Nurse* 2(2), 87–97.

2. Aristotle (2004) *Nicomachean ethics* [revised edition] [trans. J Thomson]. Penguin Books, London.

3. Callahan, S. (1988) The role of emotion in ethical decision making. *Hastings Centre Report* June/July 9–14.

4. Senge, P. (1990) *The Fifth Discipline: The Art and Practice of the Learning Organization.* Century Business, London.

5. Boud, D., Keogh, R., Walker, D. (1985) Promoting reflection in learning: a model. In D. Boud, R. Keogh, D. Walker [Eds.] *Reflection: Turning Experience Into Learning.* Kogan Page, London.

6. Salovey, P., Mayer, J. D. (1990) Emotional intelligence. *Imagination, Cognition and Personality*, 9, 185–211.

7. Rosenberg, L. (1998) *Breath by Breath.* Shambhala, Boston.

8. Beck, C. Y. (1997) *Everyday Zen.* Thorsons, London.

9. Ramos, M. (1992) The nurse patient relationship: themes and variations. *Journal of Advanced Nursing* 17, 496–506.

10. Menzies-Lyth, I. (1988) *Containing Anxiety in Institutions: Selected Essays.* Free Association Books, London, 43–85.

11. Cox, M. (1988) *Structuring the Therapeutic Process; Compromise with Chaos* (revised edition). Jessica Kingsley Publications, London.

12. Puzan, E. (2003) The unbearable whiteness of being (in nursing). *Nursing Inquiry*, 10(3), 193–200.

13. Blackford, J. (2003) Cultural frameworks of nursing practice: exposing an exclusionary healthcare culture. *Nursing Inquiry*, 10(4), 236–2424.

14. Williams, R. (1999) Cultural safety – what does it mean for our work practice? *Australian and New Zealand Journal of Public health*, 23(2). 213–214.

15. Nursing Council of New Zealand. (2002). *Guidelines for Cultural Safety, the Treaty of Waitangi, and Maori Health in Nursing and Midwifery Education and Practice.* Wellington: Nursing Council of New Zealand.

16. Sacks, O. (1976) *Awakenings.* Pelican Books, London.

17. Blackwolf, J. G. (1995) *Earth Dance Drum.* Commune-E-Key, Salt Lake City.

18. Clandinin, D. J., Connelly, E. M. (2000) *Narrative Inquiry: Experience and Story in Qualitative Research.* Jossey-Bass, San Francisco.

19. Cooper, M. (1991) Principle orientated ethics and the ethics of care: a creative tension. *Advances in Nursing Science* 15(2), 22–31.

20. Parker, R. (1990) Nurses' stories: the search a relational ethic of care. *Advances in Nursing Science* 13(1), 31–40.

21. Johns, C. (1999) Unravelling the dilemmas of everyday nursing practice. *Nursing Ethics* 6, 287–298.

22. Seedhouse, D. (1988) *Ethics: The Heart of Health Care.* John Wiley & Sons, Chichester.

23. Parsons, T. (1951) *The Social System.* Free Press, Glencoe, IL.

24. Benjamin, M., Curtis, J. (1986) *Ethics in Nursing* (second edition). Oxford University Press, New York.

25. Gilligan, C. (1982) *In A Different Voice*. Harvard University Press, Cambridge, MA.

26. Logstrup, K. E. (1997) *The Ethical Demand*. University of Notre Dame Press, Notre Dame.

27. Loxley, A. (1997) *Collaboration in Health and Welfare: Working with Difference*. Jessica Kingsley Publishers, London.

28. Margolis, H. (1993) *Paradigm and Barriers: How Habits of Mind Govern Scientific Beliefs*. University of Chicago Press, Chicago.

29. Moorcock, M. (2002) *London Bone*. Scribner, London.

30. O'Donohue, J. (1997) *Anam Cara: Spiritual Wisdom from the Celtic World*. Bantam Press, London.

31. Fay, B. (1987) *Critical Social Science: Liberation and Its Limits*. Polity Press, Cambridge.

32. Johns, C. (2017) Engaging the reflective spiral: the second dialogical movement. In C. Johns [Ed.] *Becoming A Reflective Practitioner* (fifth edition). Wiley Blackwell, Oxford, 35–58.

33. Stockwell, F. (1972) *The Unpopular Patient*. Croom Helm, Beckenham.

34. Johnson, M., Webb, C. (1995) Rediscovering unpopular patients: the concept of social judgement. *Journal of Advanced Nursing* 21, 466–475.

35. Trexler, J. C. (1995) Reformulation of deviance and labelling theory for nursing. *IMAGE: Journal of Nursing Scholarship* 28(2), 131–135.

36. Johns, C. (2024) Holistic or person-centred vision for practice. In C. Johns [Ed.] *Holistic Practice in Healthcare: The Buford NDU Person-centred Model*. Wiley Blackwell, 1–18.

37. Stewart, I., Joines, V. (1987) *TA Today: A New Introduction to Transactional Analysis*. Russell Press, Nottingham.

38. Thomas, K., Kilmann, R. (1974) Thomas Kilmann Conflict Mode Instrument. Xicom Toledo.

39. Blackwolf, J. G. (1996) *Earth Dance Drum*. Commune-E-Key, Salt Lake City.

40. Johns, C. (1993) Professional supervision. *Journal of Nursing Management* 1(1), 9–18

41. Dewey, J. (1933) How we think. J.C> Heath, Boston.

42. James, N. (1989) Emotional labour: skill and work in the social regulation of feelings. *Sociological Review* 37(1), 15–42.

43. Bolton, S. (2000) Who cares? Offering emotion work as a 'gift' in the nursing labour process. *Journal of Advanced Nursing* 32, 580–586.

44. Taylor, B. (1992) From helper to human: a reconceptualisation of the nurse as a person. *Journal of Advanced Nursing* 17, 1042–1049.

45. Jourard, S. (1971) *The Transparent Self*. Van Nostrand, Newark.

46. Hall, C. (2003) *Nurse Shortage in the NHS Is Near Crisis Point*. Daily Telegraph 29th April.

47. Wall, T., Bolden, R., Borril, C. (1997) Minor psychiatric disturbance in NHS Trust staff. *British Journal of Psychiatry* 171, 519–523.

48. Pike, A. (1991) Moral outrage and moral discourse in nurse-physician collaboration. *Journal of Professional Nursing* 7(6), 351–363.

49. Wilkinson, J. (1988) Moral distress in nursing practice: experience and effect. *Nursing Forum* 23(1), 16–29.

50. Cherniss, G. (1980) *Professional Burn-out in Human Service Organisations*. Praeger, New York.

51. Maslach, C. (1976) Burned-out. *Human Behaviour* 5, 16–22.

52. McNeely, R. (1983) Organizational patterns and work satisfaction in a comprehensive human service agency: an empirical test. *Human Relations*, 36(10), 957–972.

53. Benner, P., Wrubel, J. (1989) *The Primacy of Caring*. Addison-Wesley, Menlo Park. 53.

Notes

i. Blacklivesmatter.com.

ii. Google.com.

iii. The Oregon Primary Care association term empathic inquiry. They note – 'In the growing movement in health care to address the social determinants of health, system changes have largely focused on the tools for social needs screening, rather than the communication skills required to effectively guide these interactions with patients. In order to create primary care environments that provide patient-centred, whole person care, we must build our systems and prepare our workforce to approach these delicate topics with an emphasis on sensitivity, compassion, and patient empowerment.

Empathic Inquiry was created through the synthesis and application of motivational interviewing and trauma-informed care approaches, along with input from patients and other stakeholders.

We call our approach *Empathic Inquiry* because these words describe how we hope to relate to patients, from a place of non-judgmental curiosity and understanding. Empathic Inquiry is intended to facilitate collaboration and emotional support for both patients and health centre staff through the social needs screening process, as well as evoke patient priorities relating to social determinants of health needs for integration into subsequent care planning and delivery processes. https://orpca.org/empathic-inquiry/.

iv. https://plato.stanford.edu/entries/kant-moral/.

v. https://www.gov.uk/data-protection.

vi. https://dictionary.cambridge.org/dictionary/english/do-as-you-would-be-done-by.

vii. http:// www.vocabulary.com dictionary > sensibility.

viii. https://www.dictionary.com/e/slang/the-proof-is-in-the-pudding/.

ix. https://www.google.com/search?q=communicative+competence&oq=communicative+competence&aqs=chrome..69i57.7885j0j15&sourceid=chrome&ie=UTF-8.

x. Poise is fundamental to the practitioner being available to the other, where patient or colleague (see Figure 5.3).

xi. https://www.rcn.org.uk/news-and-events/Press-Releases/nhs-sickness-data-shows-average-nurse-took-entire-week-off-sick-last-year-stress-apr24#:~:text=NHS%20England%20data%20shows%20that,driving%20the%20pressure%20on%20staff.

xii. The 2023 survey showed an improvement in staff morale reflecting the Trust's efforts to improve morale. https://royalcornwallhospitals.nhs.uk/2024/03/08/results-of-the-2023-staff-survey-paint-an-improving-picture-for-rcht/.

CHAPTER 5

Framing Insights

Introduction

Working through the MSR cues, whether sequentially or intuitively, the practitioner's attention is focused on drawing tentative insights, prompted by the MSR cue – 'What tentative insights do I draw from this experience?' (Figure 2.2).

Insights are learning that changes the practitioner in some way through understanding, empowerment and transformation. Understanding can be one's reality, finding meaning in one's vision, problem-solving, appreciating different ways of responding, one's attitudes and feelings, all towards realising the practitioner's vision as a lived reality. Understanding leads to empowerment, acting on one's understanding and whether one *can* act considering barriers that might constrain the practitioner. Empowerment leads to transformation, responding differently in tune with one's vision with desired outcomes as evidenced in subsequent reflection on experience.

Insights inform and develop the practitioner's knowing in practice within the hermeneutic spiral (as noted in Chapter 2). Insights are tentative because the practitioner may be uncertain of their substance. They may not necessarily be new, but a reinforcement of things already known or sensed to some degree but with deeper understanding and lifted more consciously into mind.

Insights are not necessarily easy to pinpoint. Indeed, the practitioner may not initially recognise them as such. The challenge for the practitioner is to penetrate 'beyond what is superficial or obvious' [1]. Insights may emerge later when reading through the reflective journal, or linked to subsequent reflections. They are not easily forced but may come intuitively to mind as something of a revelation at unexpected times rather than from a more rational or logical approach. It is like playing around with emerging ideas and then suddenly the insight is realised as if a kind of creative play.

Okri [2, p. 21] writes –

> 'Creativity, it would appear, should be approached in the spirit of play, of foreplay, of dalliance, doodling, messing around – and then, bit by bit, you somehow get deeper into the matter. But if you go in there with a businessman's solemnity or the fanaticism of some artistic types you are likely to be rewarded with a stiff response, a joyless dribble, strained originality, ideas that come out all strapped up and strangled by too much effort'.

Dallying suggests giving the mind free rein to explore. Perhaps as you rest or walk, or indeed at any time of the day, perhaps at work the next day or next week triggered by another experience, an insight will emerge. It is as if the mind has subconsciously churning over the reflection, as if the insight has been germinating within your mind.

The Wood from the Trees

It may be difficult to discern insights because the practitioner cannot see 'the wood for the trees', whereby the whole picture is not clear, because you are looking too closely at small details, or you are too closely involved [3]. The practitioner needs to stand back enough to see the whole picture and the pattern of issues within it. This is where a guide is helpful to guide the practitioner to view the whole picture and offer a different perspective in contrast with the practitioner's perspective leading to co-creation of insights (see Chapters 8 and 9.) Looking too closely, the practitioner may have blind spots and miss the insight.

Single Lines

Breaking the reflective text into single lines may help the practitioner to see the wood from the trees simply by opening up the text. The practitioner can scroll down the 'opened text' to read between the lines where insights may be revealed. In scrolling down, imagine pulling away the veneer of normal practice to see self from a new, less familiar perspective in tune with your vision [4].

Framing Insights

As I have noted, identifying insights may not be easy. Some guiding framework may prove helpful. When first constructing the MSR I utilised Carper's 'Fundamental ways of knowing in nursing' [5] as a framework for insights.

Carper's Fundamental Ways of Knowing

Carper identified four fundamental ways of knowing: the empirical, the ethical, the personal and the aesthetic. I interpreted the aesthetic as the core way of knowing because it is the knowing the practitioner uses in practice, informed by the ethical, empirical and personal ways of knowing. Aesthetics is concerned with performance. Observe a health care practitioner go about their practice and you witness a performance that integrates all aspects of their practice. Perhaps it flows with grace and perhaps it stutters awkwardly. Like dancers, practitioners move about the patient and their colleagues. Like sculptors, practitioners shape their practice. Like actors, practitioners play out their dramas. Like poets, practitioners sense the urgency and intimacy within each unfolding moment. Like joiners, practitioners chisel to create perfect joints.

Carper's ways of knowing offered an approach to appreciate the breadth of knowing in practice. It attracted much attention. White [6] suggested the 'socio-political' way of knowing to contextualise the ways of knowing within societal norms. Munhall [7] suggested 'unknowing' as a way of knowing, that influences the clinical response. I developed 'reflexive knowing' as a fifth way of knowing to term the knowing (insights) emanating from reflection reflexively fed back to inform and deepen the practitioner's existing knowing in practice with the hermeneutic spiral [8]. Identifying reflexivity as a way of knowing added a dynamic movement to Carper's work. Reflecting further on Carper's extended framework, I have added

Ethical knowing: Responding to the situation in terms of what is the best or right action [or non-action].	Empiric knowing: How theoretical sources did or could have informed my response to the situation	Personal knowing: Understanding the impact of myself on my practice
	Aesthetic knowing: Understanding how I acted within the particular experience	
	Anticipatory knowing: Envisaged knowing how best to respond differently in tune with my vision of practice in future experiences.	
	Reflexive knowing: Picking up insights in subsequent reflections – Was I able to respond as envisaged? If not, why not?	

FIGURE 5.1 Carper's fundamental pattern of knowing in nursing.

a sixth way of knowing – 'Anticipatory knowing' (Figure 5.1). Basically, Personal, Empiric and Ethical knowing inform Aesthetic knowing, which in turn informs Anticipatory knowing to inform subsequent experiences. Reflexive knowing is the knowing picked up in subsequent reflections within a continuous flow of being and becoming towards realising one's vision of practice.

Utilising Carper's framework, the practitioner asks 'how has this experience enabled me to:

- Understand how and why I acted within the particular experience (the aesthetic)
- Appreciate how drawing on theory informed my response (the empiric)
- Understand myself and its impact on my practice (the personal)
- Understand whether my actions were for the good or best (the ethical)
- Anticipate how I could respond differently in tune with my vision of practice to inform future experiences (the anticipatory)
- Draw insights between this particular experience to inform future practice (the reflexive)

The Framing Perspectives

Practitioners struggled to utilise Carper's framework because of its abstract nature. As such, I developed 'The Framing Perspectives' as a more practical approach (Figure 5.2) to offer a more pragmatic and expansive approach to identifying insights.

Developmental Framing

Developmental framing is converting theory into a framework, whereby the practitioner can visualise and monitor their development towards realising their vision of practice. So, if the practitioner's vision is to realise patient-centred practice how might they frame this

In using the framing perspectives note:

1. Each framing perspective has the precursor question – 'what insights do I draw from….
2. All framing perspectives feed into anticipatory framing towards realising my vision as a lived reality.

Visionary framing: Inquiry into the meaning of my vision as something lived rather than words?	*Aesthetic and ethical framing:* Understanding why I responded as I did from skilful and ethical perspectives?	*Reality perspective framing:* Understanding the barriers that constrain realising my vision?
Parallel process framing: Making connections between guidance to inform and develop my knowing in practice?	*Anticipatory framing:* Anticipating of how I could respond differently in tune with my vision of practice in future experiences?	*Theory framing:* Drawing on theory (in its broadest sense[i]) that did or might have informed my experience?
Temporal framing Reflecting on the extent past experiences influenced my clinical judgment and response?	*Developmental framing:* Utilising developmental frameworks to frame and monitor my development?	*Role framing:* Reflecting on the significance of my role and relationships with others?

Reflexive knowing: Picked up in subsequent experiences -

1. Did I respond as envisaged?
2. If so, what insights can I draw?
3. If not, what insights can I draw

FIGURE 5.2 Framing perspectives.

realisation? If the practitioner's vision is to become a transformational leader, how might they frame this realisation? Besides outcomes such as person-centred practice and leadership, processes of becoming can also be framed such as empowerment.

The Being Available Template (BAT)

The being available template is an inductively derived framework to enable practitioners to visualise person-centred practice and monitor their development towards realising it. The template was initially developed through analysing the dialogue between the guide and practitioners in guided reflection, whereby practitioners strove to realise person-centred practice [9]. Being available is the irreducible core essence of person-centred practice whereby the practitioner is available to work with the person[s] to enable them to find meaning in their experience as the basis for negotiated decision making about their health-illness needs and to assist them as appropriate to meet those needs'.

The extent the practitioner can be available is influenced by the pattern of six inter-related attributes: holding the intent to realise a valid vision, concern for the person, knowing the person, the aesthetic response, poise and creating a practice environment where it is possible to be available (Figure 5.3).

The first five attributes are related to the individual practitioner working with persons. The sixth attribute 'creating an environment' challenges the practitioner to consider the extent the practice environment is conducive to person-centred practice. Thus, reflection extends into the structure and culture of the organisation and the practitioner's ability to shift the organisation towards enabling person-centred practice.

The use of the BAT in guided reflection is illustrated in Chapters 10–12 and 24.

Dimension	
Core	The practitioner is available to the person to enable the person to find meaning in their experience as the basis for negotiating decision making about their health and to assist them as appropriate to meet those needs'.
Elements	The extent the practitioner can be available is determined along six inter-related influences:
The practitioner intends to realise a vision of practice	Holding intent, the practitioner is more likely to realise their vision in practice. Through reflection, vision is constantly scrutinised for its lived meaning in practice and value to frame practice.
The practitioner 'knows' the other	Through empathic inquiry the practitioner appreciates the pattern of the person's wholeness and the meanings they give to health by tuning in and flowing with the unfolding pattern of the person's experience [wavelength]. Knowing the person is guided through the Buford NDU model nine reflective cues (see Chapter 6).
The practitioner is concerned for the other.	Concern is an energy that creates possibility within the caring relationship. The greater the practitioner's concern for the other the more available the practitioner is and the more the person receiving care knows this leading to trust and relationship.
The aesthetic response	The practitioner is effective in meeting the person's needs. Four abilities constitute effective performance: 1. The ability to grasp and interpret the clinical moment. 2. The ability to make most appropriate and ethical clinical judgment in response to the patient's needs. 3. The ability to respond with appropriate skilful, ethical and creative action. 4. The ability to evaluate one's effectiveness.
Poise	The practitioner knows and manages self within relationship so that their personal concerns do not interfere with being available to the person. It is having balance, awareness, foresight and a dignified, self-confident manner or bearing.[ii] Poise is the flip side of concern for the person. Concern tends to make the practitioner vulnerable to the other's suffering, whereas poise enables the practitioner to manage their vulnerability without diminishing concern. Being poised one is 'ready and prepared to do something [10, p. 785].
Create and sustain an environment where being available is possible	Dimensions 1–5 above relate to realising person-centred practice between the practitioner and the patient. This practice takes place within a clinical and organisational environment. Hence, the practitioner necessarily works towards: 1. Creating a learning environment to enable practitioners to flourish and sustain collaborative and dialogical patterns of relationships with other health care workers towards realising person-centred practice. 2. Being assertive and political to ensure a clinical and organisational culture to support person-centred practice. This includes being able to confront aspects of organisational practice that constrain realising effective person-centred practice. 3. Congruent person-centred leadership and organisational systems.

FIGURE 5.3 The being available template.

The following attributes cannot be viewed in isolation. They are parts of a conceptual whole way of being and doing:

1. Leaders are mindful; mindfulness is the hallmark of leadership.
2. Leaders are visionary [10] with shared values congruent with its purpose.
3. Leaders are moral [11, 12] acting with integrity towards creating better worlds for others no matter what resistance is encountered, yet yielding graciously as appropriate.
4. Leaders have foresight [13] always on the front foot and anticipating the next move. Foresight is a reflection of wisdom in simply knowing what to do within a complex and largely indeterminate world.
5. Leaders are of service in working collaboratively with colleagues to accomplish what needs to be done towards realising a collective vision for practice [13].
6. Leaders invest in people to enable them to grow and fulfil their potential.
7. Leaders are poised and emotionally intelligent in the face of disturbance and uncertainty, with the ability to sustain self within mutually supportive networks.
8. Leaders are authentic; necessarily transparent for deep trust, mindful of walking the talk of leadership, without being hooked on ego.
9. Leaders are inspirational, energetic and creative; they lift themselves and others to higher levels of motivation and achievement within an acknowledged learning community where nothing is taken for granted.

FIGURE 5.4 Person-centred leadership template.

Person-centred Framework for Leadership

The person-centred framework for leadership is based on:

- Reflection on my personal leadership as a hospital general manager and clinical lead towards realising person-centred practice.
- An analysis of leadership theories – transactional, transformational and servant-leadership.
- Reflection on developing and directing the MSc Leadership in Healthcare.
- Analysis of more than 100 leadership dissertations on becoming a leader.

My analysis led to extrapolating the following attributes in constructing the 'Person-centred Leadership' template [14, p. 28]. These have been revised as shown in Figure 5.4. I initially termed it 'Mindful Leadership'. However, being mindful is just part of being a person-centred leader. The framework is offered as a model of reflection, for the practitioner to consider the extent they realise each of its attributes within the whole notion of being a leader yet always mindful of the threat that a trait or attribute approach to practice is viewed either in isolation of the other attributes or as authoritative.

Kieffer's Framework for Participatory Competence (15)

This framework guides practitioners to view the development of empowerment towards taking necessary action. Kieffer identified four distinct and progressive phases of involvement as individuals construct the skills and insights which constitute a fully matured attainment of participatory competence (Table 5.1).

Kieffer [15, p. 27] noted that the process of empowerment involved

'Reconstructing and re-orientating deeply engrained personal systems of social relations. Moreover, they confront these tasks in an environment which historically has enforced their political oppression and which continues its active and implicit attempts at subversion and constructive change'.

Kieffer's words reflect the difficulty practitioners may face striving to realise their vision of practice because it involves such a radical culture shift in disrupting normal ways of doing things. The framework is apposite because of its focus on contradiction, dialogue and empowerment. Kieffer acknowledges the necessity of a continuing constructive dialogue or

TABLE 5.1

Kieffer's Framework for Participatory Competence

Phase	Development
Era of entry Birth of struggle against conflict	Birth of emergence of participatory competence. Integrity violated provoking and mobilising sense of frustration and powerlessness towards an empowering response 'when realising that they can change things'. The de-mythification of power and reorienting the self in relation to authority is the central developmental demand of this initial post-mobilisation phase. During this period, participation is exploratory, unknowing and unsure. Individuals are first discovering their political muscles and potential for external impact' [p. 19] finding their voice.
Era of advancement	Maturation of empowerment through extension of involvement and deepening understanding through intensive self-reflection with the help of peers and external enabler. Three major aspects of empowering evolution in this phase are: • the centrality of a mentor relationship • the enabling impact of supportive peer relationships within a collective organisational structure • cultivation of a more critical understanding of social and political relation.
Era of incorporation: 'The sense of growing up' [p. 23]	Reconstructs sense of self as author and actor in environment. Learning to confront and contend with barriers to self-determination leads to a sense of mastery and competence in the individual's sense of being.
Era of commitment: Adulthood of participatory competence – integrates new abilities and insight into reality in meaningful ways.	Those who develop a fully realised participatory competence are those who succeed in reconstructing their sense of mastery and awareness in relation to the political world ... continuing to struggle with integrating new personal knowledge and skill into the reality and structure of their everyday life-worlds [p. 24].

the maintenance of the creative force of internal contradiction – people must feel the confrontation to respond [sense of constructive conflict]. The constructive dialogue takes place on different levels. Most significantly is dialogue with one's colleagues towards a collective empowerment but also with a guide as within guided reflection. As Jane noted (Chapter 24):

> 'I am aware I have not yet explored attitudes to DSH patients with my colleagues and yet that is vital to change our collective practice. I accept that responsibility bat a later stage. But first I must get my own house in order'.

Jane's comment points to the truth that she needs to feel empowered as an individual before tackling others. Through reflection comes insight of contradiction. Through guided dialogue comes insight of understanding. Through understanding comes insight of empowerment. Through empowerment comes insight of transformation. It is the journey towards becoming a reflective practitioner and realising vision.

Kieffer adds [15, p. 27–8]

> 'Throughout the proposed developmental model reflective experience is the irreducible source of growth ... there is no substitute for learning through experience. More passive forms of training and instruction may be useful in instances where specific information is required: but the didactic approach apparently has little relevance in promoting the most critical elements of empowerment. As a participant remarks –

'People can't really learn the things I've learned through workshops or through classes or courses. You have to experience it yourself to really know'.

Beck's words of 'running in place' return to mind (Chapter 1)'.
In Chapter 26, I expand Kieffer's framework by suggesting an 'era of enlightenment'.

Summary

Gaining insight is the aim of reflective learning. The framing perspectives guide practitioners to summarise their learning. As with all reflective frameworks, they are to be viewed as a heuristic, a means to an end, rather than a rigid framework to force insights into arbitrary boxes. Holding tentative insights, the practitioner can dialogue with extant sources of knowledge to inform, deepen their tentative insights and open possibility for new insights (Chapter 7), and dialogue with guides and peers in guided reflection to co-create insights (Chapters 8 and 9).

In Chapter 6, I set out a reflective approach to 'knowing the person', an element within the 'Being Available Template' within the broader context of the Buford NDU Person-centred Model.

References

1. Carson, J. (2008) *Spider Speculations: A Physics and Biophysics of Storytelling*. Theatre Communications group, New York.

2. Okri, B. (1997) *A Way of Being Free*. Phoenix House, London.

3. Nicholls, D. (2015) Seeing the wood for the trees: beware organizational blindness. https://dannicholls1.com/2015/04/01/seeing-the-wood-for-the-trees-beware-organisationalblindness/

4. Winterson, J. (2001) *The Powerbook*. Vintage, London.

5. Carper, B. (1978) Fundamental patterns of knowing in nursing. *Advances in Nursing Science* 1(1), 13–23.

6. White, J. (1995) Patterns of knowing: review, critique and update. *Advances Nursing Science* 17(4), 73–86.

7. Munhall, P. (1993) 'Unknowing': towards another pattern of knowing in nursing. *Nursing Outlook* 41(3), 125–128.

8. Johns, C. (1995) Framing learning through reflection within Carper's fundamental ways of knowing. *Journal of Advanced Nursing* 22, 226–234.

9. Johns C. (1988) *Becoming A Reflective Practitioner Through Guided Reflection*. Unpublished PhD thesis, The Open University.

10. Senge, P. M. (1990) *The Fifth Discipline: The Art and Practice of the Learning Organization*. Century Business, London.

11. Bass, B. (1985) *Leadership and Performance Beyond Expectations*. Free Press, New York.

12. Bass, B. (1990) From transactional to transformational leadership: learning to share the vision. *Organizational Dynamics* Winter, 18, 19–31.

13. Greenleaf, R. K. (1977/2002) *Servant Leadership: A Journey into the Nature of Legitimate Power and Greatness*. Paulist Press, New York/Mahwah, NJ.

14. Johns, C. (2016) *Mindful Leadership: A Guide for the Health Care Professions*. Palgrave, London.

15. Kieffer, C. (1984) Citizen empowerment: a developmental perspective. *Prevention in Human Sciences* 84, 9–36.

Notes

i. In the broadest sense I draw on the following definition of theory – 'a formal statement of the rules on which a subject of study is based or of ideas that are suggested to explain a fact or event or, more generally, an opinion or explanation: https://dictionary.cambridge.org/dictionary/english/theory (see also Chapter 7).

ii. https://www.dictionary.com/browse/poise.

CHAPTER 6

The Nine Reflective Cues to Appreciate 'Knowing the Person'

Introduction

If practitioners are committed to becoming a reflective practitioner and realising their vision of practice, then it is essential that organisational systems are developed to facilitate practitioners to achieve this. This was the challenge at Buford Hospital. Based on its collective vision of person-centred practice, the Buford Nursing Development Unit developed the Buford NDU person-centred model comprising five inter-locking systems to create the reflective organisational environment to facilitate practitioners realising the hospital's vision [1].

These five systems are:

- System for tuning practitioners into the person-centred vision (reflective cues).
- System for communicating practice (dialogue and narrative).
- System for organising delivery of practice (primary nursing and servant-leadership).
- System for enabling practitioners to realise person-centred practice (guided reflection as expounded throughout the book).
- System to enable practitioners to live quality (guided reflection and standards of care).

System for Tuning Practitioners into the Person-centred Vision (2)

Fundamental to realising person-centred practice is 'knowing the person'. It is an acknowledged attribute of 'being available' (Figure 5.3). Given this understanding, how might practitioners be guided to know the person from a person-centred perspective?

The Buford solution was to devise nine reflective cues to tune the practitioner

- into seeing the person from a person-centred perspective,
- into appreciate the pattern of the person's being and needs,
- into themselves so as to see the person clearly.

The nine cues:

- Who is this person?
- What meaning does this health-illness experience have for the person?
- How is this person feeling?

- How do I feel about this person?
- How has this event affected their usual life pattern and roles?
- How can I help this person?
- What is important to make their stay at the Day centre comfortable?
- What support does this person have in life?
- How does this person view the future for themselves and others?

Pattern Appreciation

The notion of 'pattern appreciation' rather than 'assessment' is to deflect from the idea of assessment as something done on admission. Reading a person's pattern is viewing the person as a whole [3, 4]. The practitioner appreciates the person by tuning into the person by being fully present in the moment as a continuous process throughout the person's stay.

Becker writes [5, p. 13.] –

> 'The point to bear in mind is to know your own feelings about the person you are addressing, to accept the person exactly as he is – a person as worthy as yourselves. Listen and respond to him without making judgments about him. People feel a lot freer around someone who is quietly accepting them for what they are. It is for you to remain relaxed in the presence of nothing going on. Simply to be present in an atmosphere like that is a healing thing. It is actually this caring listening response, and not a showing or doing response, which makes the osteopathic manipulation treatment work'.

Of course I am not writing about osteopathic manipulation, but the same principle applies to making the healing connection of person-centred practice work. Thus, the practitioner approaches the person with this curious attitude with the intent to know the person and establish a relationship.

The cues follow a line of inquiry that flows naturally with the way the person-centred practitioner thinks. The cues are easy to appreciate. The cue – 'How do I feel about this person?' – is perhaps more challenging because it tunes the practitioner into their own feelings, thoughts and attitudes, and how these might impact on perceiving the person. It resonates with the MSR cue 'Did my feelings and attitudes influence me?' (Figure 2.2).

With experience, the cues are internalised as a natural and intuitive reflective lens to tune into the unfolding clinical situation as a continuous process of assessment, response and evaluation. Thus, the cues are always at work moment by moment. They do not require direct answers. I emphasise this point because the practitioner who has embodied a reductionist systems approach may miss the reflective point and view the cues as yet another set of boxes to complete.

As Sutherland [6, p. 96] noted –

> 'Although at first I did find myself going back to the Roper model[i] headings to make sure that I had not missed anything, omitting what was physically important, I did not need to do this for very long'.

Sutherland further noted the impact of the reflective cues in changing her mind-set [6, p. 96] –

> 'Because the emphasis is centred on feelings and the total picture of that person's situation rather than on their ongoing physical needs, it forced me to move away from a need to find things out, fill things in and get things done as soon as possible in an orderly fashion. It forced me to start listening to what patients themselves were saying was important to them and then to plan care with them from this basis. It gradually became a welcome release for me'.

There is something astonishing in Sutherland's words about the way she thought the Burford cues forced her to listen to the person, as if she hadn't really listened to the person before. As she suggests, the 'old model' became the task – hence the effort was to complete it rather than really listen to what the patient or family were saying. As Sutherland suggests, the key is listening and connecting and then working with the person towards meeting their healthcare needs.

The practitioner's skill is to create the dialogical conditions whereby the person can reveal their experience, what Patterson and Zderad [7, p. 23] described as a 'lived dialogue'. Only when the practitioner is in tune with the person can they appreciate and respond appropriately to the person's unfolding needs. Newman [3, p. 13] writes –

> 'The task is not to try to change another person's pattern but to recognise it as information that depicts the whole and relate to it as it unfolds'.

My use of the Buford cues is evident in my experience working with Tony in my role as a bank staff nurse working within a hospice to illustrate the Buford cues in action, the way they shape my perception and response within the clinical moment.

Knowing Tony

Susan [a staff nurse] asks me to help get Tony up for lunch. I have not met him before. I am informed that he is 53 years old, that he has primary lung cancer with liver metastases. He has been in the hospice for respite care four days.

I ask Susan 'Is there anything in particular I should be mindful of?'

'He's bit moody'.

'Why's that?'

'He's unhappy here and wants to go home. He finds it difficult to co-ordinate himself but doesn't want help'.

I knock on the closed door. No reply. I knock again and enter the room. The hand-drawn cards fixed to the bedroom wall immediately catch my attention.

'Hi Mr Birchall, I'm Chris. How are you this morning?'

He looks at me but doesn't answer. I sense his irritation. Susan's words come to mind. I gaze at the cards pinned to the wall – 'Who made these lovely cards?'

'My grand-daughter'.

'She has talent. Tell me about her?'

'Her name is Michelle. She is four years old'.

He becomes animated talking about her. She is very special to him, adding to his sadness and restlessness. I have opened a door to connect with Tony, talking about the thing that he cares most deeply for and grieves for its forthcoming loss. I reveal I have two young children. We talk about schooling and about his work – he had been a plumber. He knows he is not going to work anymore and accepts this. All the while his anger simmers. Do I let him know I sense this? Such catharsis might prick the tension and yet it might embarrass him. I take the risk 'You seem irritated being here?'

In doing so, I release my own anxiety. As if I have pressed a button, he pointedly says 'I want to be at home. Not that it's unpleasant in here but …'.

His words drift off. Patiently I wait.

He adds 'I want to be at home'.

'I sense that … so why are you here?'

'I had no choice because my daughter is away for the week and I need her support'.

He relaxes. He has expressed his irritation – a potent cocktail of anger at the hospice, at me, at himself, at the cancer, at his daughter, that he is dying, grief of anticipatory loss, indeed at the world at large. He moves out of the shadow of his despair more willing to engage with me.

He asks 'Tell me about yourself'.

I sense he needs to know me to accept my presence. I explain I work at the hospice to maintain my credibility as a palliative care teacher. He is intrigued. He stands and takes off his pyjamas. His nakedness exposed. I hold him steady as he moves into and out of the shower. Slowly he dresses. I help him with his socks and shoes. I have been with him over an hour.

I ask 'Do you have any pain?'

'No'.

'That's good ... I can see you need help with washing and dressing. Do you get this support at home ok?'

'My daughter helps me. We do have a nurse who comes in and monitors me so if things get any worse she's on hand to help'.

We go to lunch in the communal dining room. It is empty. We are late. Everybody else has gone. He invites me to join him for lunch. I stay with him until he has finished. There is something normalising about having a meal with someone. He tells me he was a keen cyclist. I tell him I am a morris dancer. By the time we finish, I am on his wavelength and sense his ease. I too am easier, having worked through my own anxiety. I sense the way feelings are reciprocated. It highlights for me the fundamental need to know people in order to respond appropriately to them on a level that is meaningful. We got there, but it took an effort.

I imagine it must be difficult for him to deal with yet another nurse. I imagine he would rather have Susan help him, someone he knows. He doesn't say that, at least not in words. Perhaps I could have said to him – 'I'll get Susan to help you', acknowledging his initial discomfort with me. But then as Susan said he's moody with everyone. Do patients have the right to choose their nurses in hospice? It is a profound question because I cannot impose my idea of relationship on patients. The very nature of suffering and facing dying must always make relationship precarious. In getting to know someone who is suffering I trip along a fine edge of raw emotion.

Perhaps I could have simply connected superficially with him by helping him to wash, dress, escort him to lunch, administer and monitor his pain medication and other symptom relief. But this was not the level of help he really needed. On a deeper level, I knew he was in crisis. I could read that, but that was my difficulty. I could not respond easily to the superficial caring issues outside that deeper context. Hence helping him wash and dress became difficult once I had touched his suffering. He also knew that and perhaps resisted me because he needed to protect himself from this intruding stranger. On the other hand, he might have preferred my superficial attention. I felt as if I had pushed his limits and challenged his control of the situation.

Later, I share this experience with Susan. She affirms my experience, acknowledging Tony's struggle in facing death. She feels I shouldn't worry unduly as Tony is 'difficult'. In other words, my experience is normal. Sensitivity flattened in order to cope with the stress of the day. The patient is the problem not the inadequacy of the nurse.

Before I leave the hospice, I go and shake hands with Tony and thank him for accommodating me. He reciprocates my thanks, for having the patience to stay with him. I sense he is lonely here without his daughter and grand-daughter visiting. A week can seem a long time when time is running out and when such relationships are precious.

Applying the Reflective Cues

'Who Is This Person?'

On approaching Tony, I brought myself present to the moment. I asked myself 'who is this person?', to know him within the context of his world. His family and culture are brought into focus and scope of care. In acknowledging Tony as a person, I also acknowledge myself as a person that sets the basis for a person-centred relationship. The most meaningful way to know a person is to listen to their story.

Krishnamurti's words are challenging [8, p. 178/179] –

> 'Very few of us listen to what is being said, we always translate or interpret it according to a particular point of view. We have formulations, opinions, judgments, beliefs through which we listen, so we are never actually listening at all; we are only listening in terms of our own prejudices, conclusions or experiences. We are always interpreting what we hear, and obviously that does not bring about understanding. Whatever we listen to is always apprehended through the screen of this conditioning; therefore, we can never approach any problem with a fresh mind ... where the mind's conditioning is imposed by society'.

Listening carefully immediately communicates concern and availability. It is putting aside any filters that obscure knowing the person and making judgment.

This may be challenging when that person's story is uncertain, for example, with people who are distressed, mentally disturbed or terminally ill, situations where their story may be chaotic.

To know Tony, I must tune into his wavelength and flow with his story. Then, I am available to work with him to sort out his diverse needs and to perhaps find a healthier wave length (Figure 6.1a). When people experience crisis in their lives, their wave patterns become chaotic. Practitioners normally expect the patient to fit into the stereotyped 'good patient' mould – a symbolic straight line that flattens humanness (Figure 6.1b). The reward is to be accepted and cared for. Failure to 'fit-in' often leads to censure as characterised by the image of the 'unpopular patient' [9, 10]. Such relationships lack harmony and feel flat.

The key to tuning into Tony is to attentively listen [11] and be empathic to Tony's experience beneath the surface signs and assumptions that might lead me to assume what it means. It means being prepared to self-disclose as appropriate, challenging the professional barriers that practitioners may prefer to hide behind [12].

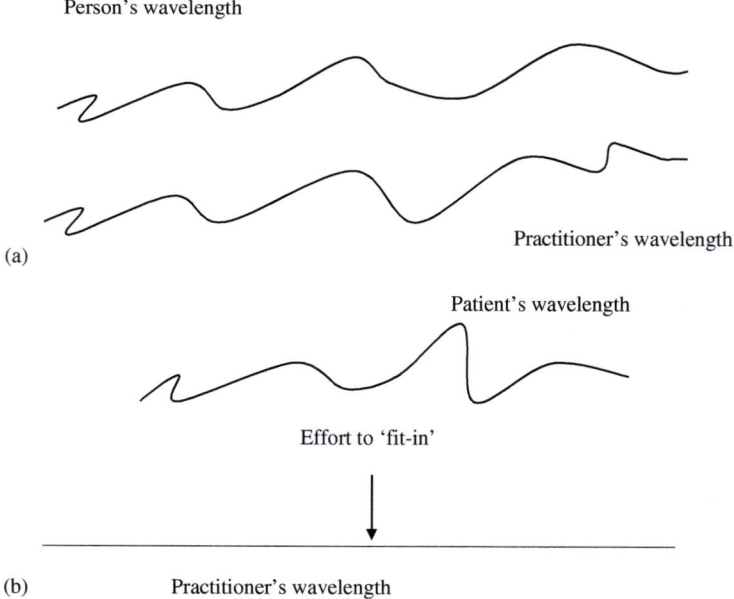

FIGURE 6.1 (a) The practitioner tuning into and flowing with the person's wavelength. (b) The practitioner expects the person to 'fit-into' their wavelength.

He needed to know me. This understanding challenges the practitioner adopting a 'bedside manner'. Jourard [13] observed the way the nurse dons a bedside manner when she dons her uniform, and that the uniform encourages stereotypical behaviour that diminishes the individual. Jourard notes [13, p. 180] –

> 'It is acquired as a means of coping with the anxieties engendered by repeated encounters with suffering, demanding patients'.

Unfortunately, such a manner becomes rigid over time. The patient will recognise this, limiting their willingness to tell their story. It is a controlling behaviour designed to reduce the possibility that the patient will behave in ways that are likely to threaten the professional person. As Murray Cox [14, p. 51] puts it –

> 'The therapist must at all times be himself. It has something to do with a genuine emotional engagement, rather than an adoption of a professional role'.

'What Meaning Does This Health Event Have for the Person?'

Having gained an appreciation of who Tony is, I then tune into the particular health issues that bring Tony into the hospice. My intent is to enable him to make sense of his bewildering experience. Newman [15] describes this as a rhythm of relating, acknowledging that the patient's rhythm may be in turmoil due to the illness experience. As Newman [15, p. 227] notes –

> 'Nurses should develop a tolerance for ambiguity and uncertainty and 'hang in there' with clients until a new rhythm emerges more compatible with health'.

Appreciating the meanings, he gives to his experience I also find meaning in my approach to him.

'How Is This Person Feeling?'

Tony revealed a cocktail of distressing emotions that bubbled to the surface. I tripped along this cue cautiously, not wanting to intrude inappropriately into his private world but mindful of opening a space whereby he could express these emotions safely and discharge as appropriate. Until these emotions were released, it was difficult to talk through his experience in any meaningful way.

The obvious response to this cue is to ask the person 'How are you?'

However, as Cameron [16, p. 53] noted

> 'How are you? is a question that turns us back to who we are as health care professionals and calls us to be more deeply attentive to the moment. When we *sincerely* ask 'how are you', we enact our ethical commitment to one another'.

Sincerely differentiates the therapeutic from the merely sociable. Indeed, *how are you?* as a social ritual is likely to disengage rather than engage the person if interpreted as merely a social nicety.

'How Do I Feel About This Person?'

Initially, I felt both concern and uneasy with Tony. Susan's report that Tony was difficult had made me wary. Her comment reveals how quickly practitioners can label patients when they exhibit certain types of 'difficult' behaviour and fit into what is deemed as acceptable behaviour. It would have preferred if she hadn't disclosed this fact to me beforehand then I might have been less uneasy and less guarded. In telling his story, I sensed his anger lay thick on the surface despite his compliance. I endeavoured to be poised and open to his experience rather than defend myself to manage my uneasiness in order to be fully present and available to Tony.

'How Has This Event Affected Their Usual Life Pattern and Roles?'

Serious illness can prompt a radical reassessment of lifestyle and what people consider significant within their lives. Disruption of normal patterns can have detrimental consequences if not carefully managed; hence, knowing Tony's normal lifestyle was essential so I did not disrupt it unnecessarily or disturb his control over events, and perhaps, to help him find new, more beneficial life patterns and roles even as he faced dying.

'How Can I Help This Person?'

How can I help this person can be viewed on three levels:

- Help to meet Tony's immediate needs.
- Help to meet Tony's longer-term needs.
- Help to enable Tony grow through his experience.

These needs are all set against the background of my intention to help ease Tony's suffering within the broader vision of person-centred practice. To do this, I needed to understand his suffering as best I can. He did not reveal himself to me easily so to help him I first had to create the conditions where he could reveal himself. Of course I needed time to do this and fortunately I had it. In the fast pace of clinical practice, such time might be at a premium creating a dilemma for the practitioner in prioritising time for such work. Hence, how I prioritise time is always a practical and ethical issue for myself.

Responding to Tony is viewed in terms of what he needs, not what I think his needs are, although I may have an opinion about that. Clearly, as an experienced nurse and therapist I have an almost innate sense of knowing Tony's experience and his likely needs. Thus, I must suspend my opinions to hear Tony so we can discuss and negotiate my response to his needs.

Murray Cox [14, p. 101] notes –

> 'It is the gauging of what the client (person) needs and not what the (therapist) wishes him to need that is the guideline for optimal structuring of the therapeutic process (p. 81). It is a matter of profound importance that the personal views of the therapist must not set limits on the person his patient is becoming'.

As the narrative reveals, his suffering expressed itself as multifaceted anger. Acknowledging his anger was the first step to easing it using the communication skills of catharsis, catalytic and confrontation within our dialogue [17] – see Chapter 8.

My poise was pivotal in not absorbing his anger but dissolving it through understanding his predicament. Having lunch with him and talking about our interests normalised the environment for him, taking him out of the 'being treated' experience. It was journeying with him rather than doing things to him – the very essence of person-centred practice.

Murray Cox [14, p. 107] gives pause for deeper reflection:

'Every experience is the opportunity for growth when I pay attention to it with learning intent. Reflection opens the learning space. Ontological insecurity is the condition for learning. Such tensions always exist, they can never be resolved within the mystery of the human-human encounter. Security would simply be an illusion'.

Did Tony grow through his experience of being cared for? I hope so. Our respective ontological insecurity was at the core of our encounter. Did I grow through the experience? Yes. Reflection always leads to insight and growth.

'What Is Important for This Person to Make Their Stay in the Hospice Comfortable?'

Tony did not want to be at the hospice but felt obliged to because of his social circumstances. The cue raises issues of comfort and control, especially those 'little things' that make a significant difference to the person's comfort and perception of being cared for [18]. For Tony I suspected that being understood made his stay more comfortable, enabling him to flow more easily in this potentially hostile environment. Talking about his granddaughter was clearly significant.

Perhaps I could have challenged Susan's analysis and labelling of Tony as 'difficult'. Labelling is such a perverse act and disrupts any therapeutic potential. I recognise that my avoidance to confront Susan verbally reflects a deeper need to avoid conflict, reflecting how practitioners also conform to a social norm of the harmonious team [19]. Mindful of creating a care environment where people are comfortable reflects and communicates a deep sensitivity to the person as befits any claim to person-centred care.

'What Support Does This Person Have in Life?'

I tentatively queried his support at home. I did not meet his daughter so did not gain her perspective. However, the hospice is geared up to social and psychological aspects of care. My role is to collaborate with others if aspects of supporting Tony emerge through our conversation. From a pragmatic perspective, support is vital to mobilise and develop with a view to eventual discharge especially where the person requires support in the community with the risk and associated impact and cost of the person blocking the bed.

'How Does This Person View the Future?'

Tony knew his condition was terminal. His anticipatory loss rippled through our whole encounter. His imminent death was present between us even if we did not overtly mention it. Perhaps I could have explicitly used this cue as knowing him would have made this an easier topic to broach. Other, more specialist practitioners would also broach this cue with him. As such, I was mindful of not over-stepping my role in that moment.

The nine reflective cues illustrate how reflection can be built into the fabric of person-centred practice. In doing so, the cues enable practitioners to live reflection moment by moment in journeying with persons and mindfulness. No longer are patients viewed as boxes to fill in or assessment a task to do on admission.

Communicating Tony's Care

Part of knowing Tony is communicating his hospice journey in the most meaningful manner. As I have noted [20, p. 41] –

> 'Communication is the beating heart of holistic practice through dialogue with persons and colleagues reflected in written notes (narrative) to ensure consist and congruent practice'.

The written notes are written as an unfolding narrative. I wrote in Tony's notes – 'Tony's anger is an expression of his suffering and loss at being in the hospice. It is understandable although difficult to respond to. I feel he needs to have control of being in the hospice. After helping him wash and dress we lunched together and shared many common interests that helped to lift his despair at least for the moment. He acknowledges he needs to be here as difficult as that is for him. In particular he misses his granddaughter'.

My use of the word 'suffering' was to challenge the staff's prevailing idea that Tony was difficult. It is an evocative word central to WHO definition of palliative care. Using the word thus confronted the predominant symptom management attitude that prevailed at the hospice. My notes were also a subtle confrontation of the label 'difficult', intending to help other staff see him as I did.

Knowing Lorna

Tony was able to respond to me. Yet many people are unable to communicate and thus require a deeper sensitivity to knowing them and their needs.

The doctor approaches me to ask if I might help Lorna to lift her out of her flatness. She is 37. She has cancer of her ovary and now a stroke resulting in a dense left hemiplegia. Her speech is affected and there is a question about her cognitive ability simply because she only says 'yes'. I know she is a scientist. She is married to David and have two young children aged 4 and 6.

Framed with this information, I enter her orbit. A blue head scarf covers her head. I question myself – 'Does she wear it to hide her hair loss due to chemotherapy? It doesn't matter. She wears glasses and looks very young. Just gazing at her, I sense her tragedy. She takes my offered hand and smiles weekly. I say who I am and what I do. She seems open to my approach. 'Would she like some therapy?' I ask expectantly. She says 'yes' but I am uncertain because, as I have been told, she always says 'yes'. How knowledge structures the view; that if I had not known she only says 'yes' would I have responded differently? Less from my body and senses, more from my head filled as it is with knowledge? How do I read the signs? I move to touch her hand yet mindful of my touch. She does not resist my continued hold. My inclination is to give some reflexology and therapeutic touch. I sense reflexology would help stimulate and balance her body and ease her despair. I say this and she says 'yes'. She returns my smile. I sense her permission. Oils mixed. I guide Lorna to relax. Being at her feet feels remote. Perhaps holding her occiput would have felt less so. But would that be for my need? I must be wary of over-concern and pity for her intense vulnerability and tragedy.

Her husband David arrives and quietly slips into the room and sits by her side, holding her hand. Afterwards I ask how she feels and she says 'yes' but there is a glint in her eyes and she utters a cry as David embraces her. I show David the small kitchen and offer a therapy if he should need it. He shrugs off his own despair. Yet he acknowledges it is tough, very tough for him right now. Lorna died the following Thursday.

Reflection

Knowing Lorna and responding to the Buford cues is much more intuitive than knowing Tony. It is sensed. Under such circumstances, it is easy to feel pity. Certainly, I had no idea how she must be feeling. I might imagine it was deep fear and sadness. Intuitively I sensed that reflexology would be helpful. I know it is deeply relaxing and eases suffering. I have been told many times. I also know that presence connects her to the world. It gives a message she is not alone. Holding her hand, holding her feet with concern I am reminded of the words of Blackwolf and Jones and [21, p. 184] –

'Touch is the harmonic healing the grieving spirit craves'.

Knowing David is part of knowing Lorna. He is her support. Indeed, responding to Lorna is also responding to him when he sees the glint in Lorna's eye he knows she is comforted. I explicitly offer to support him sensing his own suffering. But he wanted no distraction from Lorna.

People Are Not Numbers to Crunch

Returning to Sutherland's words, my own experience of accompanying Otter for an angio-gram is a sobering reflection of task-focused nursing where Otter was not viewed as a person and myself excluded from the nurse's vision. Clearly the nurse was 'unreflective', not aware of her impact on us.

I reflected on the experience [22]

Enter the First Blind Mouse

She saunters into the bay dressed in blues, clipboard in hand. She positions herself at the end of the bed as if keeping her distance surveying the work to be done. No introduction. No recognition of me. 'Hello – I'm here' I say to myself.

She wears a name badge on her chest. The writing is too small to read from where I'm sitting. My eyes strain to make out her name … No, I can't make it out. I cast my eyes aside. God forgive – she might think I'm staring at her breasts. I imagine her comment 'right pervert in there'; but I want to know her name. I strain again to no avail. My eyes turn away fearful of judgment. Maybe I should simply ask – 'what is your name nurse?

But I don't. Why am I rendered silent? Am I merely a bystander outside her gaze?

She does the talking, firing questions, scribbling on her clipboard. In response to each answer she exclaims 'fantastic'.

Check your date of birth? Fantastic!

When was the last time you had anything to eat or drink? Fantastic!

Have you had your medicines this morning? Fantastic!

Did you bring your medicines in with you? Fantastic!

Are you allergic to anything? Fantastic!

Patient identity confirmed. The name bracelet fixed. A final fantastic and then she goes, no doubt pleased she has been both efficient and friendly. I look at Otter. She looks at me.

'Fanbloodytastic!' I laugh.

I name her 'little miss fantastic'. Roger Hargreaves eat your heart out.

'Shooosh' Otter says anxiously, 'they'll hear you. We might get thrown out'.

Otter anxious not to make a fuss, to be the good patient.

My laugh turns to a frown.
No empathy for someone admitted for an angiogram and possible stent insertion
No inquiry how Otter is feeling or if she is anxious about anything.
No information of what to expect.

Otter is simply an object being processed. But surely, this is a specialist cardiac unit. There is something very wrong here. No Oscar for her performance, unless of course, it's a horror movie. I am a bystander outside your gaze.

> Outside your gaze you do not see me.
> Yes me, sitting over here anxious about my partner
> Her life on edge
> Tell me your name at least
> Greet me with a smile
> Ask me how I am
> Not a lot to ask really or perhaps it is
> Wrapped up, as you are, in the machine
> Perfunctory responses *fantastic, fantastic, fantastic*!
> I wonder how you would respond if I had said
> Excuse me – what is your name nurse?
> Or hello, I'm Chris and stood to shake your hand
> I didn't so I don't know.
> Tick the box nurse fantastic.
> ☐   I am a robot'.

On further reflection, readers may ask why I didn't introduce myself and ask the nurse's name. It was because I was caught up in the task. How do you communicate with a bright and breezy robot? The whole experience reflects how little the nurse knows the person. Indeed, Otter was merely an object being processed where humanness was filtered out. The nurse is merely a technician unreflectively going through the motions. I wonder how she would have responded to Otter using the Buford cues and what difference Otter's care might have made as a consequence.

Summary

The nine Buford cues offer a reflective system to know the person from a person-centred vision. The cues guide the practitioner to live reflection as an active and dynamic process, reinforcing what it means to be a reflective practitioner whereby reflection is lived as an unfolding narrative towards realising their vision moment by moment.

References

1. Johns, C. (2024a) Setting out the Buford NDU Model. In C. Johns [Ed.] *Holistic Practice in Health Care: The Buford NDU Person-centred Model.* Wiley Blackwell, Oxford, 19–31.

2. Johns, C. (2024b) System to tuning practitioners into the holistic vision. In C. Johns [Ed.] *Holistic Practice in Health Care: The Buford NDU Person-centred Model.* Wiley Blackwell, 35–40.

3. Newman, M. (1994) *Health as Expanded Consciousness.* National League of Nursing, New York.

4. Cowling, R. (2000) Healing as appreciating wholeness. *Advances in Nursing Science* 22(3), 16–32.

5. Becker, R. (1997) In R.E. Brooks [Ed.] *Life in Motion.* Stillness Press, Portland, OR.

6. Sutherland, L. (1994) Caring as mutual empowerment: working within the BNDU model at Burford. In C. Johns [Ed.] *Holistic Practice in Healthcare: The Buford NDU Person-centred Model.* Wiley Blackwell, 91–100.

7. Paterson, J., Zderad, L. (1988) *Humanistic Nursing.* National League for Nursing, New York.

8. Krishnamurti, J. (1996) *Total Freedom.* Harper, San Francisco.

9. Johnson, M., Webb, C. (1995) Rediscovering unpopular patients: the concept of social judgment. *Journal of Advanced Nursing* 21, 466–475.

10. Kelly, M., May, D. (1982) Good and bad patients: a review of the literature and theoretical critique. *Journal of Advanced Nursing* 7, 147–156.

11. Smith, M., Liehr, P. (1999) Attentively embracing story; a middle range theory with practice and research implications. *Scholarly Inquiry for Nursing Practice* 13(3), 3–27.

12. Derlaga, V. J., Berg, J. H. (2014) *Self-disclosure: Theory, Research, and Therapy.* Springer, New York.

13. Jourard, S. (1971) *The Transparent Self.* Van Nostrand, Newark.

14. Cox, M. (1988) *Structuring the Therapeutic Process: Compromise with Chaos* (revised edition). Jessica Kingsley Publishing, London.

15. Newman, M. (1999) The rhythm of relating in a paradigm of wholeness. *Image: Journal of Nursing Scholarship* 31(3), 227–230.

16. Cameron, D. (2004) *Globalizing Communication.* Routledge, London.

17. Heron, J. (1975) Six-category intervention analysis. Human Potential Research Group, University of Surrey.

18. MacLeoad, M. (1994) 'It's the little things that count': the hidden complexity of everyday nursing practice. *Journal of Clinical Nursing*, 3, p. 361–368.

19. Johns, C. (1992) Ownership and the harmonious team: barriers to developing the therapeutic nursing team in primary nursing. *Journal of Clinical Nursing* 1, 89–94.

20. Johns, C. (2024) System for communicating holistic practice. In C. Johns [Ed.] *Holistic Practice in Health Care: The Buford NDU Person-centred Model.* Wiley Blackwell, 41–56.

21. Blackwolf., Jones, G. (1996) *Earth Dance Drum: A Celebration of Life.* Commune-A-Key Publishing, Salt Lake City.

22. Johns, C., Rose, O. (2022) 'People are not numbers to crunch': a performance narrative and storyboard. In C. Johns [Ed.] *Becoming A Reflective Practitioner* (sixth edition). Wiley Blackwell, 133–142.

23. Roper, N., Logan, W. W., Tierney, A. J. (1980) *The Elements of Nursing.* Churchill Livingstone, Edinburgh.

Note

i. Buford hospital had previously utilised the Roper, Logan and Tierney model [23] to assess patient need. This is a reductionist model that reduced the patient into 10 activities of living. It lacked congruence with person-centred practice. An audit of the model in practice revealed assessment was done on admission as a box-filling task rather than as a continuous process and poorly documented.

CHAPTER 7

Informing Insights Through Dialogue with Theoretical Sources: The Third Dialogical Movement

Holding tentative insights, the practitioner dialogues with theoretical sources, prompted by the MSR cue – 'How has theory informed and deepened my insights and knowing in practice? (Figure 2.2). This is evident in the previous chapter where I drew on Cox (1) to inform my 'knowing the person'. Cox's work was critiqued in juxtaposition with my experience of working with Tony and subsequently assimilated within my knowing in practice.

Brookfield (2, p. 36) writes that –

'Theory can help us name our practice by illuminating the general elements of what we think are idiosyncratic experiences. It can provide multiple perspectives on familiar situations'.

Brookfield refers to 'theory'. I reiterate (from Chapter 5) my use of the word theory in the broadest sense as meaning 'a formal statement of the rules on which a subject of study is based or of ideas that are suggested to explain a fact or event or, more generally, an opinion or explanation.[i] Thus, 'theory' includes any source of information that the practitioner considers relevant to inform their reflections and develop insights.

Cox (1) offers no proof for his assertions. They result from his reflections on his practice over many years culminating in his practice wisdom. His words resonated with me and made sense. They fitted the bill so to speak.

All theory, no matter its authoritative claim, is viewed through a sceptical eye for its authority to inform the practitioner's knowing in practice and tentative insights. It is always critiqued for its value to inform (3). However, weighing up the value of theory to inform is not just simply critique. It also requires a leap of imagination. Greenleaf (4, p. 31) quotes Alfred North Whitehead –

'No language can be anything but elliptical, requiring a leap of imagination to understand its meaning in its relevance to immediate experience'.

Not-knowing

Drawing on theory helps to moderate the helplessness of not-knowing. But it remains important that theory should be the servant to the practice and not its master. By listening too readily to accepted theories, and to what they lead the practitioner to expect, it is easy to become deaf to the unexpected. It is all too easy to equate not-knowing with ignorance, that can lead practitioners to seek refuge in an illusion that they understand' [5, p. 4]. This brings the risk of getting it wrong or fitting the patient to a misunderstanding of what they really need.

Putting Evidence-based Practice into a Reflective Perspective

Appreciating the scope of theory from a reflective perspective overturns the dominance of 'evidence-based practice' as de rigueur to clinical practice – that the evidence to determine practice is *statistically proven* as a fact. Its ethos is 'give us the problem and we will provide the solution that the practitioner can apply'. This may be true for technical aspects of care but not for aspects of practice concerned with human encounters that are unique and never having been experienced before. It is at odds with the prevalent ideology ideal of person-centred practice because it reduces the human condition where people are viewed essentially as statistics to crunch. From this perspective, people can easily be viewed as objects to be manipulated. As Schön [6] noted, everyday practice is complex and indeterminate that defies applying evidence-based solutions to its problems.

Nevo and Slonim-Nevo [7, p. 1176] give perspective on what counts as evidence based or informed practice

> 'Evidence informed practice should be understood as *excluding non-scientific prejudices and superstitions*, but leaving ample room for clinical experience as well as the constructive and imaginative judgments of practitioners and clients who are in constant interaction and dialogue with one another'.

Opening the door to practitioner and client's imagination inevitably involves prejudice and opinion. It is part of human nature, and whilst prejudice and opinion can be surfaced, explored and shifted towards a less prejudiced and opinionated perspective through reflection, it will continue to influence judgment.

The notion of excluding non-scientific evidence is restrictive. Opening up 'what counts as evidence' was highlighted by Rycroft-Malone et al. [8] to include clinical experience, local context and environment and patients, clients and carers, whilst acknowledging the pre-eminent position of evidence-based research.

Diverse Sources of Theory

From a reflective practice perspective, theory can come from any source deemed relevant by the practitioner to inform their practice; notably, the patient's story and preferences, but also sources such as newspaper cuttings, TV documentaries, adverts, philosophy, theology, non-fiction and fiction; indeed, the list of potential sources of information is endless alongside what is deemed as 'evidence' in a more traditional academic and professional perspective as something proven. It is for the reflective practitioner to discern its relevance to inform their clinical judgment and to 'test' its efficacy to inform through subsequent reflection.

As one practitioner noted [9, p. 144]

> 'Just because punk music and Native American ideology is not nursing theory, is it less relevant to inform our values and practice? I would argue that it adds flavour and new perspectives. So when Chris enthusiastically says "look what I've found in Native American dancing philosophies" why should I doubt. Get out of the box for it is a coffin'.

The reflective practitioner always has an eye open for any source of theory to inform practice. This 'eye' becomes a radar, as if insights are fine wired within the brain to receive such messages. For example, the performance narrative title 'People are not numbers to crunch' [10] was inspired by a Virgin Money poster that stated exactly that – 'People are not numbers to crunch', that was revealed in the narrative as dismally lacking in our experience of undergoing an angiogram at a specialist cardiac centre.

Beyond Horizons

Such is the value and excitement of theory to help us see beyond our normal horizons. We gobble up the words and make them our own. Infused in our minds, we return to practice with these words buzzing and germinate them into our practice.

Often, when practitioners read theory, it is 'out-there' in a space that their mind grapples with. Because of its abstract nature, it may be difficult to relate to in terms of the practitioner's experience.

Hardy (as cited in Chapter 22) noted –

> 'I have illuminated the way I am now framing my experiences within the context of theory, and holding that theory up for critique for its value to inform my practice. For example, I reject Morse's [11] idea of types of relationships. From a holistic perspective there can only be connected-type relationships; the other types are merely descriptive failures of the connected relationship'.

Theoretical Mapping

Theory can be interpreted as a framework in which the practitioner can position themself. I term this *theoretical mapping*. It enables the practitioner to visualise and judge their current reality whilst visualising and envisaging a more desirable reality. It visualises the focus of the practitioner's subsequent reflections to move towards realising their desired reality. One example of theoretical mapping is 'The Thomas-Kilmann conflict mode instrument [12] that sets out five modes of managing conflict. The instrument is almost universally applicable in all guided reflection relationships given the significance of conflict because it is uncomfortable and draws the practitioner to pay attention to it, especially as it is constantly evident, they do not manage it well with a tendency to avoid it or brush it away. Its value is evident in its utilisation in narratives throughout the book, for example, see Figure 22.1.

Another example of theoretical mapping is Transactional Analysis [13, 14]. This framework enables practitioners to position and explore their ego mode of communication in relation to others. This map is set out in Figure 17.2 whilst guiding third year nursing students.

Inductive Sources

Interpreting recorded guided reflection dialogue enabled me to construct inductive theories of guided reflection and the nature of person-centred practice. A notable example is the 'Being available template', the default framework for knowing and monitoring the practitioner's development of person-centred practice (Figure 5.2). The Buford reflective cues (Chapter 6) were initially intuitive and proved its efficacy through reflection on its use to the extent they have not changed over 30 years.

It became apparent that assertiveness was a key attribute to being person-centred resulting in the 'Assertiveness action ladder' – a step-by-step approach as if climbing a ladder. This is set out in Figures 4.4 and 17.1. Understanding and managing one's stress is significant factor in becoming poised. In response, I designed the 'Feeling fluffy, feeling drained scale'. This is set out in Figure 17.3 in context of guiding third-year student nurses.

Accessing Information

Clearly, there is much information 'out there' to inform the practitioner's experience. So much so, the practitioner may feel overwhelmed by the task. Just browse the professional journals to feel the weight of available knowledge. The librarian will usually assist, as will peers pursuing similar theories, notably within group guided reflection. Results can be shared and posted on the intranet to be available to others. As the saying goes, 'Many hands make light work'.

At Buford hospital, I established a library of information for practitioners. I scanned our journal subscriptions to pull out relevant articles to post on an information board for all practitioners to view. Our approach to living quality involved setting standards of care, whereby the practitioners responsible for monitoring and updating the particular standard established attached resource files that informed the standard ensuring the standard was informed by the latest knowledge [15].

In the educational setting, sources of knowledge have traditionally been supplied (or spoon fed) by the teacher in the form of reading lists. Such lists may be helpful but are limited in that they narrow the focus of potentially informative texts.

Guidance

Dialogue with theoretical sources benefits from guidance. The guide will point the practitioner towards accessing sources and may stock specific sources that have proved relevant and useful, to 'pull out of the bag' at the appropriate moment to input into the dialogue (see Chapters 8 and 9). The guide can help the practitioner make sense of theory and critique its relevance to inform the particular experience.

Thus, the third and fourth dialogical movements become interwoven.

References

1. Cox, M. (1988) *Structuring the Therapeutic Process: Compromise with Chaos* (revised edition). Jessica Kingsley Publishing, London.

2. Brookfield, S. (1995) *Becoming A Critically Reflective Teacher*. Jossey-Bass, San Francisco.

3. Dewey, J. (1933) *How We Think*. JC Heath, Boston.

4. Greenleaf, R. (1977/2002) *Servant Leadership: A Journey into the Nature of Legitimate Power and Greatness*. Paulist Press, New York.

5. Casement, P. (1985) *On Learning from the Patient*. Routledge, London.

6. Schön, D. A. (1987) *Educating the Reflective Practitioner*. Jossey-Bass, San Francisco.

7. Nevo, I., Slonim-Nevo, V. (2011) The myth of evidence-based practice: towards evidence-informed practice. *British Journal of Social Work* 41, 1176–1197.

8. Rycroft-Malone, J., Seers K., Titchen A., Harvey G., Kitson A., McCormack, B. (2003) What counts as

evidence in evidence—based practice. *Journal of Advanced Nursing* 47(1): 81–90.

9. Johns, C. (2013) Balancing the wind and a lot of hot air. In C. Johns [Ed.] *Becoming A Reflective Practitioner* (fourth edition). Wiley-Blackwell, Hoboken. 138–145.

10. Johns, C., Rose, O. (2022) 'People are not numbers to crunch': a performance narrative and storyboard. In C. Johns [Ed.] *Becoming A Reflective Practitioner* (sixth edition). Wiley Blackwell, Hoboken. 133–142.

11. Morse, J. (1991) Negotiating commitment and involvement in the nurse-patient relationship. *Journal of Advanced Nursing* 16, 496–506.

12. Thomas, K., Kilmann, R. (1974) *Thomas Kilmann Conflict Mode Instrument*. Xicom Toledo, San Francisco.

13. Berne, E. (1961) *Transactional Analysis in Psychotherapy: The Classic Guide to Its Principles*. Grove Press, New York.

14. Stewart, I., Joines, V. (1987) *TA Today: A New Introduction to Transactional Analysis*. Russell Press, Nottingham.

15. Johns, C. (2024) A system to enable practitioners to live quality. In C. Johns [Ed.] *Holistic Practice in Healthcare: The Buford NDU Person-centred Model*. Wiley-Blackwell, Hoboken. 81–88.

Note

i. https://dictionary.cambridge.org/dictionary/english/theory.

CHAPTER 8

Guiding Reflection: The Fourth Dialogical Movement

Guided reflection is a contracted relationship whereby a guide guides the practitioner, either as an individual or in groups, to learn through reflection on their everyday experiences to gain insight towards realising their vision of practice as a lived reality. It addresses the MSR cue (Figure 2.2) – 'How has guidance deepened my tentative insights?' In this process, the guide challenges and supports the practitioner to see their reality more clearly, filtering through and shifting contradictory assumptions and opening new horizons of practice and possibilities towards realising their vision as a lived reality.

As Flemons and Green (1, p. 90) put it –

'Opening the possibility of the practitioner looking at themselves in a different light'.

Without doubt guidance has proven to be both a necessary and beneficial aspect of learning through reflection. Boud, Keogh and Walker (2, p. 36) note

'Whilst reflection is something the student could do for themselves, the learning process can be considerably accelerated by appropriate support'.

Bolman and Deal (3, p. 53) write –

'Leaders learn most from their experience – especially from their failures. Too often, though, they miss the lessons. They lack the reflective capacity to learn on their own and have not been fortunate enough to find a guide who can help them sort things out'.

Cox, Hickson and Taylor (4, p. 385) identify reasons why guidance is both necessary and beneficial. These can be summarised as:

- Surfacing and transcending what may be the practitioner's distorted self-understandings
- Asking ourselves difficult, often self-exposing questions
- Facing the difficult answers to such questions
- Keeping the practitioner's vision directed towards new possibilities for understanding and action.

Clare Wrote in her Assignment[i]

'For me one of the immense values of this course was that the process of reflection was guidance. Being in the reflective group helped me to remain focused and motivated me to continue on my journey. If my reflective journey had not have been guided, then I feel it may well have been more of a magical mystery tour'.

The Guide as Servant-leader

Guiding practitioners in formal guided reflection was integral to my role as clinical leader at Buford hospital. It enabled me to fulfil my perceived leadership role to enable practitioners to develop the reflective expertise towards realising the hospital's collective vision of holistic practice.

In reviewing theories of leadership, servant-leadership offered the most compelling image of the guide. It has the qualities of leading from behind, being of service, guiding people to 'not-know, creating community, having awareness, contextualization and foresight' [5].

These attributes can be summarised:

- The guide leads from behind in contrast with other leadership theories of leading from the front. This reflects that learning is primarily the practitioner's responsibility. However, they will need collaborative support to live this responsibility with a little push from time to time rather than be pulled along.
- The guide is of service to the practitioner to guide their learning and growth in ways that mirror the practitioner being of service (being available) to persons. Thus, there is synergy between the learning process and learning outcomes.
- The guide is like a wise ancient master. The Tao Te Ching [6, p. 65] noted:

  'The ancient masters didn't try to educate people but kindly taught them to not-know. When they think they know the answers people are difficult to guide'.

  Dewey noted [7, p. 151] that –

  'A person needs to see for themselves, and he can't see just by being told, although the right kind of telling may guide his seeing and thus help him see what he needs to see'.

- The guide creates a community of inquiry whereby guides and practitioners collaborate through dialogue towards common purpose both within guided reflection and outside within clinical practice.
- The guide has foresight to guide the practitioner beyond their own perception and horizons towards understanding and possibility.

  Saunders writes [8] –

  'The importance of a guide cannot be fully emphasized. Had I not had a guide when I went to Egypt I would have missed the translation of hieroglyphics and their meanings. In the same way, if I had not had a guide within this course I may have missed the significance of my insights. This does not mean I cannot continue with self-exploration, but as Boyd and Fales [9] discuss, guidance guides the practitioner towards openness and lateral thinking'.

- The guide can contextualise what the practitioner has said by feeding back – 'this is what I have heard'. It demonstrates the guide has listened, perceived and come to an understanding, perhaps the fundamental aspect of dialogue.
- The guide has awareness of self in guiding the practitioner.

Greenleaf notes [5, p. 41] –

> 'When one is aware, there is more than the usual alertness, more intense contact with the immediate situation, and more is stored away in the unconscious computer to produce intuitive insights in the future when needed. The cultivation of awareness gives one the basis for detachment, the ability to stand aside and see oneself in perspective in the context of one's own experience amid the ever present dangers, threats, and alarms'.

With awareness, the guide learns to become mindful of their own assumptions, values and the suchlike and its influence on the way they guide. Thus, guiding the practitioner's reflection is a continuous learning experience for the guide as they reflect on their experience of guiding. As previously noted, such awareness is a paramount condition for genuine dialogue. This point has widespread acceptance within collaborative human inquiry research theory [10] and feminist theory [11, 12]. Paget [12] recognised how the similarity between her own and her interviewees' life experiences influenced questions she asked and entered into her understanding and interpretation of the story being told. Paget points out her approach, which gave control of the interview process to the interviewee, establishing solidarity between them as they engaged in the shared task of trying to understand significant life experiences.

The External Enabler

In Kieffer's [13] study of empowerment of grass root community leaders in the USA, participants referred with great emotional intensity to the importance of the external enabler to support their struggle against more powerful others who were motivated to maintain the status quo (see Chapter 1). The guide connects with the practitioner as a representative of the wider community, the gatekeeper and guide to this new world. To do this, the guide must connect with the practitioner in terms of their existing reality and, simultaneously in terms of a potential new reality. Kieffer's framework for participatory competence as a framework for the development of empowerment was set out in Chapter 5.

As general manager of Buford I was the 'more powerful other'. However, I was working to shift the 'status quo' to a more collaborative community. As a non-line manager guide, I find I am exactly the 'external enabler' plotting with practitioners in their struggle to realise their visions of practice against the status quo (see below regarding the organisational position of the guide).

A Developmental Approach

Ralph [14] constructed a developmental approach that I adapted for guided reflection (Figure 8.1). It reflects a movement from dependence to independence of learning. The guide's initial response to the novice reflective practitioner is directive yet always directed to liberating the practitioner from dependence.

Journal Entry 8.1

Karen, an associate nurse at Burford, reflects on her supervision 'breakthrough' [15]

> 'Sessions 1–6 were very much led by my supervisor, but in session 7 we had a sudden breakthrough and I took control. From then on I felt I was growing through supervision – I remember telling my supervisor, that I felt like a seedling in spring which has felt the sun and is now growing big and strong into a tree. I knew how much I benefited, but I also knew how much energy it took and I often felt drained afterwards'.

> Stage 1
> Providing authoritative and definitive solutions and advice to the practitioner including the application of extant knowledge in response to presenting contradictions between a vision of holistic practice and its lived reality with a primary focus on development of self in relationship with both guide and persons.
>
> Guide as Catalyst
>
> Stage 2
> Providing a facilitative response to the practitioner's increasing awareness of both the utility and limitations of their feelings and actions – reflecting the practitioner's growth to continuously monitor themselves and recognising the centrality of themselves to the effective realisation of holistic practice within the therapeutic team.
>
> Guide as Catalyst
>
> Stage 3
> The practitioner reaches 'master level' characterised by personal autonomy, insightful awareness, personal security, stable motivation and an awareness of the need to confront any problems that interfere with realising holistic practice.

FIGURE 8.1   Adapted from Ralph's developmental milestones [15].

Karen's words reflect the effort it took to attune to guided reflection. Her learning patterns had not prepared her for such a learning experience. She also felt threatened that her lack of competence would be exposed and that she would be judged as a poor nurse. She was anxious to demonstrate her competence after qualifying with a nursing degree. As such, at the time when she most needed support, she resisted it because she wanted to show she was competent. An ironic twist, yet seemingly a common response from newly qualified practitioners [16]. As such, the initial sessions were very directive and supportive as a gradual easing into Karen taking responsibility for her learning. The guide must be patient. Learning through reflection takes time. It involves peeling away old layers of learning that have become embodied so new ways can take root and flourish.

The Guide as Catalyst

The guide is a catalyst to guide the practitioner to move through Ralph's adapted developmental stages. The experiences practitioners disclose in guided reflection have often been triggered by a sense of disturbance to normal patterns of practice for one reason or another resulting in discharging negative energy.

The guide, as a catalyst, enables the practitioner to convert this negative energy into positive energy for taking action based on insights. This catalytic response is illustrated in Figure 8.2. The single curly line represents the practitioner's undisturbed practice until it they experience a situation where normal thinking and responses fail resulting in anxiety or crisis. Through exploring the experience, negative energy is dissipated through understanding and new ways of responding explored for taking future action to resolve the crisis and emerge at a higher level of consciousness.

If negative energy is stuck, one un-sticking manoeuvre is to suggest that the practitioner imagines a rope extending into her body connected to these negative feelings. I ask her to imagine I am pulling out the negative energy from her body. Hand over hand I pull the imaginary rope until it pulls free. Such visualisation has proved effective.

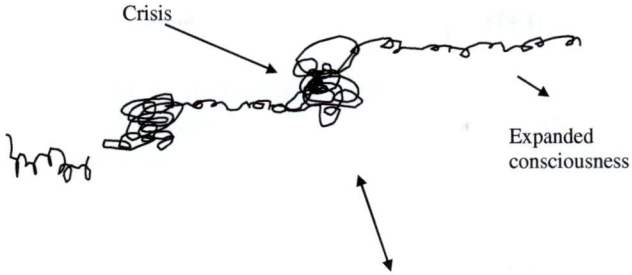

Crisis

Expanded
consciousness

Conversion of negative energy to positive energy

FIGURE 8.2 The guide as catalyst [17, p. 38].
Source: Adapted from [18].

Journal Entry 8.2

Kevin[ii] suggests the significance of converting his negative energy caused by a difficult practice situation (19, p. 142)

> 'I shared my dilemma with the guided reflection group. Waterworth [19] argues that such workshops allow nothing more than a forum for expressing negativity. In my experience this is not so. The session supported me and nurtured my creativity. So, Waterworth, stick that in your pipe! Of course Chris would argue, "Where is Waterworth coming from? What is the basis for her claim?" And it's true, I partially read stuff and draw hasty conclusions. Stick that in my pipe!'

Expanded consciousness reflects a fundamental shift in the practitioner, a new self-conception.

Fay [20, p. 265–6] writes –

> 'Coming to a radically new self-conception is hardly ever a process that occurs simply by reading some theoretical work; rather it requires an environment of trust and support in which one's own preconceptions and feeling can be properly made conscious to oneself, in which one can think through one's experiences in terms of a radically new vocabulary which expresses a fundamentally different conceptualisation of the world in which one can see the particular and concrete ways that one unwittingly collaborates in producing one's own misery and in which one can gain emotional strength to accept and act on one's new insights'.

Misery sounds an exaggeration, but I have met few practitioners who have been happy with 'their lot', especially under current working conditions of 'more for less' that has left them tired and demoralised. The guide may struggle with the trauma stories the practitioner reveals and it becomes an ethical issue to urge the practitioner to take action and then watch them stumble and fall against the hard edge of reality. The key is not to fix the problem for the practitioner but guide them to see ways they can fix it for themselves by generating new ideas and possibilities.

Margolis [21] considers that new ideas compete with existing ideas. The success of adopting new ideas depends on the robustness of existing ones and the force of argument available to support the new idea. Practitioners may feel anxious when their 'old ways' are exposed as contradictory with their vision of practice. They are caught between defending self from this anxiety and opening self to new possibilities. They may experience a crisis of isolation or separateness [22]. Isaacs [22, p. 38] notes –

> 'Such loosening of rigid thought patterns frees energy that now permits new levels of intelligence and creativity'.

Climbing Mountains

Practitioners may feel that learning through reflection is like 'climbing a mountain'. Undoubtedly, some practitioners will struggle with reflection.

Pirsig [23, p. 208] offers the practitioner some advice about climbing mountains akin to climbing towards one's vision in guided reflection –

> 'Mountains should be climbed with as little effort and without desire. The reality of your own nature should determine the speed. If you become restless, speed up. If you become winded slow down. You climb the mountain in an equilibrium of restlessness and exhaustion. Then, when you are no longer thinking ahead, each footstep isn't just a means to an end but a unique event in itself. This leaf has jagged edges. This rock looks loose. From this place the snow is less visible, even though closer. These things you should notice anyway. To live only for some future goal is shallow. It's the sides of the mountain which sustain life, not the top. Here's where things grow. But, of course, without the top you can't have any sides. It's the top that defines the sides'.

Hence, the focus of guided reflection is on the journey set against the visionary background. Each experience is a footstep paying attention to the detail. The pace of the journey cannot be determined in advance.

Communicative Competence

There are at least four key aspects of communicative competence the guide is aware of and seeks to develop both within themselves and with practitioners:

1. Dialogue
2. Six category intervention analysis
3. Development of voice
4. Asserting self

1. Dialogue

The mode of 'talk' in guided reflection is dialogue. Much of early work within guided reflection is learning to dialogue (see Chapter 2 for conditions for effective dialogue). The guide's role is to coach dialogical competence thus requiring the guide is dialogically competent.

Senge [24, p. 241] notes that

> 'In dialogue, individuals gain insights that simply could not be achieved individually. A new kind of mind begins to come into being which is based on the development of a common meaning ... people are no longer primarily in opposition, nor can they said to be interacting, rather they are participating in this pool of common meaning, which is capable of constant development and change'.

Dialogue will take time to develop and flow freely until both guide and practitioner find dialogical resonance. Through dialogue, mutual perceptions are explored towards co-constructing insights. The practitioner and guide have different roles and status that may inhibit the practitioner if they feel their performance is being directed or judged. Dialogue gets stuck when the power issue is not addressed. Hence, the guide actively works at deconstructing power so that dominant authority is left at the door. Trust develops through creating a community of inquiry to work collaboratively.

Hooks notes [25, p. 109] –

> 'Creating trust usually means finding out what it is we have in common as well as what separates us and makes us different'.

Hence, the learning space is also a social space where difference is open and respected. The guide knows that creating community is essential for, without it, practitioners will not feel secure and, as a consequence, be wary of what to reveal. It is perhaps the guide's most crucial task.

Senge writes [24, p. 246] –

> 'The facilitator always *walks a careful line* [my emphasis] between being knowledgeable and helpful to the process at hand, and yet taking on the "expert" or "doctor" mantle that would shift attention away from the members of the team, and their own ideas and responsibility. But in dialogue the facilitator also does something more. Their understanding of dialogue allows them to influence the flow of development simply through participating. For example, after someone has made an observation, the facilitator may say 'but the opposite may also be true?'

2. Six Category Intervention Analysis

Communicative competence is enhanced using intervention typology such as six-category intervention analysis [26] to structure dialogue and offer the practitioner a range of communicative interventions. Heron proposes six basic therapeutic interventions that can be either authoritative or facilitative.

Authoritative interventions are:

- Giving information – enabling the other to make a rational decision based on information
- Giving advice – helping the other see other, better ways of seeing and doing things
- Confrontation – challenging the other's restrictive attitudes, beliefs or behaviour

Facilitative interventions are:

- Being cathartic – enabling the other to express a difficult emotion so it can be resolved
- Being catalytic – enabling the other to talk through an issue
- Being supportive – communicating a sense of 'being there' for the other.

The guide chooses the most appropriate intervention to respond to the practitioner, being able to move easily between the interventions. These interventions can be manipulative or perverse when the person uses the interventions to meet their own needs or agenda.

The guide can make the use of the interventions explicit, to make them available for the practitioner to use in their clinical practice (what I term 'parallel process framing' – see Figure 5.2). In particular, confrontation, being cathartic, and being catalytic have been shown to be difficult for practitioners to use and hence tend to be avoided and yet are vital interventions for the practitioner to develop [27].

The guide's use of interventions often follows a pattern:

1. When an underlying emotion is sensed – the guide will use a cathartic response – 'you seem angry at your manager?' The intention is to surface and release the underlying emotion so it can be dealt with. At this level practitioners may fear releasing the emotion because they do not know how to respond to it.
2. Having released the emotion, the guide uses a catalytic response to help the person talk through the issue with the intention of helping them find meaning in their feelings, and through talking through it, to understand deeper underlying reasons and assumptions for these feelings. In this way, the supervisee is helped to convert the released negative energy into positive energy for taking action.
3. Confrontation can then be used to challenge, yet always within a supportive framework. Confrontation is a subtle rather than direct intervention – for example – 'Can you see other ways of responding?' implicitly suggesting that the practitioner's response was not effective, yet without direct judgment.

4. Information is useful to inform the situation. I am always wary of giving advice because it is taking responsibility for the other person. Much better to say 'What options do you have' rather than 'I would do it like this', even for novice practitioners who seek direction. In giving advice, the guide draw the practitioner's attention to the fact – 'I am going to give you some advice for you to consider'.

3. Developing Voice

Competent communication requires the practitioner to be able to voice their thoughts, feelings and opinions. The practitioner may write in their journal something like 'I wish I has said something but …' Writing thus opens the voice if just on paper. It begs the questions 'What did I want to say?' and 'Why didn't I say it?'

Being unable to voice self is an impoverished state of being. It easy away at self undermining the practitioner's confidence and self-esteem. It is a state of fear. As Audre Lorde [28, p. 21] evocatively shares –

In the cause of silence, each one of us draws the face of their own fear – fear of contempt, of censure, or some judgment, or recognition, of challenge, of annihilation. But most of all, I think we fear the very visibility without which we also cannot truly live.

Sharing their story in guided reflection gives voice to the practitioner's experience, a voice that may have been rendered silent through patterns of relationships with more powerful groups [29].

Through dialogue, the practitioner develops and strengthens their voice, giving vent to opinions and ideas. It is empowering especially when the voice has previously been dominated by silence when the practitioner had no voice or when the practitioner speaks solely through the authoritative received words of others.

Belenky et al. [30, p. 134] term this voicing the 'subjective voice'. It is a quest for self towards reclaiming self'. Its learning mode is one of inward listening and watching, valuing, and accepting one's own voice as a source of knowing. They note [30, p. 85] –

'Subjective knowing is the precursor to reflective and critical thought. During the period of subjective knowing, women lay down procedures for systematically learning and analysing experience. But what seems distinctive in these women is that their strategies for knowing grow out of their very embeddedness in human relationships and the alertness of everyday life'.

Practitioners begin to question received knowledge, no longer accepting on face value what they have been told as to their thoughts, beliefs and actions. As one of Belenky et al.'s respondents noted [30, p. 85] –

'I keep discovering things inside myself. I am seeing myself all the time in a different light'.

Such words reflect an awakening of self. Life suddenly becomes interesting with the focus on the self. Such practitioners are curious and open to new experiences. Subjectivist women value what they see and hear around them and begin to feel a need to understand the people with whom they live and who impinge on their lives. Though they maybe emotionally isolated from others at this point in their histories, they begin to actively analyse their past and current interactions with others.

The idea that practitioners might be isolated is intriguing. Does the received voice mode of being deny expression of opinion and feelings, and hence isolate the practitioner from others? My experience of guiding practitioners gives this notion substance. However, the subjective voice is tentative, vulnerable in its uncertainty and hence benefits from guidance in a community of like-minded people such as guided reflection. It may be confusing because it is competing with received voices. As such, it is easy to discount one's own subjective voice as being unsubstantiated, even ridiculed by more 'knowing' others. Listening to yourself it may seem to be an uncanny stranger on display [31].

Connected knowing		Separate knowing
is gained by listening and understanding to the experiences of others known through empathy and reflection	Synthesis V	is gained through critiquing extant sources of knowledge for its validity to inform.
The constructed voice		

FIGURE 8.3 The procedural voice.

Guided reflection is thus a sound box reverberating the practitioner's voice back to the practitioner so they can hear themselves clearly. The practitioner refines her subjective voice through dialogue towards developing firstly, a 'procedural' voice and subsequently, a 'constructed' voice.

The procedural voice has two divergent ways of knowing: connected and separate knowing (Figure 8.3)

In Chapter 22, Helen Hardy illustrates the significance of both connected and separate knowing. Yet it is connected, knowing that sets the context for critiquing and juxtaposing separate knowing. Separate knowing stems from the left side of the brain that fosters rational logical thinking, whereas connected knowing stems from the right brain that fosters creativity, imagination, perception, curiosity, intuition, spirit and wholeness.

The Constructed Voice

The constructed voice is the synthesis between the connected and separate voices. It is a fusion between the left and right side of the brain so that the mind is fully fertilised and uses all its faculties [32]. Practitioners with constructed voice speak with an informed and authentic voice. They are able to think and voice outside normal frames of reference, shifting previously abstract frames into personal frames. Through developing the constructed voice, the practitioner puts extant sources of knowledge in its place, no longer succumbing, as Visinstainer [33, p. 37] notes, to

> 'The belief that the 'soft stuff' such as feelings and beliefs and support, are not quite as substantive as the hard data from laboratory reports and sophisticated monitoring'.

Thus, the reflective practitioner seeks to develop the constructed voice as the voice necessary to become a reflective practitioner towards realising one's vision of practice. However, developing a constructed voice does not mean it is heard or listened to by those who claim authority to make decisions.

As Belenky et al. [30, p. 146] note with a salutary voice –

> 'Even among women who feel they have found their voice, problems with voice abound. Some women told us, in anger and frustration, how frequently they felt unheard and unheeded. In our society, which values the word of male authority, constructivist women are no more immune to the feeling of being silenced than any other group of women'.

As such, the development of an assertive voice is a vital aspect of becoming a reflective practitioner, as reflected in many of the book's narratives.

4. Asserting Self

I noted the significance of communicative competence in asserting self in Chapter 4. This is linked with the development of voice. The guide is assertive, and in being assertive, role models assertiveness in developing the practitioner's ability to be assertive towards ensuring their vision of practice is not compromised.

Balancing High Challenge with High Support

Guidance is the balance between high challenge and high support, enabling the guide to challenge any aspect of the practitioner's experience yet be sensitive and supportive of the impact of the challenge on the practitioner. This is achieved by the guide being mindful of creating an environment of trust by communicating from the outset a real sense of genuineness and positive regard towards the practitioner so that the practitioner feels positive given the potential threat of revealing oneself [34]. With trust, the practitioner welcomes high challenge because they know that the guide has their best interests at heart. As such, high challenge does not threaten them. In fact, they learn to welcome it.

Journal Entry 8.3

Lisa noted 'I felt that being challenged is an essential element of guidance, providing you feel comfortable in your environment and at ease with your guide. The challenge element encouraged me to think further than I had been and to deal with issues in a way I would not have considered before'.

Being challenged can create anxiety. Deeper parts of self may become exposed making the practitioner feel vulnerable. The guide, mindful of this potential anxiety, seeks to become part of the practitioner's defence system as if a holding hand across the indeterminate swampy lowlands of everyday practice [35]. It informs the practitioner that they are not alone.

The Challenge/Support Grid

The balance of challenge and support can be visualised and monitored using the challenge/support grid (Figure 8.4). Ideally, the practitioner would score their guide 10/10 for both challenge and support. Perfect balance. This is the optimum learning environment for the guide to strive realising. If the guide is more challenging than supportive, it is likely to create anxiety for the practitioner and a sense of losing control. This imbalance tends to occur if the guide becomes anxious about the practitioner's response. High challenge and low support undermine trust the practitioner may have for the guide and make the practitioner wary of further disclosure.

Bolman and Deal [3, p. 76] note –

'When you push someone to become what she's already becoming, you get in the way. You become a meddler'.

Condition of low challenge/high support reflects the guide's reluctance or commitment to be critical of the practitioner to avoid any practitioner discomfort. As such, the guide adopts a maternal mode that can make the practitioner feel like a child.

Bohm [36, p. 13/18] notes –

'If five or six people get together, they can usually adjust to each other so they don't say things that upset each other – they get a "cozy adjustment" ... 'when a dialogue group is new, in general people tend to talk around the point for a while. In all human relations nowadays, people talk around things, avoiding the difficulties'.

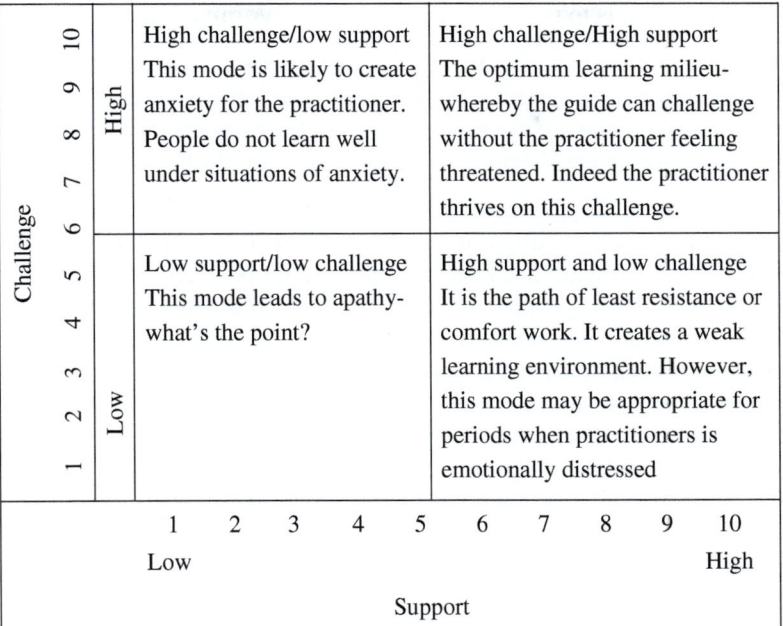

FIGURE 8.4 Challenge-support axis.

Group Versus Individual Guided Reflection

Guided reflection can be with an individual practitioner or in groups both within clinical practice or educational curriculum. Groups can be single discipline or multi-disciplinary.

Peer Support

Group guided reflection offers peer support. It can feel very supportive to be in the same boat as others who can connect with the practitioner's experiences with similar experiences. It creates a sense of 'not being alone'. However, it may not be easy to disclose oneself to others, mindful of their judgement.

Kevin noted [37, p. 2013] –

> 'I write in my journal, "They, the family, don't give a damn about Mary, they are fleecing her blind. I need to be more assertive and shed my fear of conflict". Reading this out in guided reflection, I feel embarrassed as if I am some kind of failure. The punk rocker brought to his knees. Exposed as a fraud. Yet the group are amazingly supportive. They all recognise the conflict avoider in themselves'.

Wheatley and Kellner-Roberts [38, p. 53] write –

> 'When we link up with others, we open ourselves to yet another paradox. While surrendering some of our freedom, we open ourselves to even more creative forms of expression. This stage of being has been described as communion, because we are preserved as ourselves but are shorn of our sep- arateness or aloneness. What we bring to others remains our self-expression. Yet the meaning of who we are changes through our communion with them. We are identifiable as our selves. But we have discovered new meaning and different contributions, and we are no longer the same'.

Wheatley and Keller-Rogers use the word 'communion' – resonating with the idea that group guided reflection is a community of inquiry.

Brookfield [39, p. 36] adds to the significance of being within a group

> 'Just knowing that we are not alone in our struggles is profoundly reassuring. Although critical reflection often begins alone, it is ultimately a collective endeavour. We need colleagues to help us know what our assumptions are and help us to change the structures of power so that democratic actions and values are rewarded, both within and outside our institutions'.

In groups, peers can challenge and support each other offering multiple perspectives for each other to consider thus enriching the inquiry and learning. It opens the guided reflection space as an opportunity for team learning. It enables a more overt realignment of authority within the group even though people with different positions within the hierarchy may constitute the group. It cannot be assumed that collaboration will exist, at least at first until any power issues are worked through. However, some practitioners may prefer individual guidance, because it has a greater focus on themselves with less worry about performing in a group or anxious about self-disclosure.

Rotating the role of 'guide' in groups reinforces the individual's responsibility for the group's functioning and enables individuals to develop guidance skills. If a 'peer' did impose authority on another 'peer', the guide and other peers in accordance with the group's contract will challenge the offending 'peer'.

Pragmatics

Establishing group guided reflection in clinical practice can be fraught with pragmatic difficulty. For example, who should be in the group and managing time for the group to meet, especially if the group takes place within normal hours of clinical practice when guided reflection time, no matter if allocated, becomes a victim of the exigencies of the clinical moment. One contentious solution would be to suggest that guided reflection takes place outside clinical hours. I do not think this unreasonable in terms of professional responsibility to be 'fit for practice' and CPD fulfilment. In my experience, practitioners committed to their learning easily accept 'out of shift' time for guided reflection. Resistance to this idea may stem from a traditional 'shift culture' of doing work and domestic arrangements. Despite the potential difficulties of forming group guided reflection, it does foster collaborative teamwork, shared vision, team learning, mutual support, role responsibility and quality; all advantages over individual guided reflection.

Group Dynamics

Within group guided reflection, the guide invites the practitioner to share their experience before opening it up to peers. I term this as 'opening up the space'. This then enables peers to link the shared experience with their own thoughts and experiences and draw their own insights. Dialogue around practitioners' perceptions of each other's experiences have been shown to have the potential 'to improve observational and communication skills, teaching practitioners to speak out in safe ways which may mitigate errors in patient care [40, p. 754].

The astute guide is always checking out the pattern of dialogue within the group to ensure voices are heard and issues adequately talked through. The guide is mindful of peers who are silent to draw them into the dialogue. Sharing clinical experiences that for whatever reason has compromised patient health are often difficult for the practitioner to voice and yet the practitioner is anxious to share as if carrying a burden [41]. The guide can literally ask – 'is there a situation you need to share?'

Game Playing

The guide is sensitive to the unfolding dynamics of the guided reflection relationship and able to surface and resolve any tension or game playing. Some practitioners and guides may not feel safe or comfortable in guided reflection and resort to game playing as a defence against the anxiety that revealing self might create [42]. For example, practitioners may be reluctant to be critical of peers due to a collusive strategy to make the dialogue space safe so they can avoid criticism when telling their own stories. The guide is mindful not to fall into 'the expert trap' of the all-knowing guru that the group wants to learn from. Games disrupt learning with their emphasis on playing the game. Games are minimised when the guidance process is constantly monitored. Practitioners can be informed about the nature and extent of game-playing [43] so it becomes the whole group's responsibility to tackle towards ensuring the learning process is not compromised. In a similar vein, Hawthorne [44, p. 179] revealed games that guide play to construct a 'comfortable and effective guide identity'. As with all ideas, there is a potential shadow aside to guidance.

Guidance Traps

- The guide responds to the practitioner(s) in ways that reflect organisational normal patterns of relating, reinforcing authority and hierarchy, which has no place in dialogue [37].
- The guide responds to 'fix it' the practitioner rather than enabling the practitioner to resolve her own contradictions. This is more likely when the guide views their own success as entangled with that of the practitioner or sees self as expert leading to attachment to ideas that curs down possibility. It can lead to a prescriptive/directive approach rather than a facilitative one.
- The guide manipulates the practitioner to adopt their own values and dominant perspectives. This can lead to 'moulding' whereby the guide 'shapes' the practitioner into an image of him or herself.
- The guide is anxious about the practitioner's revelations leading to inappropriate critical and nurturing parent pattern of response that breakdown the possibility of dialogue. This inevitably leads to thin trust and the practitioner's wariness of what to disclose.
- The guide is anxious of their own limitations to guide the practitioner's self-inquiry and transformation, especially when they lack experience of constructing their own narratives of self-inquiry. In response, the guide may 'hide' behind a theoretical approach that denies the creative nature of dialogue.

Considering these 'traps', the practitioner must feel empowered to challenge the guide, no matter its benevolent intent, and resist the intrinsic threat of the guide imposing an agenda and dominant meanings.

The Guide's Organisational Position

Appreciating the shadow side of guidance draws attention to the guide's position in relation to the practitioner. This is more complex in the clinical situation than in an educational setting where the guide is usually the teacher (see Chapter 14).

Within the clinical setting, a number of guide positions are possible:

- line managed
- non-line managed within the organisation
- non-line managed from outside the organisation

Analysing patterns of guidance dialogue, revealed that the shadow side of guidance (as noted above) are more likely with line management guidance due to the transactional culture of the health care organisation. This is evident in Ruth's comment where she is supervising a colleague in her role as hospital manager.

Ruth[iii] writes [45]

'Reflective writing brings everyday experiences into focus enabling the journal to act as a midwife, giving birth to new understanding [46]. My own experience has consistently proved the value of this. Regardless of the brevity of time allowed, I find the process of journaling consistently enlightening. My writing tends to take place during unplanned quiet moments at home and I am frequently amazed by the insights that just a few moments of focused reflection can achieve. Today I wrote briefly about a clinical supervision session with Ellen in which I was acting as supervisor, triggered by a distant feeling of unease'.

> 'May 2005 – Ellen spoke of the difficulties she was having with another member of staff. Initially I thought this was a helpful session but now as I look back I recognize how I took over the conversation and led the conclusions. The unhealthy relationship she described did not surprise me as its effects are obvious and causing problems for other members of staff. I can see that my strong (and rather irritated) feelings on the subject led me to give solutions rather than allow Ellen to consider her own. My responses echo back at me sounding managerial and uncompromising ...'

These insights surprised me because since I had not recognised them earlier. Ellen had been tearful during the session causing me some disquiet but that had been erased by the business of the rest of the day. Through writing reflectively on this event, my future ways of responding are challenged and changed. The possibility of journal writing is to write freely and without censure.

Ruth reveals the contradiction between her response to Ellen and her aspiration towards transformational leadership. It shows how managers can easily manipulate guidance in response to their own feelings and agenda. She also reveals the transformative significance of journaling and reflection.

In establishing guided reflection at Burford hospital, I was the line-manager guide.

At the time this did not seem a disadvantage. It wasn't until I guided practitioners as a non-line manger that I realised that a common shared topic was conflict with the manager/ organisation. Reviewing guided reflection dialogue, I further realised that practitioners at Buford had not shared experiences that concerned myself, illuminating that even with collaborative intent, practitioners viewed me with caution. Why was that? I suggest it reflects a natural suspicion of management due to practitioners being socialised into subordinate type relationships that have been embodied and not easily overthrown. Rather like the traditional image of supervision as someone looking over your shoulder ensuring you work competently. A sense of being supervised is inherently threatening, asking the practitioner to reveal their practice for scrutiny no matter the supervisor's good intention.

However, the advantages of line-managed guidance are compelling when the guide has the right transformational attitude (adapted from [47])

- The guide and practitioner share a collective vision and thus work collaboratively towards realising this vision as a lived reality.
- The guide knows the practitioner's practice and therefore has a better understanding of issues the practitioner reveals so they can be tackled together;
- Guidance talk spills over into everyday practice, facilitating collaborative ways of relating within practice.
- The guide acknowledges and values the practitioner by giving positive feedback and support so that the practitioner feels the guide's concern, boosting morale and melting stress.
- The guide actively develops and fulfils their leadership role in enabling the practitioner.

Managers may resist the ideal of guided reflection because it facilitates practitioners having a voice and developing responsibility. This may threaten line managers' sense of authority and control of the clinical area. Thus, the line manager may adopt an authoritative approach using guided reflection as a means of control, which is one reason why I avoid using the term 'clinical supervision' in clinical practice because of this legacy whereby one person (the guide/supervisor) stands over another person (the practitioner) to ensure the practitioner is competent (competence being defined by the guide/supervisor).

Weighing up the advantages and disadvantages, I advocate for line-managed guided reflection because it offers a significant role of clinical leadership to enable practitioners towards realising a vision of practice. This ideally requires motivated leaders to be engaged in supportive group-guided reflection linked to the organisation's vision of realising person-centred practice. This requires an enlightened organisational approach, even to the extent of the executive board having guided reflection. However, leadership is a rare commodity, and left to their own devices managers will tend to guide as they manage, even when they undertake guidance education, due to embodied ways of responding within transactional organisations. Often clinical areas do not have a vision and hence are not vision-driven but locked into a task approach to get through the work with limited resources. Then time to accommodate guided reflection becomes an issue, another task to do adding to stress – 'how can we fit it in?'

The non-line manager within or outside the organisation is less likely to respond personally to the practitioner's experience and thus be more objective (see Chapter 13 as exemplars of the non-line guide within the organisation). However, this type of relationship might make the practitioner's line manager anxious about what takes place within the guided reflection relationship and deprive the manager the opportunity to develop their leadership role as a guide.

The availability and potential resource cost of non-line managers is another factor to consider, especially when guided reflection has no or minimal organisational budget. Ideally, practitioners would choose their guides. Yet the organisational complexity of enabling that would be difficult and reasons for choice questionable. Put another way, if guides were skilled, it wouldn't matter who the guide was. Every guided reflection relationship must inevitably work through teething issues to develop genuine collaborative relationships.

Intent and Emphasis

Depending on the intent and emphasis of the guide, guided reflection can be a very different experience for the practitioner. In Figure 8.5, the terms 'emancipatory' and 'technical' represent two specific types of knowledge constituted interests [48]. Emancipatory knowledge intends to liberate people to fulfil their vision of practice, whereas technical knowledge intends to shape practitioners towards performing competently. Habermas [48] terms dialogue as *communicative* knowledge that mediates between the emancipatory and technical perspectives. In practice, the guide may emphasise either the emancipatory or technical. Indeed, the practitioner may prefer the guide to hold a more technical attitude because it is more objective with a focus on problem solving. The tension between the emancipatory and technical resonates with developing the procedural voice (as noted previously in this chapter) whereby the technical informs the emancipatory. From this perspective, both the guide and practitioner(s) necessarily hold emancipatory intent.

Working within transactional organisations does not prepare either the guide or practitioner for their respective roles within guided reflection. This inevitably requires a realignment of transactional authority relationships no matter the setting. However, in reality, people simply cannot just become different. It needs an active working towards.

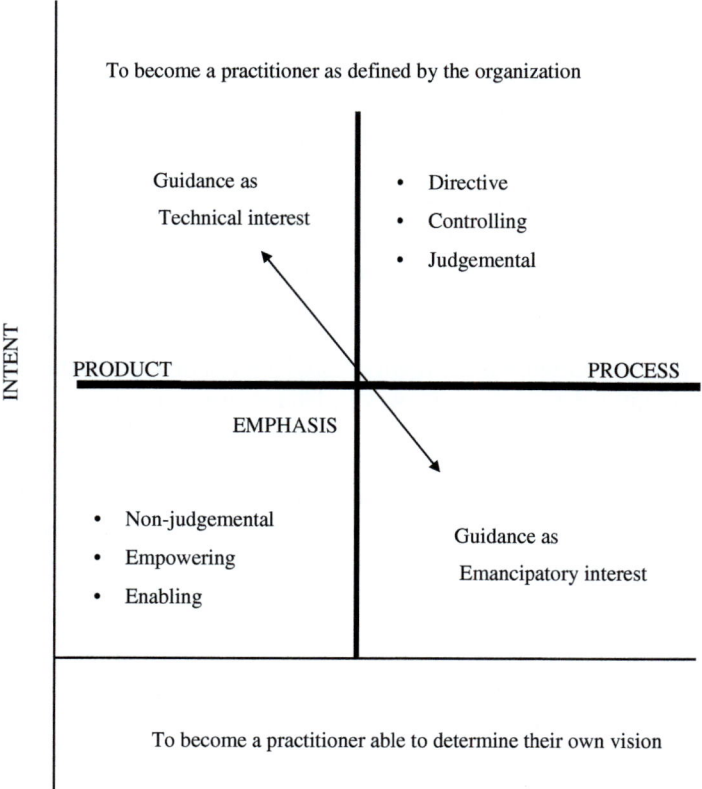

To become a practitioner as defined by the organization

Guidance as
Technical interest

- Directive
- Controlling
- Judgemental

INTENT

PRODUCT   PROCESS

EMPHASIS

- Non-judgemental
- Empowering
- Enabling

Guidance as
Emancipatory interest

To become a practitioner able to determine their own vision

FIGURE 8.5 The intent-emphasis scale.
Source: [49]/John Wiley & Sons.

Voluntary or Mandatory Guided Reflection

It was mandatory at Buford hospital for practitioners to engage in guided reflection. All new practitioners agreed to this within their contract. This reflects a leadership attitude that 'guided reflection is of significant benefit' as indeed it was proven, having been piloted over the previous 18 months with a staff nurse volunteer[iv] [50].

Guided reflection was first established at Buford Hospital in 1989, four years before the clinical supervision agenda emerged for general nursing. Clinical supervision was promoted as a professional activity rather than a managerial activity in response to increasing nursing's accountability to offset public concern. Yet clinical supervision is generally implemented as a top-down organisational approach with very little resource attached to it. From this perspective, it was perhaps inevitable that supervision became the responsibility of unit leaders to implement, leading to a managerial approach despite its 'professional' rhetoric. A mandatory approach would require significant resourcing in terms of development and sustainment. Guided reflection within clinical practice requires time out from practice itself. In the fast pace of clinical practice, time is a premium and costs money. Hence, it must be viewed as an effective legitimate staff development and support system.

Voluntary arrangements may exist both within or outside normal work hours as a reflection of professional commitment and professional patterns of working, especially when such arrangements are peer-led breaking out of a 'shift bound' transactional and subordinate culture. However, it is likely that practitioners would be reluctant to use their 'own time' where guided reflection is viewed as yet another task to be undertaken by staff already under work load pressure. Practitioners are likely to view mandatory guided reflection as a form of social control and surveillance [51, 52] and therefore resist it rather than see it as a developmental opportunity. Practitioners are more likely to be committed to their development when they choose to engage. However, a voluntary arrangement may only attract practitioners already committed to their professional development. However, NMC registration demand from 2016 may shift this perspective whereby practitioners come to view guided reflection as an opportunity to meet NMC requirements and therefore, more likely to respond to opportunities such as guided reflection, although I imagine such people will see reflection as a necessary evil and merely conform by doing the least amount of work required. In other words, it becomes just another but necessary task to fulfil.

In the narrative 'Passing people by' (Chapter 10), I took my experience to guided reflection. The group was a voluntary group open to all staff within the hospice although few attended. Indeed, those who did attend were regular. Usually six: one therapist, three nurses, a new young doctor and the senior physiotherapist. The group took it in turns to share experiences and rotated the guide.

I discussed reasons with other hospice staff about their non-attendance. A number of excuses were offered:

'I'm too busy!'
'I don't believe it will help my practice'.
'I don't like sharing myself within groups'.
'I talk with others if I have any problems'.
'I never liked reflective practice as a student nurse'.
'Navel gazing!'

Those practitioners who did attend seem more committed, more caring than others, as if they take their practice seriously and welcome the learning opportunity.

I asked staff who did attend why they attend. Some responses were:

'It's good to talk over issues with colleagues. It creates a sense of community that spills over into practice itself'.
'I realise that what bothers me is shared by others'. 'It helps me deal with any conflicts I have'.
'I have learnt a lot about ethics and ways of talking with patients'.
'It's good professional practice'.
'Rotating the group's guide facilitates guidance skills. That's useful because it actually teaches me to listen and weigh up options that I can transfer to my clinical practice'.

Spill Over into Practice

As I noted, an advantage of line-managed guided reflection is the 'spill over' into everyday clinical practice resulting in a more collaborative and dialogical approach to communication resulting in informal guided reflection whereby issues are dealt with more immediately creating a dynamic learning practice environment whereby guided reflection is built into the practice fabric.

Developing Guides

When I introduced guided reflection at Buford hospital, I had no specific preparation for this role. It was intuitive common sense 'tell me your story'. It matched the practitioner's approach to the patient within the Buford model – 'tell me your story' in getting to know the person and developing relationship. Through analysing patterns of recorded dialogue, I constructed guidance theory not in any authoritative sense but as guidance.

The most effective, pragmatic and economical way to develop guides is through being guided, notably in groups, whereby the processes of guidance are learnt. As I explore in Chapter 14, this is an explicit aim of the reflective curriculum so student nurses emerge from their undergraduate programme as competent guides.

One approach to developing guidance for post-registration practitioners is to undertake a bespoke programme like the 'Becoming a guided reflection guide' programme as outlined in Chapter 14.

A more direct programme I constructed at the University comprised a double module spanning one academic semester that met for one afternoon or morning (16 practitioners split into two groups of 8) every week over 12 sessions. Two sessions were devoted to introduction and evaluation/group dynamics. Alongside the classroom activity, each student was required to contract guided reflection with one person from their work setting to meet for an hour every two weeks.

Each session was divided into three exercises:

	Exercise	Time (mins)
1	Group supervision led by the group guide whereby practitioner students share work experiences.	60
	The group had an evaluation sheet (Figure 8.5) to evaluate and dialogue my performance. After four sessions, I invited group members to guide shadowed by myself.	
2	Break into triads rotating roles of practitioner/guide/observer (including tea). The observer feedback using observer sheet (Figure 8.6).	90
3	Plenary of exercise 2 and debrief from work-guided reflection relationship (as set out below).	30

As a formal academic course,[v] practitioners were required to present two assignments:

1. Reflection on being guided either within the group or in their triads
2. Reflection on guiding their contracted practitioner in the work setting

1	Guide is non-judgmental
2	Good balance of high challenge and high support
3	Guide introduces appropriate extant sources of information to help the practitioner frame issues and insights
4	Guide addresses Model for structured reflection cues
5	Guide checks practitioner has prepared for the session (as contract)
6	Guide prompts practitioner to consider cues for anticipatory reflection
7	Guide responds with appropriate interventions (after Heron)
8	Guide listens and picks up cues appropriately
9	Guide effectively wraps up session by checking how practitioner is now feeling
10	Guide wraps up session by asking the practitioner to summarise learning and action to take as a consequence (pick up next session)

FIGURE 8.6 Observer check list.

Summary

In this chapter, I have set out the significance of guided reflection. In the next chapter, I set out the process of guidance.

References

1. Flemons, D., Green, S. (2002) Stories that conform/ stories that transform: a conversation in four parts. In A. Bochner, C. Ellis [Eds.] *Ethnographically Speaking: Autoethnography, Literature and Aesthetics*. AltaMira Press, Walnut Creek, 87–94.

2. Boud, D., Keogh, R., Walker, D. (1985) Promoting reflection in learning: a model. In D. Boud, R. Keogh, R. D. Walker [Eds.] *Reflection: Turning Experience Into Learning*. Kogan Page, London.

3. Bolman, L. G., Deal, T. E. (2001) *Leading With Soul*. Jossey-Bass, San Francisco.

4. Cox, H., Hickson, P., Taylor, B. (1991) Exploring reflection: knowing and constructing practice. In G. Gray, R. Pratt [Eds.] *Towards A Discipline of Nursing*. Churchill Livingstone, Melbourne, 373–390.

5. Greenleaf, R. (1977/2002) *Servant Leadership: A Journey Into the Nature of Legitimate Power and Greatness*. Paulist Press, New York.

6. Tzu, L. (1999) *Tao Te Ching: An Illustrated Journey*. (Trns. S. Mitchell). Frances Lincoln, London.

7. Dewey, J. (1933) *How We Think*. J. C. Heath, Boston.

8. Saunders, A. (2006) *Transforming Self Through Transformational Leadership*. Unpublished MSc Leadership in Healthcare, University of Bedfordshire.

9. Boyd, E., Fales, A. (1983) Reflective learning: key to learning from experience. *Journal of Humanistic Psychology* 23(2), 99–117.

10. Heron, J. (1981) Philosophical basis for a new paradigm. In P. Reason, J. Rowan [Eds.] *Human Inquiry: A Sourcebook of New Paradigm Research*. John Wiley & Sons, Chichester, 19–36.

11. Acker, J., Barry, K., Esseveld, J. (1983) Objectivity and truth: problems in doing feminist research. *Women Studies International Forum* 6, 423–435.

12. Paget, M. (1983) Experience and knowledge. *Human Studies* 6, 67–90.

13. Kieffer, C. (1984) Citizen empowerment: a developmental perspective. *Prevention in Human Services* 84(3), 9–36.

14. Ralph, N. B. (1980) Learning psychotherapy: a developmental perspective. *Psychiatry* 43, 243–250.

15. Johns, C. (1998) Becoming a reflective practitioner through guided reflection. *PhD thesis*. The Open University, Milton Keynes.

16. Cherniss, G. (1980) *Professional Burnout in Human Service Organizations*. Praeger, New York.

17. Newman, M. (1994) *Health as Expanding Consciousness* (second edition). National League for Nursing.

18. Prigogine, I., Stengers, L. (1984) *Order Out of Chaos*. Bantam Books, New York.

19. Waterworth, D. (1995) Exploring the value of clinical nursing practice: the practitioner's perspective. *Journal of Advanced Nursing* 22, 3–7.

20. Fay, B. (1987) *Critical Social Science: Liberation and Its Limits*. Polity Press, Cambridge.

21. Margolis, H. (1993) *Paradigm and Barriers: How Habits of Mind Govern Scientific Beliefs*. University of Chicago Press, Chicago.

22. Issacs, W. (1993) *Taking Flight: Dialogue, Collective Thinking, and Organizational Learning*. Centre for Organizational learning's Dialogue project. MIT, Boston.

23. Pirsig, R. (1989) *Zen and Art of Motorcycle Maintenance*. Vintage, London.

24. Senge, P. (1990) *The Fifth Discipline: The Art & Practice of the Learning Organization*. Century Business. London.

25. Hooks, B. (1994) *Teaching to Transgress: Education as the Practice of Freedom*. Routledge, New York.

26. Heron, J. (1975) *Six-category Intervention Analysis*. Human Potential Resource Group, University of Surrey, Guildford.

27. Burnard, P., Morrison, P. (1991) *Nurses' Interpersonal Skills: A Study of Nurses' Perceptions*. Nurse Education Today 1, 24–29.

28. Lorde, A. (1980) *The Cancer Journals*. Spinsters, Ink, Argyle, New York.

29. Buckingham, J., McGrath, G. (1983) *The Social Reality of Nursing*. Adis, Sydney.

30. Belenky, M. F., Clinchy, B. M., Goldberger, N. R., Tarule J. M. (1986) *Women's Ways of Knowing: The*

Development of Self, Voice, and Mind. Basic Books, New York.

31. Cixous, H., Clément, C. (1996) *The Newly Born Woman*. I B Taurus Publishers, London.

32. Woolf, V. (1945) *A Room of One's Own*. Penguin Books, London.

33. Visinstainer, M. (1987) The nature of knowledge and theory in nursing. *Image: The Journal of Nursing Scholarship*, 18, 32–38.

34. Borders, L., Leddick, G. (1987) *Handbook of Counseling Supervision*. The American Association for Counseling and Supervision, Virginia.

35. Schön, D. (1987) *Educating the Reflective Practitioner*. Jossey-Bass, San Francisco.

36. Bohm, D. (1996) In L. Nichol [Ed.] *On Dialogue*. Routledge, London.

37. Johns, C. (2013) *Becoming A Reflective Practitioner* (fourth edition). Wiley-Blackwell, Oxford.

38. Wheatley, M. J., Kellner-Rogers, M. (1999) *A Simpler Way*. Berrett-Koehler Publishers, San Francisco.

39. Brookfield, S. (1995) *Becoming A Critically Reflective Teacher*. Josey-Bass, San Francisco.

40. Moorman, M. (2015) The meaning of visual thinking strategies for nursing students. *Humanities* 4, 748–759.

41. Bradbury-Jones, C., Sambrook, S., Irvine, F. (2011) Nursing students and the issue of voice: a qualitative study. *Nurse Education Today* 31, 628–632.

42. Berne, E. (1961) Transactional analysis in psychotherapy. *The Classic Guide to Its Principles*. Grove Press, New York.

43. Kadushin, A. (1968) Games people play in supervision. *Social Work* 23–32.

44. Hawthorne, L. (1975) Games supervisors play. *Social Work* 179–183.

45. Morgan, R. (2005) *Realising Transformational Leadership*. Unpublished MSc leadership in Healthcare Dissertation. University of Bedfordshire.

46. Pinar, W. (1981) 'Whole, bright, deep with understanding': issues in qualitative research and autobiographical method. *Journal of Curriculum Studies* 13(3), 173–188.

47. Johns, C., McCormack, B. (1998) Unfolding the conditions where the transformative potential of guided reflection (clinical supervision) might flourish or flounder. In C. Johns, D. Freshwater [Eds.] *Transforming Nursing Through Reflective Practice*. Blackwell Publishing, Oxford, 62–77.

48. Habermas, J. (1984) *Theory of Communicative Action*. Vol. 1: *Reason and the Rationalisation of Society*. Beacon Press, Boston, and Basil Blackwell, Oxford, in association with Polity Press, Cambridge.

49. Johns, C. (2001) Depending on the intent and emphasis of the supervisor, clinical supervision can be a different experience. *Journal of Nursing Management* 9, 139–145.

50. Johns, C. (2024) A system for enabling practitioners to realise holistic practice. In C. Johns [Ed.] *Holistic Practice in Health Care: The Buford NDU Person-centred Model*. Wiley Blackwell, 65–80.

51. Gilbert, T. (2001) Reflective practice and clinical supervision: meticulous rituals of the confessional. *Journal of Advanced Nursing* 36, 199–205.

52. Cotton, A. (2001) Private thoughts in public sphere: issues in reflection and reflective practices in nursing. *Journal of Advanced Nursing* 36, 512–519.

53. Johns, C. (1998) *Becoming An Effective Practitioner through Guided Reflection*. Unpublished PhD thesis. The Open University, Milton Keynes.

Notes

i. Clare wrote these words within her final assignment 'Life begins at 40' undertaking the 'Becoming a reflective and effective practitioner' course at the University of Bedfordshire. The course is outlined in Chapter 14. Her narrative is shown in Chapter 18 as an exemplar in weaving narrative.

ii. Kevin was a student on the Becoming a reflective and effective practitioner programme (see Chapter 14).

iii. Ruth was a student on the MSc Leadership in healthcare programme (see Chapter 14).

iv. This was the first case study within my doctoral research [53]. I met with the practitioner for 16 sessions between June 1989 and August 1990.

v. The course was worth 30 credits at degree level. For practitioners who already had a degree – the course could be offered at both Undergraduate/ Masters level.

CHAPTER 9

Unfolding the Process of Guidance

In Chapter 8, I set out some key issues of guided reflection. In this chapter, I focus on the process of guidance.

Contracting

The first guided reflection session is concerned with negotiating a contract between the guide and practitioner(s). The contract sets out the aims and the necessary ground rules to ensure mutual understanding of aims, responsibilities, process and pragmatics.

The explicit aims of guided reflection are:

- To guide the practitioner to realise their vision of self and practice as a lived reality
- To become a reflective practitioner (deemed essential to the first aim).

A third implicit aim is to enable the practitioner to develop guidance skills. This aim is explicit in guiding undergraduate students (see Chapter 14).

The contract should ideally be written by the guide and used as necessary to remind both parties of their responsibilities to ensure effective guidance.

Proctor [1] cited by Hawkins and Shohet [2, p. 29] note –

> 'If supervision [guided reflection] is to become and remain a co-operative experience which allows for real rather than token accountability, a clear, even tough, working agreement needs to be negotiated. The agreement needs to provide sufficient safety and clarity for the student/worker to know where she stands; and it needs sufficient teeth for the supervisor to feel free and responsible for making the challenges'.

The essence of contracting is to establish the conditions of trust whereby the practitioner(s) feel secure and confident to disclose themselves and reveal their experiences without caution. The guide seeks to put the practitioner at ease, acknowledging any unease the practitioner may have in entering the guided reflection relationship, for example, the status of the guide. The guide can anticipate any unease by asserting that the guided reflection is the 'learner's space and agenda' and that the guide's role is a facilitative and enabling role rather than authoritative and controlling role.

Hooks notes [3, p. 109] –

> 'Creating trust usually means finding out what it is we have in common as well as what separates us and makes us different. Hence the learning space is also a social space where difference is open and respected. The guide knows that creating community is essential for without it practitioners

will not feel secure and, as a consequence, be wary of what to reveal. It is perhaps the guide's most crucial task'.

In contracting, a number of issues are addressed:

- Roles and responsibility
- Clarifying the process of reflection
- Keeping a journal
- The practitioner's vision
- Confidentiality and trust
- Guided reflection is not therapy
- Monitoring the process
- Preparation for sessions
- Pragmatics

Roles and Responsibility

The guide explains that their role and responsibility is to guide the practitioner to learn through reflection towards realising their vision of practice. The guide can utilise Ralph's developmental model [4] (Figure 8.2) to show the practitioner how the guide's role will shift from a more directive to a facilitative approach as the practitioner's develops reflective competence.

Clarifying the Process of Reflection

The guide probes the practitioner's understanding and experience of reflection. They explain that the reflective learning space is the experiences the practitioner chooses to share towards understanding and resolving the contradictions between the practitioner's reality of the experience and their vision of practice.

   The guide introduces and talks through the Model of Structured Reflection (Figure 2.2) and suggests the practitioner explore using it in relation to an experience to bring to the next guided reflection session. The guide explains they will work through the model at the next session, emphasising that using the cues systematically will enable the practitioner to appreciate their depth and breadth of the model and, with experience, internalise the cues to become increasingly reflective in practice.

Vision

The guide emphasises the significance of holding a vision. Indeed, realising one's vision is the driving energy of reflection. As Senge notes –

> 'Vision becomes a living force only when people truly believe they can shape their future' [5, p. 231].

The practitioner may be uncertain of their vision, having not previously thought in terms of a vision or values. The guide inquires – 'what is your vision?' The guide can prompt the practitioner's thoughts by suggesting ideas such as person-centred practice. Further inquiry – 'Does your unit have a vision?' The practitioner can then be tasked to investigate for next session. The guide is mindful not to prescribe a vision. This may be difficult to resist if the guide holds a strong vision of what practice should be. If the guide is the practitioner's line manager, then the issue becomes, 'What is our vision?' establishing a collaborative inquiry.

Exploring vision often prompts practitioners to express their frustration of not being able to give care as they would wish due to the practice environment. Just talking about vision is powerful trigger for action. As Caitlin remarked –

> 'That's useful. Just talking about holistic practice and leadership strengthens my intent to realise it. It is motivating'. (cited in Chapter 12)

Keeping a Journal

The guide asserts the value of writing and reflecting on experiences in a journal prior to sharing the experience to make the best use of guided reflection. The practitioner can then add to the journal by recording insights gained and potential actions to take between sessions. In this way, the journal becomes a record of the practitioner's learning journey to become a portfolio to evidence professional development necessary for re-registration. The guide is realistic, noting that keeping a journal may not be easy to commence with (see Chapter 3).

Confidentiality

The guide acknowledges the importance of confidentiality to create trust. They emphasise that their role is not to judge the practitioner but to enable the practitioner to judge their own performance. The mantra – 'What is shared in guided reflection stays in guided reflection' with the proviso that there may be times when confidentiality may be breached in terms of patient safety, although, in my experience, this is extremely rare. If so, disclosure will always be negotiated with the practitioner.

This is the basis for security for the practitioner to disclose whatever they want to without fear of censure or being viewed as incompetent that dents the practitioner's self-esteem especially for newly qualified practitioners anxious to been seen as competent [7].

Guided Reflection Is Not Therapy

The guide emphasises that guidance is not therapy whilst acknowledging that, at times, the practitioner may link their experiences to personal events. This is inevitable and okay providing the guide draws the practitioner's attention to this linkage and the practitioner consents.

Monitoring the Effectiveness of Guided Reflection

The guide emphasises the practitioner's responsibility to take ownership of the learning process by giving the guide feedback. One approach is to ask the practitioner what they liked best/liked least at the end of each session, and more formally through using a feedback form. The practitioner may be reluctant to give negative feedback. If so, the guide can help by reflecting openly on their guidance, thus drawing the practitioner into an evaluation dialogue.

Preparation

The guide asks the practitioner to bring to each session at least one experience they have reflected on to disclose. In group guided reflection, a rota for disclosure can be established to ensure equity of time. I point out that the experience the practitioner discloses is opened up to the whole group to dialogue with and relate to with their own experiences. In doing so, the guide emphasises that practitioners benefit by listening and relating to others' experiences besides sharing their own. This creates a community of peer bonding and empathy.

Pragmatics

Having talked through the key contracting issues, the guide can set necessary practical ground rules: frequency of sessions, time, location, duration, termination and preparation. In the practice setting the guided reflection sessions will need to be pragmatic given the exigencies of everyday practice for both the guide and practitioner(s). When guided reflection is established within an educational programme, these pragmatics will have been established by the teaching team (see Chapter 14).

As a rule of thumb, I originally envisaged individual guided reflection within clinical practice for one hour every two weeks. However, in practice such a time span may slip to every three weeks due to one reason or another. For group guided reflection, I envisaged a two-hour session every four weeks planned in advance to enable practitioners to attend. The time of the sessions is negotiable. Beyond four weeks, continuity between sessions can become blurred, a case of – 'Where were we at?'

The 10 Step Model of Guided Reflection

The process of guiding reflection can be viewed as a 10 Step model (Figure 9.1).

1	Bringing the mind home
2	'Pick up'
3	What to share?
4	Listening with intent
5	Clarifying
6	Inputting information
7	Understanding
8	Options
9	Empowering
10	'Wrap up'

FIGURE 9.1 The 10-step process model of guided reflection.

Step 1 – Bringing the Mind Home

'The quieter you become the more you are able to hear'

Rumi[i]

Bringing the mind home is the preparation phase of the MSR (see Figure 2.1). The guide from the very beginning can help the practitioner relax and clear their mind of distraction through using the breath. Practitioners lead busy lives and drag the concerns of the day with them that, if dealt with, may be a barrier to learning. Hence, it is good practice to clear the mind of distraction to become fully present to the guided reflection session. This is also true for the guide and a helpful precursor for effective dialogue. The guide, in cultivating the practitioner's bringing the mind hole, also cultivates his or her own mind. It isn't a one-way street!

Blackwolf and Jones note [8, p. 90] –

> 'We must slow down or we will all that has meaning. Meaning is revealed when you pause, when you stop, when you pay attention. Learn the lessons of the tribal people. Put your busyness on pause, eliminate distractions, and allow the meaning of life and living return to you. Slow down in order to connect to the meaning of life'.

It is a too easy to be wrapped up in 'busyness' where people lose sight of what has meaning. Taking time out to reflect sounds easy, but when our lives are addicted to being busy, it may be hard to focus one's thoughts within rather than be scattered outside. Generally, people do not take time to slow down and press the pause button.

Using the breath can simply be breath in, breath out.

Thich Nhat Hanh [9, p. 15] offers a breathing exercise that I often use with practitioners

- Breathing in, I calm my body
- Breathing out, I smile
- Breathing in, I dwell in the present moment
- Breathing out, I know it is a wonderful moment

Breathing out a smile allows a release of any pent-up emotion. Dwelling in the present moment is to bring the practitioner fully present to this moment of learning within guided reflection knowing it is a wonderful opportunity to learn. Using the breath to bring the mind home is a useful technique for the practitioner to use in practice to bring themselves fully present to the situation.

As De Hennezel writes [10, p. 11] –

> 'I always take a split second to compose myself before walking into the room of a new patient. Each encounter I know is a new adventure'.

Bringing the mind home is also a precursor to developing mindfulness as it leads to a greater sense of awareness of self. Thus, guided reflection becomes a quiet eddy out of the fast current of life, to pause, muse, to clear the mind of distraction to recall and create a space where they can recall and focus the experience with all their senses alert.

Gradually, with practice, focusing the mind home becomes natural, achieved in seconds although it may feel strange at first. Habits are hard to break especially when the crowded mind is a defensive mechanism to not paying attention. Thus, to bring the mind home requires effort but it is worth it. It is a liberating structure to free the practitioner to pay attention to experience. Breaking free from our habitual ways of seeing and responding is at the core of reflective practice.

It is ancient wisdom. Lao Tzu (571 BC [11, p. 15]) wrote

> 'Do you have the patience to wait till your mud settles and the water is clear?'

Susan Brooks recognises the value of bringing the mind home [12]

'One of the most priceless skills learnt over the last two years of study on the MSc leadership pro-gramme[ii] is 'bringing home my mind' – slipping out of the noose of anxiety, releasing all grasping and relaxing into my true nature. By relaxing in this uncontrived, open and natural state we obtain the blessing of aimless self-liberation of whatever arises [13]. This has certainly been my experi-ence and the joy of feeling able to distance myself from the daily pressures of work by bringing my mind home is immense and a practice that, I believe, will stay with me indefinitely. Hatha yoga has become an element of my daily practice as a means to 'bring my mind home' and to promote my own physical and mental well being in a meditative context. Such practice has revealed to me that I do matter as a person and am not simply a faceless cog in the healthcare organisation. How many times have I said or heard the comment, 'I am just a nurse'? Nurses generally have not trusted their own sense of self-importance enough and yet the fact that nurses do matter is a fundamental truth [14]. Bringing my mind home focuses me on me, underpins my own sense of self-importance but also emphasises my crucial need, as a transformative leader, to recognise and encourage the development of the personhood and thoughts of others. Reflective thought has become a pleasure rather than a threat and as I sit to review the period of this study and my journey so far, I am con-tentedly aware that my mind is unshackled by the contradictory voices, dictates and feelings that usually fight for control over our inner lives (Rinpoche 13). Being available to self in this way has implications for my leadership, support and development of others since I would argue that unless I am truly available and knowing to self, transference of such availability would be problematic'.

Susan evidences the idea that 'bringing the mind home' is a precursor to becoming mindful. It enables her to become focused on realising her leadership vision by bringing her attention to her experience within practice. Of course, you do not have to do Hatha yoga or formal meditation to achieve this although such practices are beneficial.

Step 2 – 'Pick Up'

'Pick up' is the reflexive link between sessions. It picks up the 'wrap up' from the previous session (see Step 10). Insights and envisaged actions noted from the previous session are picked up and developed. Reasons why envisaged actions were not taken are explored.

Not being able to respond as envisaged can feel like banging your head against a brick wall, causing headache and frustration. The guide seeks to release the practitioner's tension by reassuring the practitioner its 'ok', and exploring the factors that actually constrained the practitioner. Sometimes the envisaged response is a 'bridge to far'. It is important the guide notes that yielding is not failure. It is a high rung step on the assertiveness action ladder yet to be climbed (see Figure 4.4). The guide may feel uncomfortable seeing the practitioner struggle with reality, to stumble and fall against the hard edge of reality. The key is not to fix the problem for the practitioner but guide them to see ways they can fix it for themselves. The reality wall can be further understood, and new strategies explored, to overcome it or just to endure it until the time is ripe to shift these forces.

Step 3 – What to Share?

The guide invites the practitioner to share an experience. This might be read from the journal or of the top of the practitioner's head. It may have been reflected on beforehand or not, although the guide constantly reinforces the value of written reflection prior to sharing as a more productive use of guided reflection time.

If the practitioner does not bring an experience to disclose, as may often the case in initial guided reflection, the guide can inquire ask – 'Tell me about one patient you cared for on your last shift?' This usually gets the ball rolling. The guide constantly reinforces keeping a journal by asking the practitioner to bring a written experience to the next session.

Step 4 – Listening with Intent

The guide attentively listens to the practitioner's disclosure with an open and curious mind and feedbacks to the practitioner what they have heard. The guide must try and refrain from interrupting the practitioner's disclosure because it disrupts the flow, even though the guide may be twitching to respond. Analysis of guided reflection dialogue [15] revealed how easy it is for the guide to disrupt the practitioner's story with questions the practitioner would have addressed.

Liehr and Smith [16] term 'story theory' whereby the guide attentively listens to the practitioner's story with the view of enabling the practitioner to find 'ease'. This is notable in that most experiences shared by practitioners are laden with trauma of some description. By listening attentively, the guide opens up a secure space for the practitioner to first tell the story, secondly to find meaning in the story, and thirdly to contemplate moving to a more desirable outcome. The parallel with the practitioner attentively listening to patients is obvious. As with all parallel framing, the guide can comment on it as simply happening or feed it into the practitioner's shared experience, for example – 'Did you attentively listen to the patient?' In doing so, story theory is examined and seeds planted for future use.

When individual tells their story to one who truly listens, a change in perspective takes place [17]. Smith and Liehr, citing Campbell [18, p. 5] they state –

> 'Self-discovery is embedded in story. Through story, persons search for clues and messages that potentiate understanding and the experience of being alive described as resonance within one's innermost being and reality'.

Revealing Woozles

In listening to the practitioner's story, the guide can be likened to Christopher Robin sitting in the tree observing Winnie-the-Pooh Pooh and Piglet go hunting and nearly catch a woozle [19]. Piglet joins Winnie-the-Pooh as he was walking and round the tree 'thinking of something else'. As they do, they become aware of their own tracks but misinterpret the tracks, thinking that they might be woozles. Round and round the tree they go, becoming increasingly anxious, until Christopher Robin, who is sitting up the tree observing, points out to Pooh his behaviour. Pooh realises what he has been doing. The guide helps Pooh to see things as they really are and to reassure Pooh. He doesn't tell Pooh what to think or do but points out Pooh's flawed thinking. Of course, the guide cannot usually observe the practitioner's actual behaviour. This has to be imagined from the practitioner's story. Often practitioners get so caught up in things 'on the ground' that they miss the bigger picture. They lose track and panic. The guide helps the practitioner put things into a new perspective. The practitioner can see their reality more clearly and more readily expose contradiction between desirable and actual practice. As Wheatley [20, p. 118] notes –

> 'Just how do I sort the wood from the trees to see clearly?'

The practitioner cannot learn if the basis of understanding is built on distortion. Lather [21] terms this self-distortion as 'false consciousness'. Brookfield [22, p. 33] writes –

> 'An intrinsic problem with private self-reflection is that when we use them, we can never completely avoid the risks of denial and distortion. We can never know just how much we're cooking the data of our memories and experience to produce images and renditions that show us off to good effect'.

Step 5 – Clarifying

The practitioner pauses in disclosing their experience. At this point, the guide can feed back to the practitioner what they have heard, asking the practitioner to clarify any points of their disclosure and probing deeper by picking up cues from the story and drawing on the MSR cues. Often the practitioner's story is loaded with emotional tension the guide cues into and helps the practitioner work through this tension to explore and help the practitioner understand the causes of the emotions to put them into perspective so as to view the experience more rationally.

Journal Entry 9.2

Lucy shares an experience. It is very descriptive. I challenge her with the MSR cues – notably 'How did she and others feel within the situation'? She laughs nervously. Her feelings are not easily expressed.

'Perhaps anger?' I suggest, picking up the cue from her description and from the way she recalled the experience.

'Yes, I did feel angry at my colleague' she reluctantly confesses.

'So why is it difficult to admit?'

'I don't know'

'Well?'

'Well anger isn't easy to admit'.

'What do the group think?' I ask expansively

Someone says 'Could you not be angry given the situation again?'

'I don't know. This woman gets under my skin'.

I say 'Anger is an embodied response. Obviously, not to be angry within this situation it is necessary to understand the reasons that made you angry. Better still the whole group consider this and put yourself in Lucy's shoes.'

In the ensuing dialogue a culture of conflict and conflict avoidance emerges.

Someone asks 'Why does so much conflict exist?'

Someone responds 'So why does it?'

Lucy responds 'Perhaps because we are frustrated in trying to realise our visions of practice as a reality. That's a problem with vision- it makes you think and when you think you get frustrated and see all these people blocking you. Perhaps it's better not to have a vision and put your head down. Turn a blind eye to injustice and rationalise it's not my responsibility'.

In responding to emotional tension, the experience becomes more coherent as if the emotional content smudges the mirror of reflection. Dealing with the tension, the practitioner is at more at ease and focused. Smith and Liehr [17, p. 10] note –

> 'As the disjointed story moments come together as a whole, there is a simultaneous anchoring and flow through recognition and meaning, which empowers release from the confines of the old story. This is ease. It is calmness and vision even for a moment. It is a powerful moment creating possibilities for human development'.

Planting Seeds of Doubt

The guide disturbs the surface of normal practice, planting seeds of doubt. Such questions as: 'Can you see another way of looking at this?' 'Perhaps the person viewed it differently?' Or more directly – 'Have you thought about it this way?'

Through dialogue these seeds are watered to grow and blossom, whilst guiding the practitioner to weed away old ideas that are no longer tenable. If the seeds don't take then the conditions why are explored until the moment when the new seed takes hold.

Step 6 – Inputting, Exploring and Juxtaposing Sources of Information

The guide can input theoretical sources to help the practitioner frame emerging issues and expand the practitioner's perspectives. As a guide, I usually carry a stock of useful literature in my briefcase that have proven helpful for input on particular aspects of practice that commonly crop up. The guide asks 'How does this theory inform you?' drawing the practitioner into a dialogue with the theory.

Following the session, the guide can attach theory discussed in the session or other sources that spring to mind and might be relevant to pick up next session as appropriate.

Step 7 – Understanding

Clarifying is a constant process of coming to an understanding of the significance of the experience towards drawing out tentative insights.

Step 8 – Options

This takes reflection into its anticipatory phase. The guide guides the practitioner to see beyond their existing horizons of knowing to reveal and explore possibilities for responding in new, more effective ways to similar situations [23]. The guide is mindful *not to impose* their perspectives but throws it into the mix for the practitioner to consider. In this way insights are co-created. In co-creating insights, the guide helps the practitioner become aware of any factors that seem to distort their reasoning or intuition, reviewing the issues raised by anticipating how the practitioner might respond differently, more in tune with their vision.

In group-guided reflection, a dynamic strategy for generating options to involve the whole group (Figure 9.2).

Facing the Reality Wall

In envisaging responding with the best option, the guide challenges the practitioner to consider any barriers that might prevent them responding as envisaged guided by the four cues set in the MSR (Figure 2.2). I term this facing 'the reality wall' (see Chapter 4).

1. The guide prompts the group to listen carefully to the practitioner's experience.
2. The guide, at the appropriate moment invites the other group members to relate to the shared experience from their own experiences.
3. The guide then invites the group members to put themselves in the practitioner's shoes to consider how they might respond in the situation, including the guide's option.
4. The group members offers their options to the practitioner to weigh up alongside the practitioner's own options.
5. The practitioner reviews the options, given feedback to each group member'
6. The practitioner states their preferred option and reasons for choosing this particular option.
7. The guide then invites the whole group to consider barriers that might constrain them responding as envisaged.

FIGURE 9.2 A strategy for generating options for responding in future situations involving the whole group.

The ideal response is one thing, acting it out is quite another. These potential constraining factors from responding as envisaged can be explored and understood and worked at overcoming.

Step 9 – Empowering

Envisaging how best to respond differently is ultimately rational. It is also empowering. What started out as vague, confusing and emotional is now understood with a clear path forward. As Johns and Butcher [24, p. 92] noted –

> 'Kate and Chris had now spent an hour discussing this experience. As Chris commented at the end of the session, "we started vaguely and have now forged a clear pathway to a clear understanding of this experience and action".

Barriers to responding differently have been revealed and ways to overcome them explored, the consequences to be picked up in the next session.

However, as Smyth [25, p. 40] notes –

> 'Most of us, unless we feel uncomfortable, shaken, or forced to look at ourselves, are unlikely to change. It is far easier to accept our current conditions and adopt the least line of resistance'.

The practitioner may sense they lack the power to respond differently.

One empowering tactic is to ask the practitioner to imagine facing the situation that made them feel anxious. Then to challenge them to 'measure your personal power by positioning your hand at a point on your body between your feet and top of head. Feet represent minimal power whereas top of head represents full power.'

Journal Entry 9.3

Keri, one of the leadership students, places her hands at the level of her knees. She laughs slightly shamefully, judging herself. She senses how those administrators and doctors take her power away.

I guide her – 'Take deep breaths as you imagine projecting your full power in contact with a particular administrator or doctor'.

With each inhalation Keri pumps up her power until she is full of it. She is amazed that just imagining power can have an effect – 'I am a powerful person. I demand respect. I no longer feel intimidated'.

Two weeks later, she shares an experience that involved attending another unit meeting. She used the technique and now positions her hand at hip level: 'It worked!' she exclaims, 'I still felt a sense of fear ripple through me but I took courage and found my voice. The projection was astonishing, I couldn't believe how it made me feel so different. I am now more mindful of my power'.

Just imagining her power empowered her. We explored a parallel technique of giving someone back their intimidation. 'I think this is your stuff not mine- have it back'.

Keri laughs 'I can't do that!'

I laugh in response 'Oh yes you can! Just imagine you hold the moral high ground and he is below you and cannot touch you'.

Two weeks later. Keri looks different, more self-assured. She says – 'I couldn't believe it! The medical director was sarcastic as usual. I asked him why he felt it necessary to put people down. The room went quiet. He was non-plussed. He apologised and said he hadn't realised he came across that way. My power surged. I felt triumphant and thanked him. The meeting took a very different turn. It was so good. I think I can begin to put my hand on my shoulder at least. Not the top of my head yet because I still felt fearful he could retaliate'.

Realising the power was the most significant part of Keri's leadership journey. Slowly she inched towards the top of her head, where all great leaders must position their hands. Only then could she be truly dialogical with her colleagues. This is true for every practitioner in guided reflection and perhaps the guide's greatest task- to help people believe they can take action, overcoming their own embodied disempowerment.

Role-play offers a way to rehearse and play out a new way to respond differently. The guide can say – 'Imagine I am that person'.

Step 10 – 'Wrap up'

'Wrap up' is de-briefing and summarising the session. At the end of the guided reflection session, the guide asks the practitioner to summarise the insights they have gleaned and what actions they envisage taking as a consequence, and to write these into their reflective journal as a record and reminder to pick up next session.

The guide asks the practitioner 'How do you do feel now?' cuing the practitioner to discharge any residual emotion left over from the session dialogue to enable the practitioner can leave the session feeling positive.

As a way for the practitioner to reflect on the effectiveness of the session the guide invites the practitioner to consider what they 'liked best' and 'liked least' about the session. The practitioner may initially feel uncomfortable in giving feedback unaccustomed to evaluating the learning process. In appreciating this difficulty, the guide can respond by saying what they liked least and liked best about their guidance. This enables the practitioner to see that giving feedback is okay and a significant aspect of the guided reflection process. A more structured approach is to utilise the 'Observer check list' (Figure 8.5).

Summary

Whilst I have set out the 10-step model, the actual practice of guidance is much more chaotic and creative, veering between steps, following the flow of dialogue especially as practitioners become more experienced and competent reflective practitioners and with the guide becoming increasingly less directive.

Chapters 11 and 12 are exemplars of guiding practitioners within clinical practice.

References

1. Proctor, B. (1988) *Supervision a Working Alliance.* (video training manual) Alexia Publications, St Leonards-on-Sea.

2. Hawkins, P., Shohet, R. (1989) *Supervision in the Helping Professions.* The Open University Press, Milton Keynes.

3. Hooks, B. (1994) *Teaching to Transgress: Education as the Practice of Freedom.* Routledge, New York.

4. Ralph, N. B. (1980) Learning psychotherapy: a developmental perspective. *Psychiatry,* 43, 243–250.

5. Senge, P. (1990) *The Fifth Discipline: The Art & Practice of the Learning Organization.* Century Business, London.

6. Gray, G., Forsstrom, S. (1991) Generating theory from practice: the reflective technique. In G. Gray, R. Pratt [Eds.] *Towards a Discipline of Nursing.* Churchill Livingstone, Melbourne, 355–372.

7. Cherniss, G. (1980) *Professional Burnout in Human Service Organizations.* Praeger, New York.

8. Blackwolf, J. G. (1996) *Earth Dance Drum.* Commune-E-Key, Salt Lake City.

9. Hanh, T. N. (1993) *The Blooming of a Lotus*. Beacon Press, Boston.

10. De Hennezel, M. (1997) *Intimate Death: How the Dying Teach us to Live*. Warner Books, London.

11. Tzu, L. (1999) *Tao Te Ching* [Trans. S. Mitchell]. Frances Lincoln, London.

12. Brooks, S. (2004) *Becoming A Transformational Leader*. Unpublished MSc Leadership in healthcare dissertation. University of Bedfordshire, Bedford.

13. Rinpoche, S. (1992) *The Tibetan Book of Living and Dying*. Rider, London.

14. Tschudin, V. (1993) *Ethics in Nursing*. (2nd ed). Butterworth Heinemann, Oxford.

15. Johns, C. (1998) *Becoming A Reflective Practitioner through Guided Reflection*. PhD thesis. The Open University, Milton Keynes.

16. Liehr, P., Smith, M. (2008) Story theory. In M. Smith, P. Liehr [Eds.] *Middle Range Theory for Nursing*. 2nd ed. Springer, New York, 205–221.

17. Smith, M., Liehr, P. (1999) Attentively embracing story; a middle range theory with practice and research implications. *Scholarly Inquiry for Nursing Practice*, 13, 3–27.

18. Campbell, J. (1988) *The Power of Myth*. Doubleday, New York.

19. Milne, A. A. (1926) *Winnie-the-Pooh*. Methuen, London.

20. Wheatley, M. (1999) *Leadership and the New Science*. Berrett-Koehler, Oakland.

21. Lather, P. (1986) Issues of validity in open ideological research: between a rock and a hard place. *Interchange*, 17, 63–84.

22. Brookfield, S. (1995) *Becoming A Critically Reflective Teacher*. Jossey-Bass, San Francisco.

23. Cox, H., Hickson, P., Taylor, B. (1991) Exploring reflection: knowing and constructing practice. In G. Gray, R. Pratt [Eds.] *Towards A Discipline of Nursing*. Churchill Livingstone, Melbourne, 373–390.

24. Johns, C., Butcher, K. (1993) Learning through reflection: a case study of respite care. *Journal of Clinical Nursing* 2(2), 89–93.

25. Smyth, W. J. (1987) *A Rationale for Teachers' Critical Pedagogy*. Deakin University Press, Melbourne.

Notes

i. https://www.goodreads.com/quotes/6822193-the-quieter-you-become-the-more-you-are-able-to.

ii. Susan Brooks was a student on the MSc Leadership in health care programme at the University of Bedfordshire.

CHAPTER 10

Applying the Model for Structured Reflection: 'Passing People by'

In the previous chapters, I set out the Model for Structured Reflection (Figure 2.2) to guide the practitioner towards drawing insights from experience. In the following narrative 'Passing people by', I apply the Model for Structured Reflection (MSR) cues sequentially to my experience with Peggy to illustrate their utility in accessing and exploring the breadth and depth of reflection. With experience of using the cues, the practitioner internalises them to use them more intuitively.

The MSR's utility is reflected in the words of Priest and Johns (1, p. 200) –

'My scalpel and instrument of investigation are manifested in the Model of Structured Reflection. However, like any new tool, it's only as good as the user. I found myself repeating the same answers to different questions. I also became impatient in reaching particular reflective cues, or going through the motions with others. The model was a skeleton key, opening previous locked complex events. Instead of jumping to conclusions, I found myself considering details which allowed for much richer experiences. By envisaging alternative outcomes or responses, I could intertwine my desired transformational leadership ideology with personal and ethical values'.

Note the technique of recalling dialogue in the description. It enlivens the description and is more mimetic with the lived experience.

Bringing the Mind Home

Sitting at my desk, my fingers poised over the laptop. Before pressing the first key I pause and use my breath to bring my mind home to the experience with Peggy that took place earlier today.

Writing Self

Another Monday. Arriving at the hospice day care centre, I looked about the sitting room. Some people were already present sitting in their usual chairs. People become territorial. On the surface, a normal day judging by other Mondays during the six weeks I have been working here as the 'Monday therapist'. Can any day be described as normal without immediately deflating it?

The morning briefing. The room filling. 20 people attending. As has become my routine, I go round and say hello to each person and take requests for therapy. I am surprised when Peggy smiles and calls out 'I'm first on the list'. I am surprised because I had not previously given Peggy a treatment. In fact, I had rarely spoken to her beyond the usual social pleasantries. She had not requested a therapy and other patients claimed my time. Caught off guard the pang of guilt hits! I struggle to frame her demand and my emotional response.

I respond 'What treatment would you like Peggy?'

She replies 'Some reflexology please'.

Caught off guard I reactively say 'OK, lets do it', as if compensating for my sense of guilt.

She walks with her stick to the treatment room. As she walks, she talks about her grief for her partner who died of cancer in March. This grief lay thick on the surface, a grief made more poignant with the death of her dog a few months later.

She cries 'I'm sorry for the tears', as if her tears might burden me.

I respond in a somewhat facile manner 'better the tears out than in'.

She is gracious 'I know. Many people tell me'.

And perhaps it is true. Opening a floodgate for the grieving heart. Opening a healing space for her raw grief wound.

I say 'Tell me about your partner Peggy?'

She tells the story of his cancer diagnosis and death just a few weeks later. Such a contrast from her own prolonged treatment from breast cancer and bone metastases in her pelvis. Her story was limited to his cancer. I do not push her to tell me more about him.

'How do you feel about coming to the Day Centre Peggy?'

She confesses she has mixed feelings, that it isn't easy sitting with other people but on the other hand she does like the company.

I respond 'I think so ... as if part of you wants to come and another part doesn't. Do you feel alone?'

She says 'Yes I do, even though I'm surrounded by well meaning friends and neighbours. I miss him so much and my dog'.

Her dog's name was Alfie.

I say 'I'm sorry about him. I don't have a dog but I imagine he must have been great company'.

Silence between us. I feel her aloneness. I sense she has lost her significant connections to life. I notice she said she was surrounded by well-meaning friends and neighbours but not family. But I do not pursue this. Thinking about what support Peggy had in her life, I inquire 'Are you religious Peggy?'

She says 'I do believe in God but have no strong religion. I mean I don't go to church. Believing in God doesn't comfort me'.

I say 'I can see you limp and grimace on walking. Do you have any pain?'

'Oh yes. My pain is managed well enough with *paracetamol* and *diclofenac*. I also take some tummy protection tablets'.

We reach the therapy room. She sits on the edge of the therapy couch and surprises me by easily removing her boots and getting herself onto the couch.

'I bought these boots recently for the winter' she says as if reading my mind.

I placed a blanket over her and ask 'What smells do you like Peggy?'

She isn't fussy. I mix lavender, frankincense and grapefruit essential oils into my reflexology cream. Grapefruit is described as a sunny oil bringing sunshine into grief's darkness. Lavender lifts the veil of sadness while Frankincense helps to slow the breath and be calm. Informing Peggy about the oils intends a placebo effect.

Peggy says 'Sounds good. Umm, the aroma is lovely. I've always loved grapefruit and lavender. Frankincense was one of the gifts of the Three Kings'.

I know that aromas hold memories. The aroma of the oils will linger with her through the day. I play some music to help her relax.

Peggy closes her eyes as I hold her feet and guide her to relax. She falls asleep. Halfway through the treatment she cried out. When she woken, she said 'I feel a weight has been lifted from me'.

My response is rather a cliché 'Grief is a heavy burden'.

But Peggy responds graciously 'Yes. It feels like that'.

It made me think how much health talk is grounded in platitudes or clichés that fill empty spaces or spoken to ease the health giver's anxiety concerned with any negative talk.

On our return to the sitting room with Peggy on my arm, faces turned to stare. I sense that two of the more demanding patients seem frustrated with me for not following the normal pattern, probably anxious about their own turn in the schedule. Mrs Perkins shouted out 'ah there you are'. I feel the pressure to conform to the normal routine but I can now see the bigger picture, my gaze no longer so focused on those with the loudest voice. I look around the room and wonder – 'Is there anybody else in the room I have "passed by"'?

What Is Significant to Reflect on?

- My routine and not paying attention to what is happening around me have careless consequences, like passing by Peggy each week when she wanted a therapy. She must have suffered when others with loud voices received a therapy with her left on the sidelines.
- How I assess people attending the day centre?
- Am I poised enough?
- Is my therapy effective?

Why Did I Respond as I Did?

Responding spontaneously to give Peggy a therapy at that particular time was a gut response triggered by a sense of guilt, rather like a naughty child being caught out.

Did I Respond in Tune with My Vision?

My vision as a holistic therapist is to help ease suffering and enable the person to grow through the therapeutic experience. This fits within the wider WHO definition of palliative care. The contradiction between my vision and my practice is evident through my reflection, notably my lack of knowing Peggy, my awareness, poise and the routine I had established in the sense of taking things for granted and its consequences.

Did I Respond Effectively in Terms of Consequences?

Peggy was pleased with her therapy and probably pleased with confronting me to get her therapy. Through talking with her, I got to know her and the sadness and loneliness in her life and a sense she felt less alone through sharing her story.

Did My Feelings Influence Me?

My sense of guilt triggered my response. She knocked me off my complacent shelf.

Did Past Experiences Influence Me?

The saying – 'those who ask get and those who don't ask don't get' rings true. People are passed by simply because it is easier to manage workload from this perspective. As I wrote in the story – *it was a normal day*. I saw what I normally saw and responded in my normal way.

The notion that aromas hold memories is based on one particular experience with the daughter of a woman who died in the hospice. The mother was agitated, and the family were agitated in response. They begged me to help. I used a cream mixed with oils to massage her hands. She became calm and lucid, enabling the family to have a positive death experience. The daughter asked if she could have a small pot of the cream I had used to remember her mother by. When I met her again, she said how much the cream had helped her deal with her grief. I gifted her a small pot of the lotion as a remembrance [2].

Did I Respond Ethically for the Best?

I was faced with a dilemma of how to respond to Peggy in the moment. My response was intuitive but was it for the best? Ethical mapping guided me to reflect on this dilemma to arrive at the most appropriate ethical response as outlined in Figure 10.1. There is always a tension between what is ethically correct according to ethical principles and the personal moral response and the perspectives of other people concerned either directly or at a distance. I put Peggy's demand first irrespective of any consequence, both to meet her need and ease my guilt.

Did Other Factors Influence Me?

Peggy's outburst was a result of my routine of persons asking for a therapy. My modus operandi being – 'if they didn't ask I assume they don't want'. Yet, I had always thought I was available to be asked exposing the contradiction.

Considering influencing theory, I am always scrutinising my choice of aromatherapy oils yet relying on Worwood's descriptors to guide me and the patient's responses.

My reflection raises assumptions based on experience, for example, aromas hold memories and music helps people relax. Worwood informs [3, p. 95] –

> 'Is it any wonder that smell has such a profound effect on us, or that extended memory can be triggered by certain aromas? Aroma is one of the means by which memory is laid down by its yet mysterious recording mechanism'.

I know that certain music blends with the movement of my hands and that my hands blend with the rhythm of the music. I also know that the music will enable Peggy to blend into the therapy. These things are not known for certain but known tacitly through experience [4].

Given a similar situation, how could I respond more effectively, for the best and in tune with my vision?

Firstly, by 'knowing the person' I would be prepared for the person's needs and their knowing what therapy was on offer. Then Peggy wouldn't have demanded "I'm first on the list"?

Patient's/family's perspective	What ethical principles inform this situation? :	My perspective
Peggy wanted to be 'first on the list' for a therapy this morning. Clearly, she felt passed by on previous days. Other patients may have had perspectives as it disrupted the normal pattern of offering and giving therapy.	Peggy's autonomy in tension with my own. Utilitarianism – potential conflicting needs of the many versus the individual Integrity – acting with best therapeutic intention	Ease my guilt by immediately offering therapy. I could have offered to give Peggy a treatment later in the morning.
Is there is conflict of perspectives/values - how might these be resolved? Potential competing need from patients with possible recrimination. The system for giving therapy must be transparent and fair.	*Did I respond ethically and morally in the moment?*	*Consider the power relationships that determined response* I controlled giving therapy although influenced by 'loud voices'
Other health care worker[s]' perspective Other health care workers were not directly involved although may have repercussions for therapists who work on other days.	How can a similar situation be responded to most ethically? Holding an attitude of 'not passing people by'. Establishing a new system for managing therapies.	The organisation's perspective Smooth running without complaint – probably fitting Peggy into a work schedule

FIGURE 10.1 Applying ethical mapping.

Perhaps I could have responded 'You should have asked Peggy'. But would that have put the onus on her when her natural inclination is not to ask, not to be a burden. I know from my hospice experience that women who care deeply for others, as she has for her partner, do not find it easy to ask for their own care. It would have increased the burden on her, to make it seem as if it was her responsibility to ask rather than mine to offer. Responding like this would be me projecting my anxiety at having been caught out, as if a naughty boy anxious to shift the blame.

Another option might be to say something like 'OK- I'll fit you into the schedule'. At first glance, this response seems reasonable. It acknowledges that I plan a schedule of therapies for the day. Yet such a formulaic response might seem insensitive. It would not have acknowledged her desperate cry. It might have put her in her place, reminding her that I control the environment not her.

Another possible response might be an act of apology 'I'm sorry Peggy I hadn't realised'. In doing so, I acknowledge my responsibility and that I can get it wrong. Humility. But by apologising, would I have burdened her with my guilt and made her feel she needed to care for me? The repentant child seeking forgiveness?

My actual response to Peggy 'let's do it now' still feels the most appropriate because it acknowledged her desperate cry. It was intuitive, a response in the moment.

Creating my practice environment was clearly flawed. I had fallen into an inappropriate routine at the beck and call of the loudest voices. What are my options?

1. Get people to put their name down for a therapy on arrival. I can then review and plan a schedule based on fairness, recognising I cannot give a therapy to everyone who wants one in one day.
2. We have two therapy rooms. If demand is greater than supply- then perhaps seek a second volunteer therapist?
3. Shorten the time span of each therapy – to enable more patients to have a therapy.

Option 1 is promising. But first I must speak with the hospice manager to get her viewpoint. I can also discuss option 2 with her. Perhaps option 3 might work but would the therapy benefit be compromised with shorter treatments? I sense my integrity as a therapist would be compromised.

What Might be the Consequences of Responding Differently?

Actions have consequences! In the above description, I contemplated the consequence of responding differently. Not just short-term consequences but also long-term consequences. I know that every action is a moral and political act towards creating a better state of affairs. For example, by responding to Peggy as I did, do I set a precedent that any patient could just grab me and demand a therapy now and then? Would I lose control of the environment?

Am I Able to Respond as I Envisage?

- Am I skilful and knowledgeable enough to respond differently?
  If I had *known* Peggy the situation would not have arisen. My approach to knowing the person is structured through the Burford NDU reflective cues (see Chapter 6). I needed to know her and all persons attending the day centre prior to planning how best to help them. However, in our conversation walking towards the therapy room, I was able to rectify my not knowing Peggy by using the Buford cues to know her adequately to give her reflexology. Our conversation was itself therapy. My skill was to communicate my knowing Peggy to the wider team and dialogue regarding issues arising from knowing Peggy.
- Am I powerful enough to respond differently?
  As a therapist, I have autonomy to go about my practice as I see fit. However, I do work within a team and plan accordingly. Reviewing my plan with the practice manager validates my action and secures support. It gives me greater authority knowing my response is now collective. I am not a lone ranger!

  It is a sobering thought to consider I might be unable to resist demand from the loud voices of patients who dominate the day centre. Am I afraid of upsetting them if I say 'No, not today- that others need my service'? I am mindful of a need to accommodate others not simply because I want to be of service but to avoid any discomfort of conflict in saying no.
- Do I have the right attitude and assumptions?
  My experience reveals to me just how easy it is to get caught up in routine as a way of organising practice. Indeed, without routine would there be chaos? I am reminded my vision is made manifest through my actions. My experience with Peggy confronts me with

the contradiction between my vision of person-centred practice and my actual practice. A wake up call! Yet I like to think my attitude was person-centred. Reflection is humbling to confess that I don't always get it right and that I took Peggy for granted. It tells me that attitude and assumptions are deeply rooted formed through years of socialisation. Person-centred practice is an ideal I strive towards and this experience is a positive step towards realising it.

- Am I poised enough to respond differently?
  I am more aware of the quality and significance of poise. Poise is such a vital aspect of being available to the person and has now become a constant focus for my reflections, especially as it is not easy at times to be poised in the face of the other's suffering and colleagues' attitudes and behaviours. Perhaps that is why practitioners wear suits of armour as protection from emotional fall-out. Yet do I wear armour?
- How does extant theory/ ideas inform and deepen my insights?
  The crux of this experience is that I had not listened to Peggy's story. I didn't know her and took her for granted – just another patient quietly sitting there without demand. How easy to 'pass her by'. The idea of attentively listening to the person's story is given theoretical weight by Liehr and Smith in their 'story theory' [5] and its impact on creating ease for the patient. As I walked Peggy to the therapy room, I did attentively listen to her story. She realised this and responded openly. It enabled her to release her feelings of sadness and loneliness that eased her suffering. It may not be easy to understand our negative emotions. They may stem back to earlier unresolved issues in our lives. Blackwolf and Jones write [6, p. 56] –

'When I fill up with negative thoughts, inside I am more worried and distracted. We cannot escape from our worrisome mind unless we unravel the mental fibre that we have erroneously woven. Take the time to reweave new patterns ...'

I sense how Peggy's terminal illness on top of the loss of her husband and dog has trapped her between the world of the living and the world of the dead [7]. Being able to talk about him and Alfie is vital so she can put them to rest in her heart as a loving memory. Just writing that I sense the significance of the 'continuing bonds theory of grief' [8]. Peggy's confessions of feeling alone and lonely are complex elements of suffering that are not easily understood and perhaps not easy to explore with someone. Although Peggy is not at the terminal stage of dying – she is terminally ill. Elias's [9, p. 84] words ring in my ears, words I have often read and yet always seek to find deeper meaning as something lived –

'Perhaps people in this situation [of dying] have a special need of other people. But for some of the dying it may be right to be alone. One must sense what they need'.

Understanding Peggy's story requires sensibility, to sense beyond any logical interpretation of her story. Yet it is listening to her story that opens myself to sensibility.

Reflection is a constant inquiry to expand my knowledge base. The experience makes me think more about routine and control. Is this done as a defence against the suffering health care practitioners face on a daily basis? I have often drawn on Blackwolf's vision to inform my practice away from more healthcare texts. He offers words for deeper reflection [6, p. 183] –

'Uncomfortable with the griever's uncertainty about life, deep sadness, encounter with death, and changed self, we turn away when we are needed most. Look at times when, perhaps, you have turned away - what were you avoiding? Most likely it was your own uncertainty, your own sadness, your own changes, your own mortality'.

Blackwolf's words are challenging. Do I unwittingly turn away? I don't think so but it is a timely reminder to be mindful in my practice.

Delving further into non-healthcare texts, Moore [10, p. 235] informs me –

> 'Day by day we live emotions and themes that have deep roots, but our reflections on these experiences tend to be superficial ... not only are our reflections often insufficient to account for intense feelings, but we may have been living from a place that is too rational and dispassionate. Rainer Maria Rilke advises the young poet to "go deep into yourself and see how deep the place is from which your life flows". We could all take note of this advice, go deep into ourselves and discover how deep is the source of our everyday lives'.

All very well, but what would *going deeper* mean? Is it sometimes better to swim in the shallow end rather than risk of deep water? How deep did I go in talking with Peggy? How deep did I go reflecting within myself? I am mindful of drawing a line between holistic therapy and grief counselling. Saying that, it challenges my perception of role and perhaps why I term myself a holistic therapist rather than a complementary therapist like my other therapy colleagues.

How Has Guidance Deepen My Insights?

Talking the experience through with my practice manager was beneficial. She guided me to talk through a feasible alternative schedule [the word routine is banned!]. She doesn't know how the other therapists go about their practice. She has left them to organise themselves, cautious of stepping on their toes as they are all volunteers. However, my experience was a wake up call for her to give more attention to organisational issues to ensure the best person-centred practice. She also responded positively to my idea of creating a collective day care vision. I intend to share this experience within my multi-disciplinary group supervision. It will be interesting to note their response and whether they have similar experiences.

What Insights Do I Draw From This Experience?

These can be summarised using the Being Available template (Figure 5.4).

Realising My Vision

The lack of the Day Centre's organisational vision is something I recognise as depressingly normal and reinforces my view that practitioners do not work consciously as a collective towards realising a person-centred vision. My personal vision as a hospice therapist is to help the person ease their suffering by being available to them.

Knowing Peggy

The reflection has made me rethink how well do I know patients and how well do I need to know patients? For example, if I had known Peggy as a person would I have responded to her differently weeks ago? The depth of her sadness and loneliness added to my guilt but also my satisfaction that I eventually helped to ease her suffering through attentively listening to her story and the actual physical therapy. The satisfaction erases the guilt. The value of the Buford BNDU model cues is both evident and reinforced.

Theories of terminal illness stimulated my perspective as a holistic therapy that listening and enabling the other person to find meaning in their grief is vital aspects of my holistic role. Listening, concern and knowing the person are reinforced as vital to realising person-centred practice – *not*-listening means that I cannot know patients as people well enough with the consequence of not being person-centred.

Concern

Without doubt, knowing Peggy's story engenders concern. Indeed, without concern, therapy is ineffective simply because concern is the healing energy.

Skilled Response

The whole experience is a reflection of responding to Peggy in tune with my vision of person-centred practice within the context of my role as a holistic therapist of being available to the whole group of persons attending rather than just the individual. Peggy's needs were met on a number of levels:

- Having her voice heard
- Having her story known gave her a sense of identity as a suffering person rather than someone attending the day centre.
- Having reflexology that she very much appreciated

Poise

The reality is, that under certain conditions, I lose my poise. If I had interpreted Peggy's demand as a threat to my control, reminding her that I was in control not her, that I would determine my schedule not her, what would have been the consequences? Ramos [11] identified the need to be in control as impasse to developing therapeutic relationships. If I had put Peggy 'in her place', I sense she would not have felt slighted and not asked again and probably refused if I invited her for a therapy in the future. Exploring the potential alternative responses to Peggy, especially the child mode perspective as a response to guilt. Using transactional analysis [TA] [12] as a theoretical map it is vital, I stay in adult mode and enable the other person to respond likewise no matter the situation unless it is therapeutically necessary to be otherwise. Just for a moment Peggy became the critical parent, admonishing my neglect of her and just for a moment I became the naughty child. But just for a moment until I regained my poise and responded in adult mode that quelled her parental edge.

Poise is vital in making good clinical judgements within the moment, acknowledging my lack of poise when emotionally challenged through conflict. The experience draws my attention to the way feelings impact on decision-making, challenging the idea that decision making is rational and that feelings distort reason [13].

Creating a Conducive Environment

I am aware of the clamour of demand for my service each week and my response – that those who ask get and those who don't ask don't get. I can see that, in the crowded room, I only paid attention to those with the loudest voices. It is certainly the route of least resistance. Perhaps meeting so many new people in my new role, it was easier for me to be approached as a way to control my anxiety. The issue of control was not something I was mindful of, yet I am now aware that a loss of control leads to a loss of poise.

Perhaps I see the fear of conflict as huge and immovable boulder. It is something I can challenge through developing a new system. Hence, I can assert the system rather than make it a personal issue. The value of systems as long as they are person-centred rather than organisationally centred. Writing this, the boulder seems to loosen and fall away. Amazing! My attachment to fear weakens and, as Rosenberg [14, p. 145] notes, 'little by little, we're not so enslaved to things'.

The tyranny of routine is to lose sight of one's vision. It leads to mindless practice. Systems must be our servants rather than our masters. The ethical use of my time to ensure justice for all persons attending is served by all persons knowing the system and by constantly evaluating the system for its appropriateness. The experience is a reminder to be mindful of routine and habit that only serve my best interests to manage my day rather than the patients' best interests with the consequence of being careless and passing people by.

'How Do I Now Feel About the Situation'?

Looking back at my experience with Peggy I am amazed that a seemingly innocuous situation emerged as so insightful. It just goes to show the power of reflection. I feel I have purged my guilt constructively. However, it wasn't easy facing up to my unsatisfactory performance and yet I have learnt so much from it. It feels as if someone wiped my reflective mirror a little cleaner! I feel the veracity of the idea that the more you try and control something the less you actually do so.

The Following Monday

My gaze takes in the whole room. I am more mindful of the bigger picture. Peggy smiles at me from across the room. I sit with her a while and ask how she's been. Not so bad. 'A therapy today Peggy?'

'No, not this week. Maybe next week'.

A new lady sits alone. I focus my breath. I go and sit with her. I introduce myself and invite her story. I feel no demand on my time.

Becker informs my approach [15, p. 13]

> 'People feel a lot freer around somebody who is quietly accepting them for what they are. It is for you to remain relaxed in the presence of nothing going on. Simply to be present in an atmosphere like that is a healing thing. It is actually this caring listening response, and not a showing or doing response which makes therapy work'.

I introduce the register for people to schedule therapy appointments. It seems to be accepted (watch this space).

Clinical Supervision Session Three Weeks Later

I share my Peggy experience with my multi profession clinical supervision group that currently meets every two months. Connie, a physiotherapist, is the group facilitator today.[i] It seems a common story. Everyone recognises 'passing people by' and how such self-management becomes embodied and hence invisible. Everyone feels the tension between involvement and detachment with patients. It becomes uncomfortable when we pay attention to this tension as if somehow we are lacking. But then involvement is not easy. Being detached we can surf through the day not oblivious to suffering but keeping it at a distance. Such approach is governed and sanctioned by the medical model with its primary gaze on the person as symptom management whereby social, psychological and spiritual issues become problems to solve rather than being seen from a holistic perspective reflected in suffering.

I had expected Marie, a doctor, to be defensive but she surprises me by agreeing that 'easing suffering', as enshrined within the WHO definition of palliative care should be emphasised as the Hospices' primary value.[ii]

Someone challenges me with the MSR cue – 'Did you act for the best?'

'No, not directly. I always think this cue is implicit? What do you think?'

'Well, consider Peggy's autonomy?'

'I know I should always respect her autonomy. To do so I need to put Peggy in a position of making a decision. Umm, that's interesting. As such, a fourth response might be - *'Would you like a therapy now Peggy? I have time'.* By saying 'I have time' frees Peggy to accept. I can see this response would be better. It acknowledges and respects her autonomy'.

The group concur. Perhaps I should not have offered any of my own alternatives but asked them to generate alternatives before sharing my own – for example, 'if you were in my shoes how might you have responded?' I sense it would have been a better learning curve.

Someone says 'You can really see the utilitarian ethic at work in your experience- the demand on time and its influence on the way we set priorities'.

Connie feeds in some theory concerning defences against anxiety stemming from the work of Menzies-Lyth [16], notably the assertion of the need for practitioners to develop a necessary professional detachment as a protection from not being overwhelmed by the other's suffering. If concern for the person is vital in opening a healing space, then I must rewrite Menzies-Lyth [16] as 'the need to develop a necessary professional involvement' to fit within my vision of person-centred practice. Marie emphasises 'We need to be emotionally intelligent or poised in order to be fully available to the other within the moment by managing one's vulnerability to the other's suffering'.

The group concur and share experiences of emotional disturbance with both patients and colleagues. I share my reading of papers by Paley [17] and Rolfe and Gardner [18]. Paley's paper in particular challenges me as to whether I had a case of 'situational blindness', which led me to pass Peggy by. I find his argument compelling. Rolfe and Gardner challenge this perspective. I can see that my need for order was a reaction to my anxiety faced with an anticipated busy workload. Anxiety, when it becomes overwhelming can create situational blindness. It narrows the focus. But does it diminish my concern? If I am wrapped up in concern for myself, does it diminish my concern of the other? Yes, if I am not mindful enough. But then I have become doubtful about compassion, as noted in the Rolfe and Gardner paper, as a feasible attribute simply because the word is bandied about without due appreciation of what it implies. I prefer 'concern for the person' as set out in the 'Being available template'. I give copies of the papers to the group to consider.

Connie, in summarising the group's work today says 'I will share this story at the next senior clinical team meeting. Wake them up a bit!' Like throwing a stone into a still pond, creating ripples to disturb.

Talking through my experience with Peggy reinforced the value of multi-professional group reflection. It is a secure place to openly dialogue about our experiences. The issues raised will stimulate deeper reflection and benefit all attending.

References

1. Priest, J.-M., Johns, C. (2010) More than eggs for breakfast. In C. Johns [Ed.] *Guided Reflection: A Narrative Approach to Advancing Professional Practice* (second edition). Wiley-Blackwell, Oxford, 195–214.

2. Johns, C. (2006) *Engaging Reflection in Practice: A Narrative Approach.* Blackwell Publishing, Oxford.

3. Worwood, V. (1999) *The Fragrant Heavens.* Doubleday, London.

4. Johns, C. (2009) Journeying with Alice: some things I do not know for certain. *Complementary Therapies in Clinical Practice* 15(3), 133–135.

5. Liehr, P., Smith, M. (2008) Story theory. In M. Smith, P. Liehr [Eds.] *Middle Range Theory for Nursing* (second edition). Springer, New York.

6. Blackwolf, J. G. (1996) *Earth Dance Drum.* Commune-E-Key, Salt Lake City.

7. Walter, T. (1994) *The Revival of Death.* Routledge, London.

8. Klass, D., Silverman, P., Nickman, S. (1996) *Continuing Bonds: New Understandings of Grief.* Taylor and Francis, Washington.

9. Elias, N. (1985) *The Loneliness of the Dying.* Basil Blackwell, Oxford.

10. Moore, T. (1992) *Care of the Soul.* HarperCollins, New York.

11. Ramos, M. (1992) The nurse-patient relationship: themes and variations. *Journal of Advanced Nursing* 17, 496–506.

12. Stewart, I., Joines, V. (1987) *TA Today: A New Introduction to Transactional Analysis.* Russell Press, Nottingham.

13. Callahan, S. (1988) *The Role of Emotion in Ethical Decision-making.* Hastings Centre Report, June/July, 9–14.

14. Rosenberg, L. (1998) *Breath by Breath.* Shambhala.

15. Becker, R. (2006) In R.E. Brooks [Ed.] *Life in Motion.* Stillness Press, Portland.

16. Menzies-Lyth, I. (1988) A case study in the functioning of social systems as a defence against anxiety. *In Containing Anxiety in Institutions: Selected Essays.* Free Association Books, London.

17. Paley, J. (2014) Cognition and the compassion deficit: the social psychology of helping behaviours in nursing. *Nursing Philosophy* 15, 274–287.

18. Rolfe, G., Gardner, L. (2014) The compassion deficit and what to do about it: a response to Paley. *Nursing Philosophy* 15, 288–297.

Notes

i.   The group planned to meet for 60 minutes every two months. Yet in practice it is often 3 months for one reason or another often with poor attendance. It was planned that practitioners took turns to facilitate the sessions.

ii. Palliative care is an approach that improves the quality of life of patients and their families facing the problem associated with life-threatening illness, through the prevention and *relief of suffering* by means of early identification and impeccable assessment and treatment of pain and other problems, physical, ... (www.who.int/cancer/palliative/definition/en/).

CHAPTER 11

Guiding Alexia to Realising Her Leadership and Vision of Person-centred Practice with Head and Neck Cancer Patients and Families

Prologue

I met Alexia when she was a student undertaking the clinical supervision module. She was enthused with the idea of learning through reflection on experience and approached me, inquiring whether I could continue working with her in a guided reflection relationship. At the time she was the ward manager and clinical nurse specialist for the regional head and neck unit, a position she had commenced six months earlier.

We met for nine sessions, meeting each month for one hour. Our relationship was discontinued by her maternity leave.

Session 1

In our first session, we contracted our relationship (see Chapter 9). As part of the contract, Alexia agreed for me to write notes of each session for her agreement that they reflected our dialogue. The notes remind her of what we had explored, enabling a deeper level of reflection and reflexive continuity between sessions where insights can be built upon and action taken. She agreed I could use the notes for purposes of research and publication.

Chris: 'It all starts with vision and stories. So what is your vision – what do you seek to realise in your practice?'

Alexia: 'I believe it is about caring for the whole person and family and enabling myself and the unit nurses to achieve this. I haven't yet facilitated constructing a "holistic" vision with the staff but feel this is imperative so we are all pulling in the same direction'.

Chris: 'Do you feel some nurses might not hold a holistic vision?'

Alexia: 'I don't know. It is not something we have discussed. It is something I have assumed all nurses would value. I must check this out. Maybe I'll ask at the beginning of each shift "what do we value about our nursing". Get a conversation going. Lift it to the surface'.

Chris: 'I think that's important- it will make the nurses think more about what they are doing and what they are striving to achieve'.

Alexia: 'I do have an experience I would like to share. Three weeks ago I was upset about a situation. I unwittingly took it home with me and it impacted on my home life. I didn't know what the reason was at first. I also know it will happen again. This patient, Paul, he had had a malignant melanoma removed from his ear in the past. His neck had become swollen and he required a 13 hour operation – a radical neck dissection that involved pulling muscle up from his chest. Body image was a problem for him. I knew it would be. I didn't admit him. A staff nurse did but I wish I had done so. I would have been better prepared to respond to his needs. He was very British – "chop the bugger out and I'll be fine" attitude. I challenged him 'and what happens if it is not fine?' He discarded this. I felt the family dynamics were 'odd'. His wife only visited at visiting time although relatives of patients who have had such surgery have open visiting. This made it difficult for me to talk to them as a couple. Then on Sunday afternoon the ward was very quiet and I could chat with him without guilt! I felt I had a good rapport with him. He was going to Addenbrookes on the Monday for radiotherapy. This made a good opener to the conversation. I chatted about myself, I think that's important so they get to know something about you. I asked him about his children. He said his son had committed suicide a year ago. He said that matter of factly. I acknowledged my shock at this news and how difficult that must be when we expect our children to bury their parents not the other way round. This had happened when he and his wife were on holiday. He was angry at his daughters for letting this happen. The son had been depressed. I noted the coincidence that it happened when he was on holiday, that the son would have done it if he was determined to. He said the son's death coincided with the Princess of Wales's death and how angry he felt when people were grieving for someone they did not know when he was grieving for his son. I noted I found the family dynamic strained. He admitted this – that he had never shed a tear. I feedback my perception that his wife didn't seem to know. He agreed – that he didn't want her to know, didn't want to bother her with it. I then picked up the "what if" question that had hung answered between us, linking it to Addenbrookes. He said "It won't happen to me"'.

Chris: 'Patients tend to respond to imminent death in three ways: to deny it, to be stoic about it, or to fight it, which as Bolen [1] suggests often leads to the best outcome'.

Alexia: 'Yes, I can see he is a "bit of denial" and a "bit stoic". No sense of "fight". I did challenge his denial of events, going out on a limb prodding him to respond, to get his to show some emotion. I felt guilty about doing that. He just said 'I don't want to talk about that'.

He was going the next day, that's why I wanted him to talk to him about it. He went back to talking about his son. He felt that somehow his stress about his son had caused the recurrence of his melanoma. Then his family came in – he didn't want to talk in front of them. At handover, I raised the need to enable Paul to talk about his feelings. The next day, Monday, we had two hours to go before he left to go to Addenbrookes at 9 am. It was really busy. I couldn't create the opportunity to be with him. And then the transport arrived – he was about to go when he burst into tears and gave me a hug, thanking me. I asked the ambulance men to have some tea for 15 minutes so I could spend some time with him. They agreed. That was all they could spare. We went into the office. He was distraught. He's coming back in one week, but I felt I hadn't done my job. I felt bereft. Sad for him and sad for me. I was thrown back into my job. At handover, the staff asked me how it had gone with him. I didn't handle that well. They said 'we know he would crack at some time, but when?'

I rang Addenbrookes each day to see how he was. He was isolated in a side room, which made it impossible to speak with him. My husband picked up the vibe and suggested I visit him. That put me in a dilemma whether I should visit him or not – where to draw the line between taking work home and becoming involved with patients and families. I do have some regret about not visiting.

Chris 'I sense your "regret" reflects your sense of involvement and the dilemma of where to draw the line. Yet you are only human and need to accept that sometimes you become drawn unwittingly into the other's suffering. That's a consequence of your concern for Paul and other patients as a part of your everyday practice. Perhaps you need to accept that's OK rather than punish yourself. It is a learning concern to balance concern with poise – the ability to know and manage yourself within relationship without diminishing your concern'.

Alexia: 'I know, but that doesn't make it any easier'.

Chris: 'But at least you can appreciate the dilemma in realising your holistic beliefs and begin to work towards "holistic balance" because, as your experience reveals, your practice is entrenched in emotional work. Another aspect of "being available" (linking to the being available template) is knowing the person, and that knowing the person engenders concern for the person'.

Alexia 'I feel that knowing Paul was paramount – "Who is this man?" "What were his feelings and thoughts?" "What meaning did he give to this illness experience?" Tuning into what was significant for him. It might have been assumed that his melanoma was the most significant issues for Paul and yet his unresolved feelings about his son most occupied his mind'.

Chris 'I can relate that to an experience shared with me by a surgical ward sister about a woman with breast cancer whose greatest concern was being made redundant from her job. In other words, nothing can be assumed. Reflect whether your assessment tools enable knowing the person well enough?'

Alexia: 'I don't know. I haven't given that any thought. I feel I am very perceptive but other staff? I need to consider this. I feel very attached to Paul. It's important to understand his sense of loss and unresolved sorrow ... to know where he is coming from'.

Chris 'I'll send you a paper on chronic sorrow [2] that may help you reflect deeper on Paul'.

Alexia 'Now, I do feel I responded appropriately to Paul, although having turned it over with you maybe I did absorb Paul's distress and become distressed myself?'

Chris (smiling): 'You pose this question? It wasn't easy to manage your work priorities differently, yet you did create the space to be with him and your concern for him enabled him to cry and communicate his distress. It's good to become more sensitive to these processes. Reflection lifts such issues to the surface'.

Alexia: 'I desperately wanted Paul to respond I can see now that this had to some extent become my need and when he couldn't respond except at the very end I felt I had failed. When faced with such family turmoil I did become entangled. I had wanted to fix it for Paul'.

Chris: 'That's such a vital insight. Whether he responded was his responsibility not yours – we can't force people to make use of ourselves. I am going to assume that when you talk about a holistic vision you acknowledge that the nursing role is to enable Paul and his family to find meaning in their experience in order to make best decisions about his/their life'.

Alexia: 'Yes, I accept that perspective. Working with cancer patients and families that is important. The emotional, psychological, social and spiritual aspects of care are really important. Since I have been on the ward we are moving towards embracing this approach rather than our prevailing medical model. I think we are getting to know our patients well over time'.

Chris: 'In other words you nurture involved relationships with patients even if some of them, like Paul, initially resist you in their efforts to cope. It is making yourself available to them'.

Alexia: 'Yes'.

Chris: 'We have already noted that holistic practice involves the whole family. Accepting that, do you feel you were overly influenced by Paul's request not to involve his wife?'

Alexia: 'I think we are generally good with relatives. I was in a dilemma about Paul's response. I can see that perhaps I should have confronted him about his wife. Perhaps I could have opened a space to ask how she was when she visited?'

Chris: 'As I see it, Paul was your primary concern. I suspect issues regarding his family will emerge at a later time. If his wife had approached you then that would have been a different kettle of fish. I raise it as an issue because we may become so focused on the person that we miss the bigger picture. One other issue – did you take over Paul's care because you felt the named nurse could not respond adequately?'

Alexia: 'It's true, I hadn't perceived the named nurse's role. I simply stepped in and responded as I did. I need to de-brief that situation with the nurse involved and with the team at large about the way their comments reflected their anxiety about Paul'.

Chris: 'As a holistic leader, do you think it's vital to prompt dialogue within the team and for you to get support from your colleagues, whereby colleagues are available to each other in ways that mirror nurses being available to patients and families?'

Alexia: 'I hadn't given a thought about support for myself except that I take it home with me. In this situation I feel I need to be "professional", to be strong which means appearing to cope'.

Chris: 'So tell me, what does "professional" mean? Does it mean that professional nurses cope and don't burden their colleagues? Put that into context of the type of team you want'.

Alexia; 'I do want a team that can support each other. It would be much healthier to deal with emotional fall-out at work not just for me but for everyone. I am trying to let go and trust the staff. I can link this back to previous experience where this had not happened, where I needed to appear tough, to win respect and trust. I sense now that is just role-modelling "being tough" to other staff and that's not the team I want. You make me think about leadership. It has been something I have rather taken for granted especially as I have had no teaching to be an effective leader. Further focus for reflection!'

Chris: 'What has been significant about sharing your experience concerning Paul?'

Alexia: 'I suppose recognising and reframing my sense of failure and guilt, thinking that I should be there for my patients at all times'.

Chris: 'Before our next session, reflect on how these feelings come about. Turn them over and have a good look at them. In my experience you are not alone- so many nurses are riddled with guilt. It's as if we take responsibility for everything and blame ourselves harshly if things go wrong. Dickson [3] calls this the "compassion trap" as if we are trapped by our concern and caring ethic. You absorbed Paul's suffering as your own and suffered. You know it's not your own but you can't break free from it. To reiterate- your work is to balance your concern with poise. So let's stamp on this guilt now!'

Chris stood up and stamped on it.

Alexia laughed: 'I do feel as if I have unloaded my rucksack. I do feel better by sharing it. I will also de-brief with my team and reflect on ways we can develop the therapeutic team with them. That feels good'.

Chris: 'Let's review the session through the lens of the being available template' (see Figure 5.3)

Alexia: 'Sounds good'.

Chris: 'First vision'.

Alexia: 'I have a stronger awareness of my leadership and person-centred practice'.

Chris: 'Your concern?'

Alexia: 'My concern for practice has always been strong. However, I feel it has been nurtured and gained strength. It has become more focused'.

Chris: 'Knowing the person?'

Alexia: 'Knowing Paul and his family has gained new dimensions by reflecting on how I tune into and ride his wavelength notably is understanding the way he responds to his illness'.

Chris 'Skilled response?'

Alexia: 'My perception has sharpened leading me to view new ways of responding to Paul. Yeah- I feel more confident'.

Chris: 'Poise?'

Alexia: 'This has been the big issue- unravelling myself to see myself and my emotions more clearly. Someway to go I think'.

Chris: 'Creating a holistic Environment?'

Alexia: 'This session is the new beginning to create a unit environment to support holistic practice. It is vital. The whole session has been enlightening and empowering'.

I added to the notes a quote from 'The Tibetan Book of Living and Dying' [4]

> 'Suffering gives you such an opportunity or working through and transforming it. The times you are suffering can be those when you are most open, and where you are extremely vulnerable can be where your greatest strength really lies. Say to yourself then: "I am not going to run away from this suffering. I want to use it in the best and richest way I can, so that I can become more compassionate and helpful to others". So whatever you do, don't shut off your pain; accept your pain and remain vulnerable. And don't we know only to well, that protection from pain doesn't work, and that when we try to defend ourselves from suffering, we only suffer more and don't learn what can do from the experience?'

Session 2

Chris: 'Any issues arising from the notes?'

Alexia: 'I can relate my experience with Paul to another patient who again aroused strong emotions within the team. He's a 42 year old Asian man who has throat and tongue cancer. This is attributed to the Bangladeshi habit of berry nut chewing and smoking. I brought the nurses together to debrief the strong emotions aroused by this man's attitude. I shared my own feelings of frustration and anger at this man which I felt enabled other nurses to share similar feelings, feelings that had been bottled up. One nurse had been having nightmares about this man, which stopped after she was able to release the tension. The Rinpoche quote you added to the notes was a real revelation about facing up to suffering rather than bottling it up. I read it to the nurses and they immediately got the message'.

Chris: 'How nurses bottle up feelings, brewing self-harm reflecting what we talked about last session that nurses feel they should be able to cope'.

Alexia: 'I felt I acted as a significant role model by enabling and empowering staff to share their feelings. We agreed we must spend more time this way. I told them we will spend 20 minutes, the patients can wait'.

Chris: 'We can frame this release of tension within the metaphor of the "water-butt theory of stress" (see Chapter 4). In this metaphor, stress is like rainwater filling a water butt, fills up the body until it reaches a point where the practitioner feels she is drowning. By then it's too late to relieve it except by "blowing your top" – which makes a mess everywhere and distracts others from the issues that caused the mess. Others hurry around to mop up the mess because it makes them feel uncomfortable. Practitioners need to become sensitive to their "water-butt" filling. Now, the water-butt has a tap which enables the gardener to draw off water at appropriate times to water the plants and help them grow and bloom. In a similar way, the practitioner can draw of stressful energy and use this energy positively to grow and bloom. You could say that's my guide's role is to help you do this. That's what you did, you helped your staff open their taps and use this energy in positive ways to enhance practice. I'm sure they grew through the experience'.

Alexia: 'I can relate this back to Paul, I was reluctant to disclose myself with my staff because I felt I needed to be strong. Now I feel confident about this, letting go of this need. I can see how this worked to bring the team together, a team that could become mutually supportive acknowledging the tough work it did and that we are only human and suffer from human vulnerability'.

I acknowledged the significance of what Alexia had shared and added 'How did this man feel about what was happening to him?'

Alexia: 'He had rejected radical surgery that would have seriously disfigured him whilst only adding months to his life. This had raised ethical issues about such surgery. The surgeon had discouraged the man's acceptance of the surgery option but nevertheless had offered the patient the choice. I doubt whether he would accept the offer of radiotherapy although palliatively this would increase his comfort. He had refused a gastrostomy tube. He was in fact booked into theatre next week to have the tube inserted. He had also taken out along peripheral line for total parental nutrition. This type of line was now used more and more instead of central lines. He had Asian food brought in ... the smell filtered across the ward'.

Chris: 'How did you feel about the smell?'

But before Alexia answered Chris continued: 'the food must have deodorised the smell from his tumour'.

Alexia laughed: 'It didn't ... the two don't mingle well!'

Chris: 'I can imagine the tumour smell and how awful that must have been for the man and his family'.

Alexia: 'Yes. His wife looks about 12. She doesn't speak English. He dominates her. The nurses haven't been able to respond to her in terms of her needs'.

Chris: 'How much is that an issue?'

Alexia: 'He has a 15 year old son who acted as an interpreter. One came up but was dismissed by him. He wanted everything said through his son. It was his son who had to tell his father his prognosis. I was concerned about the son being expected to do this ... the son had been in tears'.

Alexia laughed anticipating my next question: 'Yes, I do feel maternal to protect the son'.

Chris: 'Indeed. The son may well have been in tears anyway. At least the son telling his father enabled the son and father to share the moment as difficult as that was, that such feelings can be openly expressed. I assume the son will take over the mantle of the father in the household'.

Alexia: 'I know there is a risk of us (the nurses) taking his behaviour as a personal affront and labelling him negatively with the uncaring consequence of avoiding him. I can identify the cultural issues and can make sense of this man's attitude to women and that being a white woman and nurse made little difference. The man was quite happy for a nurse to do "menial chores" like taking the urine bottles away. He had been uncooperative with his tracheostomy tube changing. I had to confront him sternly about the need for the nurse to do it. He had ceased to talk to her after that. A nurse who spoke his language had, off her own back, tried to create the opportunity for him to talk about his illness, but he rejected her approach and ceased to have anything to do with her as a consequence'.

Chris: 'Does this explain why the staff feel angry towards him? Do we expect him to be "nice" whilst he struggles to come to terms with his cancer and forthcoming death? Underneath his antagonising surface response what are his deeper needs? Maybe he responds as he does in his effort to control his environment- a proud man brought to his knees?'

Alexia: 'He had been a school teacher in Bangladesh. Now he's a cook. Perhaps that has eroded his pride? He wasn't receptive to the tales of my Indian travels. Perhaps he has a hang-up about the colonial past or perhaps it made him reflect on his death and that was too painful?'

Chris: 'You highlight how easy it is to assume "who he is". Perhaps his deeper needs are not to be prised open for him to talk about his feelings, but to shut them up in his pride – a man who must cope for his own and his family's sake. Maybe the time will come when this façade falls apart and he needs emotional support? Linking this back to Paul's experience, do we impose this need to talk and be cooperative because he and his family are suffering seeing that our role is to ease their suffering? And when the approach is rejected, and rejected in a hostile and abusive way, the reaction is hurt with the risk that we reject him. The key to "being available" is to communicate concern and availability to him so he knows and can respond when he needs to, as difficult as that maybe'.

Alexia: 'I know that's right but it is sometimes difficult to sit back and watch the suffering, especially when you know there maybe better ways. It makes me think of Rinpoche's words. I have become more sensitive to myself within the situation. This has developed quickly from the previous session. I catch myself saying to myself "this man is making me angry- now am I responding for the best?" "What is prompting his anger?" I'll use the ideas of "being proud" and "in control" in debriefing with the staff. That's really helpful!'

Chris: 'The significance of empathy- how do we know the experience of the other and what meaning the event has for him? This experience illustrates the barriers that come between knowing the answers to those questions. Let me suggest something; a useful tactic at hand-over is to pose such questions as "What meaning does this event have for Mr Ali?" "How do you know that?" if someone responds, "How is his wife feeling?" The idea is to turn handover into an opportunity for group reflection and learning rather than merely handing over information'.

Alexia: 'We work with many Asian families and I do feel we are sensitive to cultural issues, so it would be good to surface these types of questions to clear a space to see him and challenge own negative feelings'.

Chris: 'What's been most helpful this session?'

Alexia: 'Building on issues from last session releasing energy into positive action through understanding why things are as they are and ways of changing them for better care'.

Chris: 'My intent was to enable your cathartic release. Releasing negative energy opens a creative clearing for the practitioner to yourself more clearly in context of the particular situation and hence more open to understand its nature to gain insight, notably poise, into its resolution to inform future experiences'.

I added to the notes William Blake's poem [5] 'On another' sorrow'

Can I see another's woe
And not be in sorrow too?
Can I see another's grief
And not seek for kind relief?

Session 3

Chris: 'Any issue from the notes?'

Alexia: 'I really got the message with William Blake's poem! I'd like to pick up our care for the Asian man. He's back in. My approach is very different. It is very positive. I felt a much greater connection with him which opened up possibilities for working together. The nurses all said "On no, why can't he go to another ward" when they heard he was coming back in. I confronted them with their negative attitude and helped them see him in terms of his needs and what we can offer him rather than in terms of their own concerns. They accepted that. A lot our patients are coming back in with bad news – we have three in particular. I sensed that staff feel precarious at this time as a consequence. As one staff nurses said "I don't want to be here this week"'.

Chris: 'Yeah, work can certainly seem stressful at times especially with the type of patients you work with. Still it is good staff can express their feelings and release some energy'.

Alexia: 'I feel good about my own care although I did challenge myself if I should feel good working with patients and staff who were clearly suffering'.

Chris: 'But saying that, you are shifting the ward culture so staff can express their "suffering" and work through it. Is it helping people with their suffering that brings your sense of feeling good and satisfaction?'

Alexia: 'It's true. Caring for patients brings me much satisfaction. It's what I became a nurse for. This satisfaction is increasing now I've found ways of being with these people in ways I feel are caring. And now I'm not absorbing the suffering as my own so much'.

Chris: 'You highlight Benner and Wrubel's [6] assertion that realised caring is the antidote to stress. They suggest that nurses are stressed because they have lost connection to caring and need to reconnect themselves to caring'.

Alexia: 'I sense the wisdom in that. I feel that is my own experience since working with you which parallels what I'm trying to do with my nurses. I do have two positive experiences to share concerning families'.

Bob and Molly

Bob was trying to protect Molly, his wife, by not talking about his feelings about his forth-coming death. I felt very close to this man. He talks about me as his friend. When he came in, he looked awful, dehydrated. I went home and worried about him over the weekend, resisting a strong urge to phone the ward to see how he was. On the Monday he was like a changed person, the colour back in his cheeks. I took his wife aside and asked how she was feeling. She was fearful but anxious to talk with Bob about the future, but she felt she couldn't approach him with her need. I had asked Bob – 'Did he contemplate his death – what did he feel about that? I brought Bob and Molly together almost as if they had fallen in love all over again'.

Chris: 'You tuned in to them and there came a moment when the time was right to bring them together by gently confronting their restrictive attitudes rather than force the issue. The situation reminds me of Paul from our first session'.

Alexia: 'Yes. The second situation concerned a young man who had been severely beaten up and my response to his older brother. I had taken the older brother aside so his parents didn't know. I was communicating on his level, calling the attackers "bastards", helping him talk through and validate his feelings. When he left he gave me a hug to my surprise and that of his parents! Yet it felt right, a reflection of the connection between us'.

Chris: 'What has been significant in sharing these two experiences?'

Alexia: 'Umm, I'm not sure. Giving myself positive feedback ... building on the other experiences I have reflected on'.

Session 4

Alexia: 'I need to share my experience of responding to a junior staff nurse whose "wrong attitude" is threatening the well-being of the team. I've tried to understand where she's coming from so I can respond appropriately to her but it's not easy to challenge her'.

Chris: 'So you want to confront her, to be tough on the issues but soft on the person?'

Alexia: 'Yes. I have in mind the ideal of the therapeutic team- a team that can effectively support our caring work with patients and families. I realise I have to confront her responsibility to this team'.

Chris: 'I can see it's tough for you to be tough on the issues. I know from the many experiences that practitioners have shared with me, that interpersonal issues with colleagues are the most difficult type of conflict to take action on. It's as if we have become entangled with our colleagues in ways that make it difficult to express negative feelings and resolve conflict in positive ways. I named this as "the harmonious team" [7]. Consequently we avoid conflict and expressing negative feelings and they simply fester. I'll post you the paper. You feel angry at her because she spoils things?'

Alexia: 'She does spoil things and yes it does make me feel angry! And yes, I do not like conflict ... I have a bad taste with this from my previous work'.

Chris: 'It's important to acknowledge this yet you cannot let it go. Your team look to you to role model leadership'.

Alexia: 'I know. I know!'

Chris: 'would it be helpful to role model confrontation?'

Alexia: 'Ok'

Chris: 'Confrontation can be viewed within Heron's "Six-category intervention analysis [8]". Do you know this work?'

Alexia: 'No'.

Chris: 'Basically it sets out six communication interventions

Authoritative	Facilitative
Giving information	Being cathartic (enabling the other to express some emotion releasing negative energy)
Giving advice	Being catalytic (enabling the other to talk through an issue)
Confrontation (confronting another's restrictive attitude or behaviour)	Supportive (being there for another)

Research by Burnard and Morrison [9] suggests that nurses tend to use and feel comfortable giving information and advice and being supportive. They tend to avoid and feel unskilled at being cathartic, catalytic or using confrontation – all interventions vital to holistic practice. They avoid confrontation because of the risk of conflict'.

Alexia: 'I fit the bill on that one!'

Chris: 'Yet conflict needn't be emotional. Some advice – first approach her using catharsis to help her express her feelings – for example "how do you feel working on the unit?" Then using a catalytic intervention such as – "Are there any issues you would like to talk about?" You can then confront her by explaining the value of the therapeutic team and asking how she feels about that giving her feedback that she seems to struggle with being part of this team. How does that feel?'

Alexia: 'Easy talking about it. Doing it may prove more difficult'.

Chris: 'The key to confrontation is to stay in adult mode rather than be a critical parent scolding the naughty child. You want the nurse to take responsibility and grow into an adult. That's transactional analysis theory. Would it be helpful if you made the therapeutic team more explicit? For example, at Buford we wrote the need for this team in our vision statement – as such, consider writing a new vision statement with your team expressing your beliefs about practice?'

Alexia: 'You're right- she makes me feel like a critical parent. I can see that is the wrong mode to be in – it's something I have to be mindful about as with all aspect of leadership'.

Chris: 'What has been most significant about the session?'

Alexia: 'Getting my angst about the staff nurse off my chest and exploring the theory. I so want a team that works well together and she's been a thorn in the side'.

Chris: 'I'll attach my handout on TA to the notes with reference to Stewart and Joines [10] if you want more information'. (The TA template is shown in Figure 17.1)

Session 5

Alexia: 'The notes were helpful to reflect on last session. It induces another level of reflection. The theory was really relevant. I'm now looking at all my relationships through the TA framework! However, I haven't taken any action with the staff nurse as things have quietened down'.

Chris: 'In other words the conflict is contained but continued to simmer and would undoubtedly rear its ugly head again'.

Alexia: 'That's true but I do feel better prepared to tackle it more positively when that happens. I want to share my experience concerning Tom, a 47 year old man who has been readmitted with an abscess. His wife had breast cancer- she was 45. They have two daughters. His major concern was for her rather than himself. He had wanted to go home to be with her when she died. She had visited the ward on one occasion -she had clearly been beautiful and now she looked so ill. He was a night club owner, had drunk and smoked a lot. I had kept him as long as possible for rehabilitation. He went home and she died at home the next day peacefully, I've become very close to Tom …'

Alexia paused and then reflected on her connection with Tom and spoke about the way she talked with him about his feelings over what was happening to his wife. Alexia was animated and tearful in sharing this.

She continued: 'and now, this admission, he asked me yesterday whether the abscess was a reoccurrence of his cancer? I knew from the consultant that it was 98% certain, yet I have avoided telling him. I've felt uncomfortable and unprepared to talk with him even though I suspected he knew. I'm devastated by this … gone home and felt guilty and angry at myself – why hadn't I handled it well? I felt he knew because he intimated that he would be spending some time in hospital now envisaging Christmas'.

Chris: 'I can really sense your suffering. What is significant to explore?'

Alexia: 'Talking it through it now, I feel prepared to tell him, that I can leave this session and deal with it. I'm conscious of the staff's reaction – a sense of "Oh no!" that Tom should have to go through this now. I see I have to spend time enabling Tom to talk through his feelings about his wife's death. That's where his head is … he's been talking about the funeral and making connections between now and the past'.

Chris: 'That's so important making the connections between what is happening now and the past is crucial in moving forwards. Marris's theory of change [11] and loss helps us frame this temporal connection before people can move on. Indeed, what can Tom look forward to right now?'

Alexia: 'I know the significance of this temporal connection. Marris [11] certainly helps me see it more clearly, bringing it more into consciousness'.

Chris: 'So why do you feel so entangled with him? What makes him different? Is it simply the immensity of this human tragedy – his wife dying, his cancer and the depth of your connection with him'.

Alexia: 'I don't pity him, it's genuine compassion – so why do I feel guilty? Why do I blame myself? You've challenged me before to create a space to put these things. I feel I've always had an open relationship with him but I saw it wasn't the right time to respond to Tom's question and it needed to be the right time because I had to make sense of Tom's illness for myself'.

Chris: 'I may have challenged you before but the way we see and respond to these situations are not easy to change. Ways of responding and reasons for responding as we do are deeply embodied. Through reflection and dialogue we bring these things up to the surface and contemplate them. Tom would know how difficult the question was to respond to.

Can you release your guilt and pick it up with him – "Tom, that question you asked me yesterday ...." I wonder whether the abscess was a reaction of Tom's effort to work out his grief an that being in hospital was an opportunity for him to be cared for, to give up a sense of responsibility? However, be wary of making assumptions and jumping to conclusions in your effort to "know", It might give you a sense of control but it cuts down possibilities. Once we think we know we are no longer curious and explore'.

Alexia: 'Maybe that's true ... it is so easy to jump to conclusions about what is happening to patients. I'll take my feelings into the staff room and share and explore these'.

Chris (jumping in): 'And overcome your feelings of needing to protect him as a mother might for her hurt child. Remember, it's his life. You said you don't pity him but consider the difference between pity and compassion'.

Alexia: 'I can see I have absorbed Tom's suffering and feel protective towards him and suffered because of this. Yet this does not deny my genuine sense of compassion for him. I sense my compassion and pity have got entangled leaving me vulnerable and distressed'.

Chris: 'Your concern for Tom enables you to be available to him'.

Alexia: 'Yes, but should I be so attached?'

Chris: 'Something to reflect further on – it is a strong theme running through your shared experiences. Let us finish the session by imagining a space between us to put your suffering as we did before when I stamped on your guilt. Just honour your suffering and slowly breath it out with each breath ....

(after a few minutes of silence) ... this may be a useful technique to use with patients such as Tom who are distressed'.

Session 6

Alexia talked about her miscarriage, relating this to a staff nurse she had worked with on her last ward. 'She annoyed me because she didn't want the child as she had two children. I now feel guilty about my response. The nurse had needed 6 months off work for counselling. I felt she had eked it out, gaining sympathy from every quarter. I should have been caring and I wasn't. People have been so caring towards her- fantastic midwives and I wasn't so fantastic. I have spent a couple of days dwelling on it. I won't do anything about it now but at least I have worked through some of it'.

Chris again noted Marris's theory of loss and change [11], noting that Alexia was connecting her past with her present and trying to heal a broken thread so she could move on. They linked this experience to the way Alexia was endeavouring to establish the therapeutic team on the ward, a team that was mutually available to each other in ways that mirrored a holistic approach to patients and families. In working through her experience, Alexia felt she had come to terms with this dark shadow that had haunted her. She felt it was teaching her an important lesson – that to be available to the other, we need to know and manage our own concerns. Alexia immediately felt 'softer' towards the nurse she had talked about in session 4 and reflected again on whether she knew this nurse well enough and whether her irritation blocked the view.

Chris: 'It's about tuning into her wave-length and then managing the resistance between you to be available to her. I predict she will acknowledge that and feel understood and cared for'.

Alexia: 'Too often we set the wave-length and expect the other to tune into us. I can see that with patients and families. Sometimes we get close but at other times we are miles apart. As you say, they must sense that and feel uncared for as we impose our expectations without even acknowledging their own'.

Chris: 'What has been significant about today's session?'

Alexia: 'The session has been like a confessional enabling me to off-load emotional baggage yet in ways that enabled me to understand why I had responded as I did and relating that experience to staff I currently work with who resisted me in some way. I can see my concern for patients makes me vulnerable to be intolerant towards others. Big learning curve!'

Session 7

Alexia: 'I've come prepared having written and reflected on two experiences in my journal I wish to share with you. One is "frustrating" and the other one "good". I'll start with the frustrating experience as its been going on for some time about my role. I have been in post for one year this week in my dual role as ward manager and head and neck practitioner for the hospital and community. When the post was set up I was supposed to spend two days on the ward and three days in the practitioner role. However, I can't get away from the ward. I told my managers that I need a junior ward manager to support me. I have three senior staff nurses and one of them is taking a lead role. She should be paid for the role. She feels that way too. She said "I could get a sister grade somewhere else". But she loves the ward, the work. I'm frustrated for her and she's feeling frustrated. When I broached the issue with my managers they said they would look into it. My immediate manager agreed with me but the nurse executive doesn't believe I need a sister grade.'

Chris: 'Tell me more about the role split?'

Alexia: 'The reason why I am a few minutes late was because of a visit to a tracheostomy patient on another ward. I am getting a lot of consultant referrals to see patients but I'm finding I'm doing these in my own time, often in the afternoon when I'm tired'.

Chris: 'There seems to be two issues: managing your time and making a case for the junior sister. Consider managing time- can you do an analysis of the use of your time within a vision for the practitioner role. Do you have a vision?'

Alexia: 'No, but it's time I did, especially as the head and neck unit is becoming a regional centre'.

Chris: 'Okay. First task. Second task, if I may give advice, is to plan your off-duty to accommodate your practitioner role and make the case for the junior sister, linked to the development into a regional centre. Do you have budgetary control to allow for the sister?'

Alexia threw her arms in the air, clearly exasperated: 'They say you have the budget but when you say you want to spend the money differently, they say you can't!'

Chris: 'So real issue about who controls the budget. How powerful do you feel to assert yourself and make the argument?'

Alexia: 'I don't know'.

Chris: 'Stand and indicate how powerful you feel'.

Alexia placed her hand on her chest.

Chris: 'Really assertive people would place their hands on top of their head'.

Alexia laughed: 'Some room to grow then?'

Chris: 'Visualise filling this room with your presence'.

Alexia: 'It's like pumping yourself up. It feels really powerful, this sense of presence'.

Chris: 'When you next meet with your managers, or indeed anyone else, especially if you feel they are more powerful than you or intimidate you, use this technique and see how it goes'.

Alexia: 'It is true I feel intimidated by the nurse executive. She makes me feel like a naughty little girl. It's as if she has to assert her authority'.

Chris: 'French and Raven's sources of leadership typology [12] identify authoritative and facilitative sources of power. Authoritative sources are positional power, coercive power with threat of sanction, and reward power based on external rewards to those who conform to authority. Facilitative power is based on relationships, expertise and internal reward concerned with satisfaction with practice. Management within transactional organizations, such as the hospital, generally rely on authoritative power reinforced on a daily basis through "normal" patterns of relating. Subordinates are viewed as essentially irresponsible and taught to "know their place" within the system, "seen but not heard". In other words not to have a voice'.

Alexia: 'I can sense that. It rings true in my experience, feeling an undercurrent of coercive pressure. As a leader I am naturally attracted to the facilitative sources of power; being an expert in my field and using my influence to lead people rather than imposing my senior nurse status. The reward for all the team is realising our vision of holistic practice although I can the staff nurse's desire for promotion as an external reward'.

Chris: 'You can imagine managers don't appreciate assertive practitioners who would threaten their control leading to coercive responses to control the rebellious child'.

Alexia: 'Looking back on my feelings of anger at the staff nurse, I wanted to smack her for not being a good girl. That's really scary! I can see the significance of relational power in enabling and trusting the staff to become responsible. The French and Raven typology gives me a broader perspective of power I hadn't figured before'.

Chris: 'So- your task is to assertively make the good argument, to play the "rational" game or, in other words, to speak their language in ways that cannot resist or easily shrug aside'.

Alexia: 'My manager is leaving. However, the doctors do value me highly and we could bring the doctors on board with their "political clout" even though it would reflect how "small" the nursing voice is within the corridors of power. I could threaten to resign?'

Chris: 'A power-coercive tactic to call their bluff. Another tactic might be take the "moral high ground" to highlight the detrimental impact of their decisions on patient care and staff morale?'

Alexia: 'I feel like a conspirator against the empire. I feel much better about it. I no longer have a problem1 I can see what `I need to do. I'm back on the rails!'

Chris: 'That reminds me of a Bob Dylan album "Blood on the tracks" – the way conflict often ends with metaphoric blood on the floor. These sorts of issues wear us down, sap our precious energy, deplete our ability to care, erode our motivation. This experience is very significant in reflecting on your leadership role, and contemplating how you can shift the conditions of practice to support holistic practice'.

Alexia: 'The good experience concerns Tim, a 39 year old man who has a tumour of his tongue. A 40 a day smoker, social drinker, and barrister. He had a lump on his tongue for two months and he didn't do anything about it. He hadn't been to a dentist for 10 years. A friend took him there and the dentist referred him to a consultant. He missed two appointments, so eventually the dentist brought him here himself. In surgery they removed most of his tongue, just a sliver left, reconstructed from muscle. After the surgery he was transferred to another hospital because of shortage of beds. I was very disappointed because he did not get specialised head and neck care. I eventually got him transferred back when a bed became available. He was an absolute quivering wreck ... such a proud and intelligent man. For some reason or another I didn't meet him for one week after he got back. The nurses said he had been hard work. Then, last weekend I "took him" on a Saturday late shift – looked after him all shift and started the "rap".' He was used to commanding but now felt out of control. He had never been in hospital before. I felt for him, the control issue – tuning into him. He couldn't speak. He had to write everything down including his feelings. We spent four hours chatting and broke down the barriers. He bared his soul. He didn't want to die. His children. His family came in, his wife was 'stand-offish'. She went at the end of the day and we could pick up our conversation. His biggest fear was not being able to talk again in court and as an after dinner speaker. I was truthful – I never lied to him – I said that he would talk again but not with his previous voice.

Chris: 'What has he been told by the surgeons?' Alexia: 'They told him he had up to five years. The cancer had invaded neck lymph glands. He will have radiotherapy after the surgical recovery. Next day, Sunday, I blocked off the tracheostomy and asked him to say "hello". He said "hello" and burst into tears. He asked me to do it again when his wife came in. I did – he said to her "I love you". I was on cloud nine, "making a difference". It's a wonderful relationship'.

Chris: 'And the moral of the story?' Alexia: 'Reading the pattern and enabling him to take control and the mutuality of relationship. He asked about me, cared about me'.

Chris: 'You said the staff found him hard work?'

Alexia: 'Yes. I will debrief with them and use my work with him to teach staff. The time is right to move to the Buford model. I find myself using the pattern appreciation cues with him (the cues are set out in Chapter 6). They just make utter sense!'

Chris: 'If all the team use the cues it will guide them towards more holistic care especially when linked to an explicit holistic vision – nurses can then link the cues to realising the vision creating both direction and purpose'.

Alexia: 'I can see that. I get so caught up in what's happening everyday that essential practice as constructing a vision gets sidelined. I can see its value. I really can'.

Chris: 'Tell me about Tim's sons'.

Alexia: 'Tim's two youngest sons visit at the weekends, although they live a considerable distance away. His wife visits every day but always leaves after lunch to be home in time to collect the boys from school. The two youngest boys are very loving towards Tim and obviously miss him and accept their father's new body image. They run down the ward with excitement and in anticipation of seeing their dad. The youngest boy sits on Tim's lap while the other sits on the bed beside him and they recount their tales of school and play time. Tim looks forward to their visits. The eldest son has only visited once. He seemed reluctant and afraid of seeing his father. His body language was closed and his facial expression suggested that he felt very uncomfortable on the ward. Instead of greeting Tim and sitting close together as the rest of the family did, he hovered around the bed area refusing to sit down, hands in pockets, taking more interest in the television than his dad. After the family left I asked Tim about his eldest son. He told me his behaviour was nothing unusual. He had kicked against school and family, and did not seem to grasp why his father was ill. Apparently he had expressed that he was embarrassed by Tim and had to be cajoled by his mother to visit. I suggested that maybe he couldn't cope with his father being ill and this was his way of dealing with it? Tim agreed this might be a possibility. He hadn't thought of the situation in that way. Tim's wife and two youngest sons remained in constant contact throughout his stay. The sons spoke daily with Tim on the phone but the eldest son was either out or refused to come to the phone'.

Chris: 'Your work with this man is profound. We can look back over the experiences you have shared and see this thread of holistic practice. Now you are beginning to shift the conditions of practice to accommodate and facilitate holistic practice through the ward'.

Session 8

Alexia: 'Tom, the experience I shared in session 5, may be coming back in. he had an infection. I am going to see him in out-patients this afternoon'.

Chris: 'How do you feel about that?'

Alexia: 'I have a fight with myself. I'm pleased to see him again but I don't like to see them come back in. He sees us as his family now, like we are his daughters. His daughter, Claire, phoned us this morning. She said "Dad isn't very good, another infection. He's just like when mum died. What shall I do?" I felt awful because I lied to the bed manager in order to save him a bed even though he might not come in. if I had been truthful they would not understand'.

Chris: 'Is this an indictment of the system?' Alexia: 'It is. On his last admission we didn't have a bed and he went to another ward for three days before we could get him transferred back to us. He was distraught'.

Chris: 'And what did that do to his health? But can you morally justify your action to manipulate the system to ensure a bed? We can use ethical mapping to explore the dilemma of whether to manipulate the system to save the bed or be truthful to the bed manager (see Figure 4.2). Let's commence with the bed manager's perspective'.

Alexia: 'Her perspective, as I suppose it must, is to view the bed and patient as objects. They cannot see the person, even if I made the point of "showing" her Tom- he would still be an object. The system takes the humanness out of the system. I suppose it would be chaos otherwise'.

Chris: 'And Tom and the nursing staff's perspectives?'

Alexia: 'Considering how distraught Tom was before and knowing we know him and his specialized care, the neck ward is undoubtedly the best place for him'.

Chris: 'In other words he might come to harm on another ward?' The ethical principle of 'not doing harm'. Tom has no choice. His perspective is discounted by the system. Hence, your manipulation reflects a duty of care and responsibility over justice- the system. The system must view the opposite – justice over caring, otherwise the system would simply collapse.

Alexia: 'I feel awful about this'.

Chris: 'Where does this sense of "awfulness" come from?'

Alexia: 'Because I lied an feel guilty as if a naughty child afraid of being found out and punished. What I did was covert'.

Chris: 'Why be covert? Why not be up front and say No ... the bed is saved for Tom if he needs it?'

Alexia: 'Why not indeed! I don't think I'm ready to have my head shot off!'

Chris: 'Going back to the assertive action ladder- you highlight the need to make a good argument and counter any coercion to toe the line without risk of being seen as "uncooperative" with threat of sanction. If you don't challenge the system then the system is reinforced and cannot learn'.

Alexia: 'This takes me back to last session and exploring the nature of leadership power. The struggle to assert self against the transactional organization and the struggle to be "in the right place" to do best for our patient and staff'.

Alexia continued by talking about the change in Tom's illness trajectory from night club owner and that lifestyle, the way the images had been stripped from himself – flash lifestyle to a person searching for meaning and finding new meanings in a new set of values about the beauty of life and people met along the journey ... and for his daughters and personal assistant, from shiny clothes and immaculate hair to track suits and roots showing through.

Chris: 'Does Tom fear death?' Alexia: 'I don't think so. He wants to live for his daughters and yet he looked forward to joining his wife'.

Chris: 'From what you say, it sounds as if Tom has "brought himself home" to face up to and grow through his crisis?'

Alexia: 'I am just reflecting on my journey since last May when I commenced these sessions and its profound impact it has made on both my personal and professional life. My husband said I am a nicer person, less stressed and more fulfilled. I felt hat to be true but I would never have imagined the impact of guided reflection in coming to know and transform myself. I am more available to everyone and can live out my holistic beliefs with certainty'.

Session 9

Alexia: 'I confronted the staff nurse we talked about in session 4. I told her how I felt and that I wasn't going to put up with it anymore. She dissolved into tears but I didn't feel bad about it. It's a step in the right direction. Before, I would have felt bad about it'.

Chris: 'Guilty?'

Alexia: 'Yes. And now I don't. I'm proud of myself'.

Chris: 'And the consequences?'

Alexia: 'She now knows how the rest of the staff and I feel about her and the ward is not going to put up with her behaviour anymore. She knows what she needs to do. I've put it in a positive light and if she can't do that then she knows that I do not want her as a member of the team. And I don't feel guilty about that either! I couldn't have done it a few months ago. I have the strength to do that now. I'm on top of the world again!'

Chris: 'You remind me of a quote by Anais Nin[i] that says "and then the day came when the risk to remain tight in bud was more painful than the risk to blossom"'.

Alexia (smiling knowingly): 'I had been off for six days and when I returned to work I was met by a barrage of complaints about her. I asked myself – "what's going on with this nurse?" I didn't sleep last night because of it ... and then I acted today. I feel free!'

Chris: 'Now it becomes easier to deal with it again if necessary'.

Alexia: 'I feel that's true. I've started to collect evidence in a diary of events anticipating further struggle along the road. I was looking at Dickson's book [3] you shared with me concerning assertiveness and the four stereotypes of women- This nurse is an "Ivy" – the indirectly aggressive woman – the way she was saying things about me to other staff, that I was insensitive and lacked compassion, trying to set staff against each other.'

Chris: 'Reflect on the way you responded to her. Do you know where she's coming from to act as she does? Are you responding to her behaviour rather than trying to understand it? Draw links with the "difficult" patient'.

Alexia: 'I don't like her although she is a good nurse'.

Chris: 'What do you mean by a "good nurse"?'

Alexia: 'She did say last time that she had a lot of personal problems'.

Chris: 'So she gave you a cue. Do you need to show her the team does care for each other? Even if she rejects your approach at least you can say you tried?'

Alexia: 'You face me with a new dilemma having thought I had solved the problem. I felt that I had an "open door" for my staff to approach me'.

Chris: 'Saying the door is open is one thing but staff walking through it is quite another. Perhaps you need to extend a hand?'

Alexia: 'I still feel good about the situation but you have challenged me. I think I will see her again. Be more mindful of staying in adult-mode to help her grow-up and take responsibility as a member of a therapeutic team rather than as a critical parent to a naughty child'.

Chris: 'TA is certainly a useful analytical tool. How is the junior sister situation (picking up from session 7)?'

Alexia: 'I went back to the consultants. They value me highly as the senior nurse on the unit. Their support is not yet active but will be. I'm gathering information from other head and neck units to support my argument. I am meeting with the acting senior nurse about levels of role responsibility'.

Chris: 'Which is a move towards dialogue and negotiation. So, the idea is not ruled out anymore. You are mobilizing support'.

Alexia: 'Yes, to play the power game. They will not want to lose me'.

Chris: 'You are learning the "political-power game" with increasing astuteness'.

Alexia shifted the context of the session: 'Paul (from last session) has died on the ward. Seven staff have gone to his funeral, reflecting the caring between staff. He was admitted as a medical problem and was going to be admitted to a medical ward. I heard he was in A & E but anticipating his need to be admitted here I prepared a room for him. We wanted him to be admitted here as well. I knew he was dying but they said they had to sort out his problems. His wife and daughters were very distressed. They contacted me. They said he was going to the medical ward, can't he come here? I sorted it out- spoke to the medical SHO. He said Paul had arrhythmias and other medical problems that required treatment, a pneumothorax that required chest drainage. He wanted him on the medical ward for 24 hours, wanted to do everything. I accepted this and explained to his family that Paul would be transferred after 24 hours. The SHO promised that is Paul deteriorated he would not hesitate to send him to us. I went to see him in A & E- he was clutching my hand saying "take me to William Hart ... take me to William Hart". You can imagine how I felt. I handed him over to the ward staff. I returned at the end of the shift. He had taken a turn for the worse. He had none of the planned treatment. A NFR order. Just for TLC. Therefore I asserted that they transfer him to us! This led to a full blown argument. I was getting nowhere so I contacted the senior nurse and she supported his move back to William Hart- he was with us within half an hour. He sighed "I'm home". It was all I needed, a marvelous feeling. The staff were elated and the family were joyous. It was worth fighting for, to the bitter end'.

Chris: 'The way the power of caring smashed the petty politics. You took the moral high ground and triumphed. Brilliant!'

Alexia: 'I was not going home until I won it and the staff knew that'.

Chris: 'Role modelling empowerment and assertiveness. Would the staff have been able to fight like this if you hadn't been on duty?'

Alexia: 'Umm ... I doubt it'.

Chris: 'Perhaps de-briefing with the staff may help to empower them? The situation reminds me of the way you manipulated the bed system to create the conditions where becoming available to Paul and Tom became possible. That is such a significant caring factor'.

Alexia: 'I did a double shift to support the family, him and staff, to ensure he got the care he deserved. I did that as much for me as for him and the family, so I knew I had done my utmost. The staff were distressed that he was dying'.

Chris: 'Did you feel you were getting entangled absorbing the family's distress?'

Alexia (giving me a knowing look): 'I was conscious of that. The issue was knowing it and managing it. I did not feel distressed on his behalf. We did get him home for two hours so he could sit in his garden and listen to the birds in the sky. On the morning he died he said to me "I'm going home today and take a very long walk". I knew what he meant, that he was going to die but I felt contented. He had spoken to each family member and each member of staff and thanked us. He waited for his family to be out of the room before "letting go". I was deeply honoured to be in the room and that he could talk openly to me. He really touched me. I'm not grieving for him. I'm happy for him. He said something similar to his wife. She came and said to me – "what's he talking about going home? He can't go home as if he was confused and rambling"'.

Chris: 'It's easy to misinterpret what dying people are saying. For example, Callahan and Kelly [13] note the dying people often wrap up important messages in allegorical language, highlighting the importance of listening to what people are really saying, not simply what is said on the surface'.

Alexia: 'At the funeral his family were pleased to have us. I wondered if our presence would remind them of the past few days but the wife seemed to find it easier to be with us than with her family. She sought us out. She said to me "You loved Paul didn't you? You cared for him every minute as if he was your father. I always thought of you as part of the family."

It made me realise why I am a nurse and what I want to do in the future, to be a head and neck Macmillan nurse'.

Chris: 'And Tim? What happened to him?'

Alexia: 'After his discharge Tim came back to visit us on a number of occasions. Unfortunately I was either not on the ward or on days off but the nurses told me how he looked and what he had said. Then, just recently, I was lucky enough to be working when he attended clinic and on hearing I was on the ward he came up. We greeted each other as old friends. I could not believe how great he looked. He had lost around two stones and it suited him. He had also cut off his moustache. I told him he looked years younger which he reveled in! I asked him about his family. He said his eldest son was still being very difficult which he and his wife found emotionally hard. He had given up his job to enjoy family life. As he put it "we are financially secure and I just decided that my family were my life, not my job". I have to say this came as a bit of a shock as all he ever wanted when he was an in-patient was to get back to work. He asked me the latest on the nursing staff and how I was- our reciprocal relationship speaking up again! As he walked down the ward I felt proud; I felt he had made it and we had helped him. I felt positive that in the future he would set things right with their eldest son. I look forward to the next installment with him'.

Chris: 'Your story illustrates how people come to seek and find meaning in their lives triggered by the crisis of illness and the specter of death and the significance of the nursing role. It also gives meaning to the Buford NDU model cue- "what meaning does this illness have for Tim and his family". Your caring dialogue with him was grounded in responding to this cue'.

Alexia: 'I can see that's so significant. We need to set another date'.

We didn't set another date as Alexia went on extended sick leave related to her pregnancy. The span between sessions 8 and 9 had been 3 months due to circumstances. Yet it provided a space to look back and draw together the threads of the various experiences extending through the narrative and to celebrate Alexia's realisation of becoming more available to her patients and her leadership in creating a holistic and supportive clinical environment.

Reflection

The dialogue is a compelling narrative of guiding Alexia towards realising person-centred practice. As stated in the first session – 'It all starts with vision and stories'. She was very person-centred but got emotionally entangled in her involvement with patients. The dialogue is her struggle to develop the necessary poise to understand and manage her emotional entanglement and, in doing so, to trust her colleagues to do a good job.

References

1. Bolen, J. S. (1996) *Close to the Bone: Life Threatening Illness and the Search for Meaning.* Touchstone, New York.

2. Eakes, G., Burke, M., Hainsworth, M. (1998) Middle-range theory of chronic sorrow. *Image: Journal of Nursing `Scholarship* 30, 179–184.

3. Dickson, A. (1982) *A Woman in Your Own Right.* Quartet Books, London.

4. Rinpoche, S. (1992) *The Tibetan Book of Living and Dying.* Rider, London, p. 317.

5. Gardner, S., Blake, W. (1998) *The Tyger, the Lamb, and the Terrible Desert: Songs of Innocence and of Experience in its Times and Circumstance.* Fairleigh Dickinson University Press.

6. Benner, P., Wrubel, J. (1989) *The Primacy of Caring.* Addison-Wesley, Menlo Park.

7. Johns, C. (1992) Ownership and the harmonious team: barriers to developing the therapeutic team in primary nursing. *Journal of Clinical Nursing* 1, 89–94.

8. Heron, J. (1975) *Six Category Intervention Analysis* third edition. Human Potential Research Group, University of Surrey, Guildford.

9. Burnard, P., Morrison, P. (1991) Nurses' interpersonal skills: a study of nurses' perceptions. *Nurse Education Today* 11, 24–29.

10. Stewart, I., Joines, V. (1987) *TA Today: A New Introduction to Transactional Analysis*. Russell Press, Nottingham.

11. Marris, P. (1986) *Loss and Change*. Routledge and Kegan Paul, London.

12. French, J., Raven, B. (1968) The basis of social power. In D. Cartwright, A. Zander [Eds.] *Group Dynamics Research and Theory* (third edition). Harper & Row, New York, 150–167.

13. Callanan, M., Kelly, P. (1993) *Final Gifts*. Bantam Books, New York.

Note

i. https://allpoetry.com/poem/8497015-Risk-by-Anais-Nin.

CHAPTER 12

Guiding Caitlin to Realise Her Leadership and Vision of Person-centred Practice on a Medical Ward

Introduction

Caitlin agreed to be a respondent in a research project to evaluate the impact of clinical supervision on enabling clinical leadership [1]. She is a team leader on Sunflower ward, a typical medical ward within a large district general hospital. Our relationship spanned 10 sessions spanning over 12 months. I informed her I would take notes of the session for her perusal to pick up next session for agreement and continuity of the sessions.

For all intent and purposes, I approach 'clinical supervision' as guided reflection. Hence, the terms can be used interchangeably although clinical supervision by definition (see Chapter 13) has a specific agenda to safeguard the public, leading to potentially a more judgmental approach depending on the 'supervisor's attitude (see Figure 8.4).

Session 1

Caitlin noted her vision was to lead the ward team to realise 'holistic' values in the ward's everyday practice. She acknowledged that the ward did not achieve this. When asked why she revealed her frustration – 'It's difficult to say exactly why ... perhaps its because most nurses just want to get through the work, as if they don't really care. I know that's a terrible thing to say but it feels like that'.

In response to learning through reflection she said 'I've had no experience with reflection. It wasn't an approach used in my training'.

Chris: 'We can remedy that – simply bring an experience to share next session. Try and write this down in a reflective journal using the Model for Structured Reflection cues (see Figure 2.2). But don't worry too much about it. We can talk through the cues next session applied to your experience'.

Caitlin: 'That was useful. Just talking about holistic practice and leadership strengthens my intent to realise it. It is motivating. I'll try and commence the journal'.

Session 2

Chris: 'How did you feel about last session and reading the notes I sent you?'

Caitlin: 'They reminded me what we talked about. Got me thinking about myself and developing practice'.

Chris: 'Do you have an experience to share?'

Caitlin: 'Yes. I haven't written it down or really reflected on it. It feels like a confession. I feel I am a 'softy' because I failed to tell Debbie, a junior colleague, to do a ward round with the consultant'. The consultant was asking me questions he could have asked the patient, which I then had to do, questions that Debbie could have answered. I felt uncomfortable, so I asked Debbie to take over from me when she had finished handover. She offered but was reluctant. She said she didn't know the patients particularly well and was anxious about this. So, I didn't insist. I got home at 4.40 pm. Debbie got home at 3.40 pm! I asked myself – 'why did I do that?' Why didn't I insist when she asked – 'do you want me to do the ward round?'

Chris: 'So why didn't you?'

Caitlin: 'A number of reasons really. Debbie has personal difficulties right now and I was conscious that the consultant liked "sister" to do the rounds. He plays to the audience. He makes little jibes to keep the nurses in place'.

Chris: 'Familiar humiliation tactics. Chapman [2] noted how these jibes keep nurses "in their place." You suggest he is a stickler for tradition – likes 'his' sister buzzing around him enduring his humiliating wit'.

Caitlin: 'I felt guilty expecting Debbie to do the ward round but also angry at myself. I feel I am a softy. If anybody is doing the giving in I feel it's going to be me! I feel I am telling tales! Is that usual?'

Chris: 'It seems to be the cultural norm, a part of a culture that discourages open conflict in order to maintain a sense of false harmony. You're not telling tales. You're not "attacking" Debbie in any way. Neither is being a "softy" a weakness. It shows how much you care about people, wanting to make it ok for people. But a consequence for you is to take this all on board when this responsibility belongs to others. Consider- who would have benefitted if you had insisted that Debbie took the ward round?'

Caitlin: 'The consultant would have got a better deal. I wouldn't have had this frustration. For patients – probably better care. For Debbie – to help her accept her responsibility and grow in her role. Before "team nursing," the most senior nurse would have taken the ward round'.

Chris: 'Perhaps Debbie still saw it that way – that you were the senior nurse and she felt uneasy doing the ward round? Because the structure of the ward organisation has changed doesn't automatically mean that people's expectations and behaviour will change. What do you feel you need to do?'

Caitlin: 'I'm not sure'.

Chris (paused to let Caitlin think about her options): 'Ok. Let me offer some suggestions for you to consider. One option might be to debrief with Debbie so you can both learn through it?'

Caitlin: 'This would be difficult although I know I should. I don't like conflict and try to avoid it. Perhaps that's why I always give way?'

Chris: 'You highlight the barrier of conflict avoidance. You are not alone. The majority of nurses seek to avoid conflict – a paper by Cavanagh [3] will give you perspective. I'll attach a copy to the notes. How do you feel about this situation now?'

Caitlin: 'Right now, recognising I am a softy, I feel better immediately off-loading. Given the same situation I like to think I can act differently. I would phrase it as a question to Debbie – "Are you going to do Dr Grouch's ward round?"'

Chris: 'But why give her the choice if there is no choice? You want her to do the ward round. You feel this is a legitimate then tell her – "Please do the round Debbie." If you give her the choice you also allow her to say "no" then what do you do? You can either accept her refusal and experience internal conflict as you experience or confront her and risk inter-personal conflict with her. I think your concern for Debbie is "misplaced" because it is essentially about avoiding conflict rather than right practice. We need to develop open and honest relationships within the team when we can tell others what we really think in a supportive ways rather than avoid dealing with difficult issues that arouse uncomfortable feelings'.

Caitlin: 'On reflection I can see that I should have asserted to Debbie to do the ward round- that would have been the best decision. It's been an eye-opener exploring the reasons and ethics that constrained my ability to assert myself. I know better my role responsibility to support team nursing and colleagues. Being a softy is not the best place to be in!'

Chris: 'The mantra – "tough on the issues, soft on the people"'.

Caitlin: 'I'll remember that!'

Session 3

Caitlin: 'I've been saying to people "don't give people a choice if there isn't one!" And it doesn't make me think that I'm not nice to people! I tested my assertive ability in giving a 'difficult' student some feedback about her personal mannerisms that had alienated her from the team. I reflected on it in my reflective journal. I wasn't entirely comfortable doing giving her feedback. These situations, first with Debbie and now this student are difficult for me because I am anxious about upsetting people and causing conflict. I still want to avoid them. The mantra 'tough on the issues, soft on the people' rings through my ears and has really helped me move beyond viewing these situations as personally threatening. Confronting the student has enhanced my concern for my team colleagues because it enabled me to deal with an underlying sense of frustration that team members felt and looked at me to deal with'.

Chris: 'Wow. It's amazing what just one guided reflection can do! Did you read the Cavanagh paper I sent you?'

Caitlin: 'I did. I could see myself! It really confronted me with conflict avoidance. As a leader I need to move into the collaborative mode and I feel that I have made a start. Not easy. Not comfortable but it is important'.

Chris: 'How did you feel about writing about the experience in a journal?'

Caitlin: 'It felt strange at first and then I got into it. Using the MSR cues was very helpful to open up aspects of the experience. The cues made sense and were easy to use. I did mention our first two sessions to Wendy, my ward manager. She was impressed. She felt she was also a conflict avoider'.

Chris: 'It's helpful to involve her and get her support so you do not feel alone on this journey'.

Session 4

Chris: 'Any issues arising from the notes?'

Caitlin: 'I can relate my difficulty with giving the student feedback to my 'difficult' relationship with Mrs Driver, the wife of one of the patients who I feel negative towards. How do I put it? She's critical of how we care for her husband in indirect ways. She says something like – 'my husband is meant to have three fortisips a day, how do you expect him to pierce the top himself?' I responded that earlier he didn't want it and so we didn't pierce the top to keep it fresh. She drives me onto the defensive'.

Chris: 'Why do you think she's being so critical?'

Caitlin: 'Because she cares … she is the main carer at home. Maybe she thinks we don't care enough'.

Chris: 'There are theories that suggest it's tough for carers to give up their caring role to a nurse. They may feel they can care better. Dawson [4] noted that spouses in particular may perceive "giving up caring" as failure, equating failure to care with failure of marriage role with subsequent guilt. Spouses may project this "guilt" into you, the nurse, through complaining about little things that in their mind, are not good enough. Nolan and Grant's survey [5] identified that "professionals" fail to identify and respond to carer's needs within the care setting, in particular recognising and responding to the carer's emotional needs. Your experience highlights the holistic value to "see" the "whole" family rather than just the patient in the hospital bed, especially elderly people who are likely to be discharged back into the community. You've perceived this wife as a "nuisance" rather than emphasise with her. You've only seen a crabby bold woman giving you an unfair hard time. Her criticism is a projection of her anxiety. As a consequence you want to avoid her. Hawker's research [6] illustrated the way acute ward nurses responded to relatives as essentially a nuisance to be managed because they interfere with "smooth running" of the patient's management. Ask yourself- "What support does Mrs Driver need? Does that feel like a lecture?"'

Caitlin: 'A bit … but it's useful. I can relate to what you are saying. It fits the picture. I can see how I have resisted her at a time when she most needed understanding and acceptance, not to see her as a threat or feel guilty'.

Chris: 'So what would be your tactic for dealing with Mrs Driver?'

Caitlin: 'I could involve her more in care, acknowledging her role, sympathising how tough it must be for her'.

Chris: 'Try it out. Is she in today?'

Caitlin: 'Yes she will be. Okay. It feels good'.

Chris: 'I suggest we reflect on your experience with Mrs Driver's using the "Being Available Template" (see Figure 5.3). It's based on the premise that the holistic practitioner is available to the person to help them find meaning in their experience and to help meet their needs. It identified six attributes that determine the extent the practitioner, yourself, can be available: intending a vision of holistic practice, knowing the person, concern for the person, responding with skilled action, poise, and creating a conducive environment. It offers you a mirror to look at and assess yourself'.

Caitlin: 'I can judge myself harshly against all these attributes'.

Chris: 'You could but you have demonstrated insight into these attributes. Going back to Mrs Driver you can apply these insights immediately'.

Caitlin: 'I've had another run in with Claudia. I was on an early shift after a couple of days off. I noticed that all of the ill patients were in the top half of the ward – that's team A, much more than in the bottom half of the ward – team B. I decide to balance the load by moving a terminally ill patient to team B. I discussed this with Claudia in team B – she was ok about this. I said I would discuss it with his family. They were fine about it as well, in fact they were happy for him to have a single room. Later, one of the patient's relatives came to me and said the patient was wet – could we come and help him? I went with Beth, who was taking Team B after hand-over. We were appalled at his condition. He had a bottle between his legs which had filled and spilled. It made me think he had been neglected. We washed and shaved him and did his pressure area care. These were much worse than I had seen them before. The crease of the sheet was clearly indented on his hip even though he was on a 'nimbus' bed. I immediately felt guilty with moving him'.

Chris: 'But you didn't feel guilty earlier when you moved him?'

Caitlin: 'No, but he should have got a better deal! I felt I had dumped him! Beth told me I needed to speak to Claudia about this, so I asked her who was allocated to care for Mr Smith that morning. Claudia responded – "we all mucked in." She was defensive and denied my accusations. She said the family were going to wash him that afternoon and that he had been turned'.

Chris: 'Do the family normally wash him?'

Caitlin: 'No. They help him shave'.

Chris: 'So her comment probably was untrue. Is one of the dangers of a 'nimbus' bed that nurses think they can leave patients?'

Caitlin: 'But not when they're wet!'

Chris: 'Do you think your hand-over to Claudia was adequate?'

Caitlin: 'Perhaps it wasn't but she had the same hand-over as I had from the night staff. I assumed she would know what to do'.

Chris: 'Maybe as the patient was in team A she paid less attention than to team B patients, not expecting a transfer of a patient between teams? I take it you were unhappy with Claudia's response?'

Caitlin: 'She was defensive which irritated me'.

Chris: 'Let's use Transactional Analysis (TA) to reflect on the pattern of communication between you'.

Chris drew the characteristic Parent-Adult-Child pattern for Caitlin to consider her pattern of responding to Claudia:

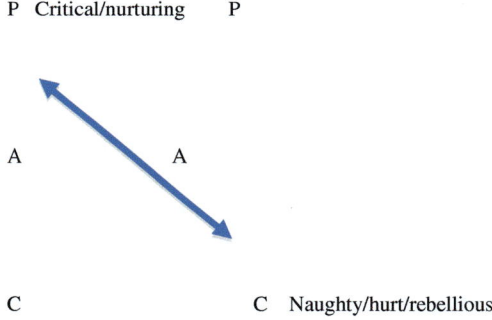

Chris: 'Ideally people respond adult- adult. However, due to anxiety people flip into either parent or child modes and talked through often forcing the other person into a reciprocal response so lines of communication do not cross. If they do cross then communication breaks down' [7].

Chris: 'Now draw a line showing how you would like to respond?'

Caitlin drew a line between adult-adult.

Chris: 'Why did you draw that line?'

Caitlin: 'Because it reflects the way I want to respond as a leader'.

Caitlin: 'I can see how I became anxious about the relative's complaint and flipped from "adult" into critical parent mode. It must have made her feel like a naughty child and squirm to escape responsibility. I need to encourage Claudia to accept responsibility for her actions without fear she was being told off. I can clearly see how I fit into that pattern. That's really enlightening'.

Chris: 'Perhaps Claudia lacks experience at planning and prioritising care?'

Caitlin: 'Probably. So how can I help her?'

Chris: 'One option might be to spend a few minutes after a morning handover helping her to plan her care? She may not feel competent- there is some research that suggests that newly qualified staff need to be seen as competent and avoid asking for support because it would expose their lack of competence [8]. Does she have preceptorship?'

Caitlin: 'No, she hasn't. I feel I've got off on the wrong foot with her'.

Chris: 'Can you see why that is?'

Caitlin: 'At least three reasons. I was angry at her because of this incident; angry at her defensive response when challenged about it; and I guess I don't like her ... Andrea, the other new staff nurse does not have preceptorship either. She's on my team so I'll set that up for her'.

Chris: 'Another option could be to set up a formal appointment to de-brief the whole situation with her?'

Caitlin: 'Go on ...'

Chris: 'You could role-model being big about making mistakes, something like "I should have handed over to you better or helped you plan your care", or "I should have arranged preceptorship for you". In doing so, she might learn that it is okay to drop any façade of competence, that it is okay to ask for support and not be defensive'.

Caitlin: 'I know I need to deal with it but not how to go about it. I just thought – I've pointed it out and she's denied it. Where do I go from here?'

Chris: 'Look at the bigger picture – consider your role responsibility as a leader to protect patient care and support staff. Perhaps she needs positive feedback when she does things well rather than just negative feedback when things go awry? That fits a culture norm of transactional organisations when people are spoken to only when something is not good enough. De-briefing might make you feel more positive towards her and towards yourself enacting your leadership role'.

Caitlin: 'I like being open and honest about these issues but it's difficult to contemplate tackling Claudia. As you know from my experience with Debra, I shy away from conflict with staff although I know I need to deal with these issues more positively. Such care wasn't good enough and neither was Claudia's response'.

Chris: 'Well, we've planted some seeds to grow. What's been useful about today's session?'

Caitlin: 'I've been really challenged about managing my feelings, dealing positively with conflict rather than avoiding it, and my role as a leader to support staff and in doing so, changing the ward culture as there is no culture for this type of work. You've been very challenging but also very supportive. It shows me how I can be the same with colleagues. I have a new mantra – "stay in adult mode!"'.

Session 5

Caitlin: 'I re-read the notes (from last session) this morning. I felt very bad not speaking to Claudia. I decided to not bring up old issues with her but as time went by I felt I should have done that because another situation cropped up. It brought it back into my mind. I felt I had opted out because she's not in my team – why me dealing with it? The ward was very busy after that over the bank holiday weekend. When I came on duty I saw how awful it had been, including Claudia. She was already stressed – I felt I would be adding to her stress. I need to be assertive but I still see myself as a softy'.

Chris: 'We've talked about this before. The culture of conflict avoidance is very powerful so you mustn't give yourself a hard time over this. We can understand the culture and the need to change to enable you to fulfil your leadership responsibility and create a healthy ward climate so conflict can be dealt with positively. The Cavanagh paper I sent you used the Thomas and Kilmann conflict management grid [9]. You positioned yourself as an avoider but desired to be collaborative'.

Chris drew the grid and talked through the descriptors for each mode

Chris: 'Where do you position yourself today?'

Caitlin: 'As before – clearly as an avoider!'

Chris: 'As I noted before, you are not alone. Cavanagh's research [3] revealed that the majority of nurses and managers respond in this mode. You noted before you would lime to respond in collaborative mode as a leader?'

Caitlin: 'Yes so as to work with people without fearing the fall-out if you don't see eye-to –eye. Maybe I mix up assertion with aggression? But when I think about it I can be assertive. There is a situation I'm thinking of where I challenged a medical decision. The patient, Elsie, was clearly dying. She had a PEG tube inserted but since the tube was inserted she had been having excess secretion following her feeds. I felt it was inappropriate to feed her. However, the consultant, Dr Pierce, said it was his duty to feed her. We are excluded from this type of decision so we need to assert our right to be involved ... to have a voice'.

Chris: 'The MSR cue – Did I act for the best draws your attention to "ethical mapping" as a way to reflect on this situation from the different perspectives of nurses, doctors, the patient and relatives, and the organisation, and then consider the ethics in terms of the "best decision" and how the decision was actually made. The dilemma is "whether Elsie should be fed"'.

Caitlin: 'Elsie had expressed her wish to George, her husband, that if she ever got like this to "let her go". George was distressed by Elsie's "bubbling" – asking why can't we deal with it? I am sitting her thinking how am I going to assert no-feeding with Dr Pierce?'

Chris: 'He intimidates you?'

Caitlin: 'In the past when his domination was threatened his response was to threaten to inform managers'.

Chris: 'Like a bully boy using coercive-positional power to get his own way and keep nurses in their place. But this power is weak when challenged because it is not grounded in the right decision. Understanding Elsie's wish you hold the moral high ground, assuming Elsie is mentally able to make the decision- then respecting her autonomy is paramount? Seedhouse [10] considers autonomy the highest ethical principle'.

Caitlin: 'Yes, she is fully aware. I can see my primary responsibility lay with Elsie and her husband rather than passively accepting the medical decision. Appreciating the "ethics" of the situation adds a new dimension to my thinking and reflection'.

Chris: 'Remember the MSR cue – "Did I act for the best?" that impacts on every decision we make. To be collaborative is to be assertive. The "Assertive action ladder" may enable you to develop your assertiveness. I have a copy in my sachel'.

Chris showed Caitlin the ladder (Figure 12.1)

Caitlin: 'I can position myself on each step of the ladder. Step 4 – making a good argument is vital. Thus an understanding of the patient's perspective and ethical theory is vital. Step 7 may need some work especially in the face of someone who generally disregards you. Remaining in adult mode is absolutely vital – thinking back to using Transactional analysis, especially when your view is resisted as with the medical staff. It is about being poised to know and manage my feelings and responsibility within the situation to remain in adult

10	Treading the fine line between pushing and yielding	
9	Playing the power game	
8	Staying in adult mode	
7	Being communicatively skilful	
6	'Just do it!' [JDI]	
5	Creating the optimum conditions to assert self	
4	Making a good argument	
3	Authority to assert self	
2	Ethically right to assert self	
1	Feeing the need to assert self	
0		

FIGURE 12.1 The assertiveness action ladder.

mode. Understanding step 10 is like a safety valve, knowing you haven't failed if you do not win the argument ... knowing that you have collaborative intent where it takes two to tango!'

Chris: 'We can pick up on Elsie's care when we next meet. Do you find it easier to assert yourself with the medical registrar than with your nursing colleagues?'

Caitlin: 'Yes, because I work with the nurses every day ... it is more personal'.

Caitlin: 'A positive experience! Mrs Driver and I have become the best of friends! I did go and see her the next day and chatted with Reg and asked how she was and how were things? She just opened up and shard her fears. She talked about the empty house. I invited her in to care for Reg. It was really easy!'

Chris: 'What do you learn from this?'

Caitlin: 'Give someone's carer acknowledgment and build relationships. It's happened a lot since then. A patient's "stroppy" daughter was talking to me ... agitated, tutting .... I acknowledged how she must be feeling. She just stopped and started talking about her anxieties'.

Chris: 'Your cathartic intervention was like bursting a bubble ... you opened a clearing for her to express her fears and feelings'. The magic of saying 'How are you?'

'With a heavy emphasis on *YOU* as concerned eyes search hers, to sense her wavelength. *How are you?* is a deceptively simple question that opens a therapeutic space'.

Caitlin: 'I really felt I tuned into her wavelength and flowed with her. I was reading about that. It was such a visual image to relate too. It makes it much easier to talk about difficult things within a relationship. For example, making a decision about whether to resuscitate a patient at the weekend. I could talk to the daughter about it as the locum doctor didn't know the patient. I could make the decision with her'.

Chris: 'It shows how working with the family makes such decisions easier. Work by Robinson and Thorne [11] may help you put your relationship with Mrs Driver into greater perspective'. They noted three ways relatives construct relationships with caring staff:

1. Naïve trusting whereby the family believe that the caring staff view the situation from their perspective and have their best interests at heart.

2. Disenchantment whereby the family realise that the caring staff view the situation differently, leading to disenchantment, conflict and potential breakdown of the relationship
3. Guarded alliance whereby the family reconstruct the relationship in order to get some of their needs met. They learn to manipulate the system to achieve this.

Caitlin: 'This experience has certainly shown me how working with the family makes decisions easier and makes me feel good. Mrs Driver was in the guarded alliance relationship having become disenchanted. I feel now she has shifted into naïve trusting, at least I hope so. Before, I had this risk of becoming involved. I linked it to controlling work time. But this was all done in ten minutes. The results were well worth it and on reflection I can see how this can save time in the long run. It brought us a long way. The only trouble is that they all want to talk to me now! The "she listens, she understands" syndrome'.

Chris: 'You note the two impasses of emotion and control to developing a therapeutic relationship identified by Ramos [12]. I'll send you her paper- it will help you appreciate these impasses more clearly. Your experience shows how available you have become to them. Imagine before- all that distress and unmet need without nurses being available to respond?'

Caitlin 'I now feel much better realising my caring self. Holistic values come alive!. Introducing the reflective frameworks and theories has been enlightening. The really help me see myself within situations and ways of responding differently. I can see that assertiveness and collaborative intent are vital to becoming an effective leader. It is a challenge though to break through being a softy and avoiding conflict'.

Chris: 'You didn't feel bombarded with theory?'

Caitlin: 'No, because it all made sense in relation to my experiences. It helped to frame our dialogue and develop my insights'.

(In my notes, I added the following related to our dialogue about asking 'How are you?')
Cameron [13, p. 53] noted

> 'How are you? is a question that turns us back to who we are as health care professionals and calls us to be more deeply attentive to the moment. When we *sincerely* ask "how are you," we enact our ethical commitment to one another'.
> '*Sincerely* differentiates the therapeutic from the merely sociable. Indeed, *how are you*? as a social ritual is likely to disengage rather than engage Mrs Driver if she interprets the greeting as merely a social nicety'.

Session 6

Caitlin: 'The Cameron quote was like icing on the cake! I felt the differentiation! Can I pick up Elsie's care?'

Chris: 'Of course. Remember guided reflection is your space'.

Caitlin: 'We reduced Elsie's feed because she was so "chesty" but 10 days later she was still alive despite all predictions! Dr Pierce wanted her feeds recommenced, well "all hell broke loose"! He discussed it with us. He was reasonable but he cited the "Tony Bland" case, noting the court ruling that the case was not to be set as a precedent and therefore each case had to be judged on its own facts. He said his hands were tied and hence we had to resume feeding her. He left it to me to tell the family. Well, I was not happy with that, so I informed the family to come in and arranged for them to see him. The family didn't want the feeding ... it was difficult for George. He was influenced by his daughter who was also a nurse. The family responded by threatening to cut the tube! They asked if another consultant could take over so Elsie could go to a hospice. Dr Pierce wanted the feed continued next day so it was arranged for her to go to the hospice that night. Dr Pierce was not happy with that in case she died in the ambulance. Elsie died the day after. This was a real predicament for me. I really cared for Elsie and George. George was being pulled in all direction and had to sign he agreed to take her own discharge. George was tortured seeing her groaning. He wanted her to live as the old Elsie, not this Elsie. He hoped she would wake up and be her old self'.

Chris: 'I can see how tough that was for you. You showed how the essence of holistic care is being available to work with the patient and family to meet their needs. In knowing the family's perspectives you were more in tune with them and worked with them to ensure the best decision and appropriate action is taken'.

We can reflect on the extent you are developing your ability to be available using the Being Available Template (Figure 5.2).

- Holding vision
- Your concern
- Knowing the people involved
- Your skilled response
- Your poise
- Creating a holistic environment

Caitlin: 'OK. I am more mindful of realising my holistic values. However, it is so easy to get wrapped up into the everyday issues that the intent sometimes slips away. Guided reflection certainly brings it back into focus.

I have always been concerned for patients, families and staff. As my reflections have shown I have shied away from involvement and conflict that seem to blunt this concern in terms of self-preservation. However, learning holistic skilled responses have certainly enabled my concern to flourish. Again, I have always prided myself on knowing my patients but using catharsis and catalytic skills have opened up this knowing regards peoples' feelings and thoughts, with staff as well'.

Chris: 'Perhaps using the Buford NDU model cues would facilitate knowing the person more-notably the first cue- "Who is this person"?' (see Chapter 6)

Caitlin: 'I agree. Our assessment of the patient is very functional with no real emphasis on how the person is feeling and thinking. I must look further into that. I have your book! [14]. Looking at my skilled responses I feel good about the way I enabled the family to assert their views and arrange transfer to the hospice. Also challenging the consultant's decision fuelled by my concern for the family I can see how my concern about the consultant's actions motivated me to take action. Yet I had collaborative intent. I didn't set out to compete. It was about doing the right thing from an ethical perspective, exposing the inhumanity in the feeding regime, the relative's distress and the inadequate analgesic response.

I definitely think I am more poised by not being so anxious about involvement and conflict by putting the person's needs as paramount in holistic care. Not sure about creating an environment?'

Chris: 'It is reflected in your actions in being a role-model for others. Your leadership is blooming!'

Caitlin: 'That's good to get such feedback. I do feel more of a leader though much work remaining notably in staff relationships'.

Session 7

Caitlin basked in a sense of achievement with her work with Elsie and her family: 'It felt really good to talk about Elsie's care. It has made me much more aware of the ethical issues involved. Dr Pierce listens to me more now than before. I can highlight that. We have a

62 year old man, Ray, who has a terminal meningioma which has been controlled by ste-roids. He was last admitted in a coma because of steroid omission. This time, we will keep him in hospital until he dies. We've stopped the steroids- this has been agreed with his wife. Lucy. She wasn't coping well with him at home'.

Chris: 'How does Ray feel about the steroids being withdrawn?'

Caitlin: 'He was not involved in that decision'.

Chris: 'Okay. That might be something you want to reflect on. Tell me, why was his wife not coping? Can she helped to cope better? Might dying at home be Ray's preferred option? Has anybody talked to him about his forthcoming death? Is he lying there wondering why his drugs have been stopped?'

   Caitlin paused before this battery of questions fired at her: 'Ray's talk is 'confused' which limits conversations with him'.

Chris: 'Is this the rationale for not involving him in his own death management? Research by Callanan and Kelley [15] considered that dying people are often labelled "confused" without adequate assessment. They challenge us to be more open and listen carefully so we can understand their messages. They claim that the dying person's messages are usually attempts to describe what they are experiencing, or requests for something they need for a peaceful death, for example reassurance that the other person can cope. What do you think?'

Caitlin: 'I'll listen to him again with "new ears." I'm uncomfortable with this idea of collusion with Lucy and excluding Ray from the decision to withdraw his steroids because I hadn't seen it and felt this was a good example of managing death, yet, if Lucy is coping should I challenge this? It would surface a potential conflict of interests between her and Ray's needs?'

Chris: 'What are Ray's rights and needs? Did we know these? Is humanness diminished by becoming an object within others' decision making process? We seem to have opened up a number of issues. What do you need to do?'

Caitlin: 'Perhaps help Lucy to explore her feelings about Ray's possible thoughts and feelings bubbling through his confused talk?'

Chris: 'You have shown through previous experiences the impact of using catharsis and con-frontation as therapeutic interventions. These are two of Heron's six category interventions; giving information, giving advice, and confrontation are what Heron notes as authoritative interventions, whilst catharsis, catalytic and supportive interventions are facilitative inter-ventions [16]. These six interventions offer you a communicative framework to reflect on and develop. The skilled practitioner draws on the most appropriate to use. Considering these interventions – how might best respond to Lucy?'

Caitlin: 'Yes, I can see that it's easier to use the authoritative interventions except for con-frontation which I find difficult because I have always wanted to avoid conflict as we've discussed previously. I can see the facilitative interventions are more therapeutic and dif-ficult to use because, as we've discussed, of the impasses of emotion and control. It would be like opening a can of worms and not knowing how to deal with it. Using catharsis and catalytic interventions, as I did with Mrs Driver, would help Lucy express and talk through her feelings and perhaps create the opportunity for Ray to respond and explore what was happening to him if he desired. Using catharsis would be subtle confrontation about pro-tecting Ray and supportive to Lucy. Wow. I can see how these interventions blend. That is so enlightening!'

Chris: 'Is she on the ward now?'

Caitlin: 'Yes she is. Perhaps I could do this tomorrow. I'm off at 3 pm today'.

Chris: 'Why not just spend five minutes with her now and ask her how she is and maybe sug-gest having a longer chat tomorrow?'

Caitlin: 'Yes. I'll do that. I feel good about that although I'm left feeling ineffective'.

Chris: 'That is the whole point of guided reflection – to take negative thoughts – "I'm left feeling ineffective" into positive thoughts through understanding for taking action. Draw an analogy with shutters – I have helped you open some shutters that limited how you saw the situation"'.

Session 8

Caitlin picked up the Lucy and Ray experience: 'I did go back to the ward. Lucy was in the dayroom with Ray's brother Len. Ray was being turned at the time. I said "Hello Lucy, how are you coping?" She became tearful. I thought "Oh lord, I've delved into it now!" She said "When I'm here it's alright, I don't cry." She was trying to keep a stiff upper lip coping at the hospital. I realised this but challenged her – "Is it important that you don't cry in front of Ray?" and then "Why would Ray think if he knew that the steroids have been withdrawn?" They both jumped in. Lucy said 'Ray has always buried his head in the sand!' I don't know if I told you last time but Ray's operation was open and closed. They never told Ray his tumour was still there. He was told the operation had gone well, that he could get on with the rest of his life. I further confronted her "Had Ray any inkling because he had deteriorated so much?" She said – "Oh no"' She was upset again. She said 'Please don't ask me about it Caitlin. It makes me cry and I don't want to cry'. I respected this.

The next day I was on an early shift. Lucy didn't come in the afternoon and therefore I didn't see her for some days. I kept thinking about it over the weekend, that Lucy didn't want to tell him but I felt she should. When I next saw Ray I asked him how he was feeling – was he feeling rough? He said something to me but I couldn't tell what it was. I got some help to sit him up and gave him some sips of water, and then asked him again but I still couldn't make it out ... you know how it is. I said something like – 'you must be feeling very sad'. I sat with him and held his hand. I asked myself – 'have I left it too late? Had I created turmoil inside him?' I was really frustrated! That evening Lucy was there with him by herself. She was crying. I went in there and sat down with the two of them. She said she was sorry, wiping her tears away. I said – 'No, its okay. Ray knows how you are feeling. I am sure you've had some very good times'. Lucy then reminisced about their times together. He knew what we were talking about. He opened his eyes but he did seem just sad really ... that air about him.

Chris: 'How do you think Lucy responded to you?'
Caitlin: 'Initially she didn't want me to see her crying but once I was in there I could see she was animated talking about their life, going through it all. It was a different kind of chat we had. I felt I got to know her much better. She came especially to see me when she went home and thanked me for the chat. Len had encouraged the suppression of feelings for her protection. She was too vulnerable on her own'.
Chris: 'You were there for her now. You were not available to her before- you had not really shown her how concerned you were for her before'.
Caitlin: 'I can accept that. I shared it with the staff as you suggested. They were very responsive. They were saying "How do start a conversation like that?" Susan, a staff nurse, came up to me later and said – "I thought about what you had shared with us. I didn't know what to do!" She had obviously picked up that we hadn't responded to this situation. She cared, she wanted to be available but hadn't known how'.
Chris: 'And therefore she avoided it'.
Caitlin: 'I felt a lot better. Ray died the next morning at 7 am. Lucy came in later for the death certificate etc. We had time to sit down. She was really pleased she had had the chance to be with him and myself at the end'.
Chris: 'So it made a difference?'

Caitlin: 'It probably did, but I wondered if it was enough. Lucy had often helped Ray, shaving, washing him but not sharing this with him'.

Chris: 'We can see two levels of involvement- one on the physical level, helping him but using this level as a way of avoiding dealing with the emotional level but fulfilling her need to feel useful. The cost of the collusion was that she hadn't said goodbye or enabled him to say goodbye. You facilitated that, that must feel very good'.

Caitlin: 'I felt I had climbed a mountain. The good thing was that all the pretence had gone. It's been really good to go through that. I have been feeling very negative. It has given me a real lift'.

Chris: 'Why so negative?'

Caitlin painted a picture of a really busy ward all summer, problems with instigating nine-hour shifts and the impact on day staff; how work was disorganised, things not being done, patients not happy.

Caitlin: 'I challenged this situation with management at a meeting but was shouted down. I was so frustrated I went home and cried. I felt like a moaning minnie1'.

Chris: 'As if somehow you are to blame for feeling like this? Once again we can see the significance of creating a practice environment to nurture and support our caring effort. It sounds as if you have "battle fatigue"'.

Caitlin: 'Yes, that's it- battle fatigue! I'm going on holiday for a week so what I like best is feeling less battle fatigued!'

Chris: 'Lets review the 'Being available template'.

Caitlin: 'I had been truly available to Ray and Lucy at this momentous time. By sharing my experience with colleagues I felt I had begun to shift the ward culture into a more reflective and holistic mode where people could talk more openly about their feelings rather than pretend to cope or bottle feelings deep inside. Caring has become more visible within the medical model, that caring is significant and did make a difference to peoples' lives. I feel more empowered to care and that was what nursing is all about. Yet the shadow of 'battle fatigue' is a dark shadow that threatens to obliterate the light of caring'.

Chris: 'I do sense your growing frustration with the environmental pressure that stifles rather than promotes holistic practice'.

Caitlin: 'It's good to let the frustration out, sharing it with you. A load of my mind'.

Session 9

Caitlin related Ray's confused talk to a new patient: 'I met him on the Saturday, He said – "I'm dying, I saw an angel ... I'm dying." I immediately identified that with what I had been reading, I confronted other staff that he might not necessarily be confused. People were saying – "Why is he so confused?" The doctors are open to what we have to say – we have a good team at the moment, but as time went on he actually thought he was dead and as time went on it develop into confusion. Doctors were saying – "He's no more likely to die than us!" Later he couldn't remember a thing except he did remember my name'.

Chris: 'It shows you are more open to possibility. How are you?'

Caitlin: 'Picking up my sense of 'battle fatigue I feel more disillusioned now. The plans to extend the staff nurse role to include reduction in doctors' hours, no extra cover and plans to take away the blood ladies and the dawning on nine-hour shifts! We try so very hard and we don't get listened to. They ask us for our comments and these just get filed away!'

Chris: 'How is this affecting you?'

Caitlin: 'I care so much for my patients and colleagues. I care nothing for management!'

Dark Clouds

Before we met for session 10, I had sent Caitlin a note asking her to contact me, which she hadn't done. So, I phoned her on the ward to make this appointment. She had seemed reluctant to do this, saying how fed up she was with everything. However, she agreed to meet.

Chris: 'You sounded desperate on the phone? Reading the notes I can see how you felt when we last met'.

Caitlin: 'It's been going on for a long time really. It does help just to feel listened to. I just want out now. The major thing is the lack of nurses on the ward'.

Chris: 'So how does that impact on how you feel?'

Caitlin: 'Let me tell you about Tim, then you can better understand my frustration. The other shift I was finishing the 6 pm drug round at 8.15 pm when a man started talking to me about his cancer. I had a million other things to do before the night staff came on, and that was wrong because I needed to sit down and talk with him when he was ready to talk'.

Chris: 'So what did you do?'

Caitlin: 'I stayed and talked with him for 5 to 10 minutes'.

Chris: 'You finished the drugs afterwards, therefore the last people to get their drugs got hem at 8.30 pm?'

Caitlin: 'Yes, and then I did the 6 pm IVs'.

Chris: 'What were your options to get round this?'

Caitlin: 'There is no other support available on the ward or from other wards. They are struggling to cope with sickness just now. The doctors could not be approached to do the IVs. They would refuse'.

Chris: 'Did the patient appreciate the 5–10 minutes?'

Caitlin: 'I say he did, yeah!'

Chris: 'He knew you were busy?'

Caitlin: 'I'm not sure because he was in a side room being reversed barrier nursed. He has "neutropenia." He's away from the hustle and bustle. Our talk came to a lull so I said "Tim, I have left the drug trolley outside, I must go and finish these"'.

Chris: 'And he understood?'

Caitlin: 'Yes. He had been on the main ward and would have seen how we worked'.

Chris: 'What was his fear?'

Caitlin: 'He was expressing how he felt in general, how he had worked hard all his life, never smoked, only drank a little, his wife had left him and now he had cancer'.

Chris: 'The "why me" feeling ... and he's going to die?'

Caitlin: 'Yes, and he has this pain which is not well controlled. I tried to explore that with him. He won't take the pain killers because he has a fear of becoming addicted to morphine'.

Chris: 'You must see a lot of people who are dying and yet afraid of addiction?'

Caitlin: 'Yes. It was the first time that he had shared this fear with someone'.

Chris: 'That's important. Does he have a family?'

Caitlin: 'None. He feels quite alone'.

Chris: 'I was just thinking of Ray and Lucy when you said – "Oh lord, I've delved into it now" and here you are under pressure of time and you open up this at this time. Did you feel guilty when you left because of time or feel good that you had spent this time with him?'

Caitlin: 'Good initially. I recognised that sitting down and talking with him at this moment was more important than finishing the drugs, but by 8.30 pm the 6 pm drugs became more pressing'.

Chris: 'So did you feel okay about leaving him then?'

Caitlin: 'I felt bad about leaving him because it was the first time he had shared that. He had been in denial. He said – "this tumour, this cancer, whatever this damn things is, why me?"'

Chris: 'Could he get more support?'

Caitlin: 'The Macmillan support nurse is already involved but I have no confidence in her. She doesn't deal with these issues well. He felt the tumour was caged in his body limiting the way he moved his trunk. He only ever had the pain killers when he was in agony. I explained to him the pain killers would loosen him up, enable him to move more easily. He then said he was worried about the addiction. I knew he needed to be given this information and to think about it for a while, so I left him to think about it. The next day I saw him. He said he had thought about it but rejected the pain killers because of the risk of addiction. I put some leading questions to him "How was he feeling today?" but he just answered these 'yes' or "no"'.

Chris: 'He was putting up his barriers again. Perhaps he felt too vulnerable admitting to the tumour at this time. There were ways you could have continued the work? For example, by reminding him of the words he had used last night and confronting his return to denial? A question of judgment?'

Caitlin: 'Yes, I can see that. But again, did I want to go through all that again when we were so busy? How much time can you give someone?'

Chris: 'He knows you are concerned for him. He knows the ward is busy. You had recognised this man's need at that moment and judged your priorities. You only have so much time- time being a precious resource. It is another example of responding for the best. How would other staff have responded?'

Caitlin: 'Most staff would think me a fool for responding as I did. It illustrates my problem of having time to be with patients like this – there is no time'.

Chris: 'I can see you're hurting with this and trying to cope'.

Caitlin: 'Going part-time and being on the ward every week will help. I'll have time to recover each time although I won't know the patients so well. I'm disappointed with myself. I saw myself climbing the ladder, becoming a ward sister, but not under these conditions'.

Chris: 'And the future of guided reflection?'

Caitlin gave me a knowing look. We left it for Caitlin to contact ne if she wished to continue.

I mused with Caitlin how quickly the glow of working with Lucy and Ray had faded. I felt that caring needed to be sustained on a daily basis not simply in peak experiences, as much as these in themselves sustaining and empowering.

Footnote

Caitlin never did contact me. She went part-time on the ward and working part-time in her own nursing home venture she had set up with two colleagues.

Reflection

The narrative reveals the reality of everyday nursing for many practitioners who know they should be person-centred rather than just getting through the work with insufficient resources. Clearly holding a vision as something to work towards is vital. It is a gathering crisis towards this climax of despair. And yet the narrative reveals the potential for Caitlin to realise herself as a person-centred practitioner and leader. Consider the extent Caitlin had become available to her patients and families. She had clarified and strengthened her beliefs about holistic practice. She had nurtured her concern for her patients. She had developed profound insights into the patients' and families' experience. She could respond with more effective action to meet patient's need. She could assert herself with the consultant. She knew herself better within relationship. And yet, overall, her despair at the system proved to be overwhelming. She was unable to create and sustain an environment whereby she could and her colleagues could be fully available to her patients. In the busyness of the medical ward, this understanding is perhaps not surprising. Her experience offers glimmers of possibility.

The narrative reveals the significance of guidance as journeying alongside the practitioner. She is no longer alone. Note Chris is a motivator and catalyst turning Caitlin's negativity into positivity to take action.

Perhaps if we had meet two-weekly rather than monthly, it would have made a difference if she could have accommodated supervision into her workload as high priority. She may well have benefitted from group supervision alongside other clinical leaders within the research project, to form a mutually supportive group [1]. At the end of the day, she was burnt-out[i] as if guided reflection had made her aware of her dissatisfaction and once, aware, could no longer be defended against. When we touch the essence of caring, nothing else can ever be good enough again.

She works within a system that doesn't listen to concerns, wrapped up as they are in their own corporate concerns proving nonsense to any claim to being 'investors in people'. As Caitlin said 'We try so very hard and we don't get listened to. They ask us for our comments and these just get filed away!'

References

1. Johns, C. (2003) Clinical supervision as a model for clinical leadership. *Journal of Nursing Management* 11, 25–34.

2. Chapman, G. (1983) Ritual and rational action in hospitals. *Journal of Advanced Nursing* 8, 13–20.

3. Cavanagh, S. (1991) The conflict management style of staff nurses and nurse managers. *Journal of Advanced Nursing* 16, 1254–1260.

4. Dawson, J. (1987) Evaluation of a community based night sitter service. In P. Fielding [Ed.] *Research in Nursing care of elderly people*. John Wiley, Chichester.

5. Nolan, M., Grant, G. (1989) Addressing the needs of informal carers: a neglected area of nursing practice. *Journal of Advanced Nursing* 14, 950–961.

6. Hawker, R. (1982) *The Interaction Between Nurses and Patients' Relatives*. Unpublished PhD thesis, University of Exeter.

7. Stewart, I., Joines, V. (1987) *TA Today: A New Introduction to Transactional Analysis'*. Lifespace Publishing, Nottingham & Chapel Hill.

8. Cherniss, G. (1980) *Professional Burn-Out in Human Service Organisations*. Praeger, New York.

9. Thomas, K., Kilmann, R. (1974) *Thomas Kilmann Conflict Mode Instrument*. Xicom, Toledo.

10. Seedhouse, D. (1988) *Ethics: The Heart of Health Care*. John Wiley & Sons, Chichester).

11. Robinson, S., Thorne, C. (1984) Strengthening family interference. *Journal of Advanced Nursing* 9, 597–602.

12. Ramos, M. (1992) The nurse-patient relationship: themes and variations. *Journal of Advanced Nursing* 17, 496–506.

13. Cameron, D. (2004) *Globalizing Communication*. Routledge, London. (p. 53).

14. Johns, C. (2004) [Ed.] *The Buford NDU Model: Caring in Practice*. Blackwell Science, Oxford.

15. Callanan, M., Kelley, P. (1983) *Final Gifts: Understanding the Special Awareness, Needs and Communication of the Dying*. Bantam Books, New York.

16. Heron, J. (1975) *Six Category Intervention Analysis*. Human Potential Research Group, University of Surrey.

Note

i. How common is burnout in nursing? Very. Results from a 2020 survey indicate that almost two-thirds of nurses (62%) experience burnout. It's especially common among younger nurses, with 69% of nurses under 25 reporting burnout. This issue affects all hospitals and health care systems in the US. https://www.nursingworld.org/content-hub/resources/workplace/what-is-nurse-burnout-how-to-prevent-it/#:~:text=to%20workplace%20stress.-,What%20Is%20the%20Burnout%20Rate%20for%20Nurses%3F,nurses%20(62%25)%20experience%20burnout.

Creating the 'Learning Organisation' in Clinical Practice Through Leadership and Clinical Supervision

Introduction

Establishing guided reflection within the clinical environment creates a learning environment for practitioners to flourish and grow towards realising their vision of person-centred practice and become reflective practitioners.

In the following narrative[i], Susan is a ward sister who aspired to becoming a transformational leader. As an evolving leader, she was inspired by the idea of establishing the 'Learning Organisation' [1] through implementing 'clinical supervision' commencing with a nurse on an adjacent ward. Clinical supervision burst upon the general nursing agenda in 1993 prompted by the Government's concern for greater professional accountability and surveillance to give the public confidence that nurses and health visitors' practice would be adequately monitored in the aftermath of the Beverley Allitt tragedy.

The Vision for the Future document (National Health Services Management Executive, [2, p. 3] defined clinical supervision as –

> 'A formal process of professional support and learning which enables individual practitioners to develop knowledge and competence, assume responsibility for their own practice and enhance consumer protection and safety of care in complex situations. It is central to the process of learning and to the expansion of the scope of practice and should be seen as a means of encouraging self-assessment and analytical and reflective skills'.

From this definition, there is little difference between guided reflection and clinical supervision. However, I reject the term 'clinical supervision' because of its connotation as meaning to watch over and control the other's performance alluded to in the explicit aim of clinical supervision to safeguard the public.

Susan's Narrative 'Liberating to Care'

The 1990 NHS and Community Care Act placed on organisations the statutory duty to provide effective quality care. In response NHS organisations have in recent years implemented a programme of clinical governance as a framework to fulfil this duty [3]. Individual practitioners are expected and required by their employers to play an active part in such local clinical governance arrangements [4]. Nurses are particularly aware of their required commitment to the concept of lifelong learning and the statutory duty to maintain professional knowledge and competence [5, 6]. Garside [7] notes a natural tension between the necessary regulatory and professional surveillance culture in the NHS and the equally necessary developmental elements of learning, where innovation and risk are welcomed. Garside admits that this tension between regulation/surveillance and learning/development is unlikely to disappear, but she does suggest that they can co-exist.

My vision, as a transformational leader, is to create the 'Learning Organisation' described by Senge [1, p. 3] as:

> 'One where people continually expand their capacities to create the results they truly desire, where new and expansive patterns of thinking are nurtured, where collective aspiration is set free, and where people are continually learning how to learn together'.

Senge identified five integrated technologies that constitute it – personal mastery, mental models, shared vision, team learning and systems thinking (Figure 13.1).

Senge notes that the state of being a learning organisation never actually exists, since the more that is learnt, the more acutely aware we become of ignorance. Statutory and regulatory

Vision	A collective consensual statement of shared beliefs that gives meaning and direction to clinical practice.
Personal mastery	Personal mastery is being a reflective practitioner, constantly striving towards resolving creative tension towards realising my vision of leadership as a lived reality. This involves clarifying my vision and seeing my current reality more clearly. Senge [1, p. 142] notes that – 'People with a high level of personal mastery live in a continual learning mode, they have a strong sense of purpose, they are deeply inquisitive thus are acutely aware of their ignorance, their incompetence and their growth areas. They are creative and deeply self-confident'.
Mental models	The discipline of working with mental models starts with turning the mirror inward, learning to unearth my internal images and assumptions of the world, to bring them to the surface and hold them rigorously to scrutiny, and subsequently shift them as necessary to align with my vision. However, assumptions and attitudes are deeply rooted. Senge [1, p. 174] notes that 'New insights fail to get put into practice because they conflict with deeply held internal images of how the world works, images that limit us to familiar ways of thinking and acting'.
Systems thinking	Systems thinking is being aware of the pattern of underlying systems that governs how the organisation operates, and shifting these systems as necessary to enable the vision to become a lived reality. Systems form a network that fuse together to work as a whole.
Team learning	Team learning guides me to work collectively towards realising 'our' vision of practice, creating a community of inquiry and learning. It takes reflective learning from an individual concern into a collective concern. This enables barriers that might block individual learning to be overcome by force of mass and organisational support. Yet it is important to emphasise my individual learning as the base line for team learning. As Senge notes [1, p. 140] – 'Organizations learn only through individuals who learn. Individual learning does not guarantee organizational learning. But without it no organizational learning occurs'.

FIGURE 13.1 Systems of the learning organisation.

documents seem to assume an innate desire in individuals to learn, and indeed Senge notes that not only is it our nature to learn, but also we love to learn. Such assumptions in the current climactic conditions in the NHS may be difficult to support. The reality of today's NHS is that nurse shortages are reportedly reaching crisis point, establishment shortfall is nationally 20%, one third of all nurses are allocated no study time, and bed occupancy is running at 98% [8]. In such an environment, Wall et al. [9] note that NHS staff suffer considerably more stress than any other workforce with 28% recording levels above the symptom threshold. Furthermore, few healthcare institutions can be described as learning organisations since, in a system largely dominated by highly structured, hierarchical and historically determined professional demarcations, it is an infrequent occurrence that norms or assumptions are challenged or that the required unlearning or relearning takes place [7]. The task of managing these tensions and inspiring and motivating people to learn and contribute to the learning organisation in such a difficult, highly pressurised arena is one that I, as an aspiring transformational leader, I recognise as a considerable challenge.

Excellent organisations are those that know how to tap people's commitment and capacity to learn at all levels of the organisation and therefore a crucial element of the learning organisation is that it pays attention to the role and development of every individual within it. This clearly suggests that the effective transformational leader should display a natural tendency to develop others and facilitate learning, wherever staff members sit in the hierarchy of the NHS organisation. Good leadership can influence an organisation to act as an effective learning organisation, one that is responsive and adaptive to changes both from within and without to build an environment for better, safer health care [10].

Malby [11] suggests that reflection can lead to new mental models about how to do things differently, and the development of the skill of reflective practice has certainly enabled me to know myself more effectively, to frame and contextualise my own mental models, and to be more available to myself and others to realise desirable practice. In the context of leading, supporting and developing the learning organisation, I would argue that unless I am truly available and knowing to myself, transference of such availability would be problematic. My developed ability to clarify my own personal perspectives on values and ethics through reflective practice combined with my understanding of the art and practice of the learning organisation has then implications for my transformational leadership capabilities within the context of organisational life and learning [12].

Utilising the disciplines of the learning organisation as the aims of supervision offers a coherent purpose for clinical supervision. Johns [13, p. 246] aligned the learning organisations systems with the aims of clinical supervision:

- To clarify and deepen personal and collective visions of best practice;
- To develop personal mastery through holding creative tension between a vision of practice and an understanding of current practice in working to realise one's vision as a lived reality.
- To develop the reflective skills to achieve personal mastery.
- To scrutinise one's mental models/assumptions and shift these in tune with realising one's vision of practice.
- To review and shift organisational systems towards creating the optimum conditions to support desirable practitioner performance.
- To work collaboratively with colleagues to develop and ensure best practice.

The role of clinical supervision in the promotion of individual learning and the development of the learning organisation seems unquestionable, but many authors have written that its implementation may be fraught with difficulties. Cottrell [14] notes that nurses existing views of clinical supervision are all too often of a hostile, pseudo-analytic process of belittlement, criticism, shaming and the attribution of blame. The tensions between emancipatory and technical interests, particularly within bureaucratic cultures have also been suggested [15]. Johns [15] opines that the emancipatory developmental and sustaining role of clinical supervision will be diminished in any interpretation of clinical supervision as a technical consumer protection methodology. A mandatory clinical supervision agenda within an organisation may suggest surveillance and lead to fear of retaliatory action from managers, and evidence suggests that some nurses covertly seek supervision outside the mandatory provision in these circumstances [16]. It seems then that though widely espoused by governmental and professional bodies and achieving a form of hegemony among some managers of the nursing profession, clinical practitioners have not embraced the concept with a similar enthusiasm [17, 18]. Furthermore, while some research evidence indicating its effectiveness exists, it seems that empirical validation is fraught with epistemological and conceptual problems [19–21].

My role as clinical supervisor within this apparently confused, indeterminate and possibly hostile arena appears loaded with complication. It is here that my skills of transformational leadership need to be clearly demonstrated if the clinical supervision agenda is to contribute to the development of the learning organisation through therapeutic interaction with another. Johns [15] notes how the intent and emphasis of the supervisor can determine the nature of the supervisory experience[ii]. Working within a transformational paradigm, I am acutely aware that I need to take shared ownership of the clinical supervision sessions that I facilitate alongside the supervisee with the consequence that I/we are in control of clinical supervision rather than being controlled by it. Without such customisation and ownership, there is always the danger that clinical supervision and the intended learning may succumb to the transactional, manipulative, managerial and oppressive agenda that arguably constitutes the reality of the NHS today [22]. Johns [15] poses a challenge when he asks whether clinical supervision can be accommodated to fit the existing culture or can the existing culture be shifted to the ideals of emancipatory supervision? For the transformational leader, a quite significant shift in the existing culture appears to be the desired state. My desire is to promote and liberate learning from experience within the clinical supervision relationship (the emancipatory element) rather than the production of a worker who can be monitored against specific criteria of what constitutes effectiveness (the technical element).

I have acted as clinical supervisor for almost two years within an advisory clinical supervision system in my current workplace. The organisation provides no formal training or support for clinical supervisors, which suggests that while it embraces the concept of clinical governance publicly, it may be covertly resisting the idea of clinical supervision as an emancipatory learning process for the organisation, since it may perceive it as a threat to established patterns of relating. There seems no reciprocal agreement between the individual willing to learn through such supervision and the current organisational culture. While commitment is currently lacking and interpretation and introduction of clinical supervision in my own organisation is minimalist, future policy directives may mean that clinical supervision will become a 'must do' in the future [18]. My role as a transformational leader will be of critical importance once clinical supervision becomes mandatory within my organisation and I am hoping to influence the clinical supervision agenda, at least in my own work area towards the emancipatory rather than technical ideal.

Sarah

I have been Sarah's clinical supervisor for six months. Sarah is a junior staff nurse on another ward and therefore outside the scope of my managerial authority. Our supervisor/supervisee relationship is mutually agreed and voluntary. Many authors write that reflective practice for both the supervisor and supervisee is intimately bound with the process of clinical supervision [23–25]. Johns [26] describes guided reflection as a way of structuring the clinical supervision space, and such reflective practice can aid the development of the learning organisation with great potential to leverage quality and effective practice. The following discussion and illumination of recent clinical supervision sessions will explore my role in Sarah's learning and demonstrate my commitment to contribute to the emergence of the spirit of the learning organisation. I had tacitly (and possibly naively) assumed that Sarah did not feel that I was monitoring her clinical performance since we do not work together but reflected recently that Sarah and I have never discussed or clarified this aspect of our relationship. Perhaps this demonstrates my lack of knowledge at the time when we commenced the clinical relationship since I now recognise clearly the need to develop formal contracts with supervisees to clarify roles and meaning in the relationship if learning is to occur [18]. I remained undecided about the accuracy of my assumption regarding Sarah's perception (although I had intended to discuss it with her) until the following incident occurred. It was the end of a clinical supervision session where a completely unrelated issue concerning drug administration was discussed. As Sarah got up to leave the room, she made some comments which, at the time, appeared almost inconsequential to her but which caused me deep reflection.

Sarah: 'Well I better get back to the ward now. It's not that I don't want to or that I don't care but I just find it so difficult to look after people like Mary with her dementia. She can't do anything for herself – she just lies there all day without doing anything or saying anything to anyone not even her husband or family. I never feed her – I can't bear it. I always get the health care assistants to do it. I can't help feeling that I don't like that sort of nursing – it's so unrewarding but I'd never tell anyone else that, it doesn't seem right does it?'.

Sarah and I parted company without further comment being made. I was immediately concerned that, in six months of supervising Sarah, I had not encountered such a forthright expression of attitude from her that I instantly felt so uncomfortable with. I was, however, aware that the prevalence of negative attitudes towards the care of older people among the nursing profession is widely reported [27, 28]. It seemed that although Sarah sensed a real tension between her professional role requirement and her personal feelings she felt comfortable enough to express them to me. This signified that she did not see me in a surveillance role but my instant reaction was to feel transactional with the desire to confront Sarah about her poor performance and attitude, as I perceived it. However, I recognised that such a stance may change the nature of our supervisory relationship and prove a stumbling block to learning in an unthreatening environment in the future. A further concern of mine was that Sarah's honest expression perhaps signified that she felt I would have no concerns about her statement and possibly shared her opinions, which I did not. I considered previous clinical supervision sessions. Had Sarah and I suffered a learning bind where we had previously missed each other's meaning in the interpretation of our practice and values? Schön [29] suggests that the ability to escape from such a learning bind depends on the supervisor's ability to reflect on the supervisor–supervisee dialogue and this I did extensively prior to the next session.

When Sarah arrived for her next supervision session, I asked her if she would like to talk about Mary, since she seemed to find caring for her difficult. Sarah's immediate agreement signified that this was indeed something that she wished to share. I was acutely aware of the need to suspend my own values and assumptions to manage the creative tensions I felt between my own vision of what nursing should be and where I currently saw Sarah's practice and attitudes. If we assume that the effective practitioner takes responsibility to ensure and monitor their own effectiveness, then the role of the supervisor is not to sit in judgement but to enable the practitioner to make such judgements for herself [15]. However, within clinical supervision there needs to be an element of challenge that needs to be managed carefully to avoid a spiral of increasing challenge from the supervisor and resultant increasing resistance from the supervisee [25, 30]. I introduced Sarah to the Model of Structured Reflection [MSR][iii] as a way of focusing self-challenge and to structure her deconstruction of her experiences to lead to new insights that could be applied to her practice.

We discussed the issues at length and some of her comments were very illuminating.

Sarah: 'Lots of old people get dementia don't they? I wonder what causes it and if it runs in families? My Grandma had it when I was little. She used to scare me and she didn't even seem to know who I was. I remember her wetting my Mum's settee one Christmas and my Dad got really cross and shouted at her. She ended up in a home and I don't remember seeing her after that. It's frightening to think anyone could end up like that'.

Guided by the MSR, Sarah and I discussed the origin and influence of her mental models at length and explored how they influenced her practice. She felt she knew nothing about dementia but thought perhaps that she should. She asked if I could recommend anything for her to read. While mindful of the need to avoid the perception that I had greater skills or knowledge than Sarah (often detrimental in the clinical supervision relationship since it may suggest supervisor authority), I provided her with some relevant references without offering any opinion on their value [24]. Sarah left the session professing a determination to think about our discussion and visit the library for more information.

When Sarah attended her next supervision session, it quickly became obvious that she had reflected quite deeply on our session, undertaken some personal learning and reading and had applied this to her practice. She related her recent experience to me.

Sarah: 'I've got to know Mary and Bill and they seem a really nice couple. Do you know Bill was telling me that during the war he didn't see Mary at all for three years. All that time she was looking after their little girl and working in a factory making aircraft parts and at night she did fire watching. That must have been so hard for her. Bill said Mary loved dancing and really missed it when the arthritis got so bad. I've seen photos of them in dance competitions and she looks lovely with her hair and make up all done'.

Sarah continued with Mary and Bill's life story, which signified that she now recognised and valued their personhood. I asked Sarah if she felt more able to nurse Mary now, and Sarah confirmed that she was happily taking a more active role in caring for Mary on a daily basis.

Sarah: 'I think I was sacred before because I didn't understand what was happening to Mary but I knew that I didn't feel right about the way I acted. Reading those articles you gave me and talking to my Mum about my own Grandma when she was young made me think that perhaps I'd missed something. It was only when I started to talk to Bill that I recognized I'd been avoiding him and Mary. She had been a patient with us for two weeks and I knew nothing about her! I've noticed other people acting the same as I did and perhaps I can do something about that. I feel like a better nurse now and I've joined the Care of the Older Person Link Group. I might even go and do a course or something'.

To me, Sarah's most significant statement came at the end of our session – again just as she was leaving the room.

Sarah: 'Thanks a lot – I feel better about it all now and I've learnt a lot but I need to think about things a bit more don't I? I'm using that (reflective) model you gave me and I'm writing things down. See you next time!'

Through the learning process, Sarah had achieved some control of the creative tension that existed, where the current reality of her practice did not match the vision of her nursing care that she professed to hold. In this way, she had enhanced her own sense of personal mastery and now felt a better nurse. She had re-examined her vision for nursing and now felt she shared and lived the vision of nursing as a profession. She had surfaced and challenged the mental models that influenced her understanding of the issues through an engagement of self with self-awareness and had accepted an internal locus of self-control and responsibility for her own actions. Sarah's personal learning had highlighted other learning needs within her team and she had resolved to join a group dedicated to learning about the care of older people and to share this with others. Senge [1] describes such team learning as vital since teams, not individuals are the fundamental learning unit in modern organisations.

My transformational approach means that I avoided the transactional, technical interest intent of clinical supervision where monitoring, surveillance and a focus on role performance are evident. Rather, the transformational skills of effective communication, honesty and empathy, development of others and risk taking, experimentation and learning were all organised to ensure that Sarah was guided on her own emancipatory learning journey of self-awareness and discovery [31]. Sarah is clearly only one person in a very large organisation – one that is not currently particularly in tune with the concept of the learning organisation, and her learning may appear insignificant to some in the larger picture.

The National Health Service has a long history of firmly established traditions and authoritarian practices. A cultural transformation will arguably be necessary if organisational learning, which embraces new and expansive patterns of thinking, leading to real service wide quality improvements is to be developed [1]. It would seem that contributing to the emergence of a learning organisation from the current cultural stance poses a considerable challenge and requires real determination from the transformational health care practitioner/leader of today. For the transformational leader, the spirit of learning and enquiry is an ever-present entity, and my contribution and commitment to the learning of both myself and others is a key aspect of my role, since the active force of any learning organisation must be the people who work there. Finally, my own sense of personal mastery has developed through this work, since I am aware that both Sarah and I have contributed to the learning organisation. We have created a more effective practice environment by working through an experience, identifying areas for growth and generating the learning needed to achieve positive results.

Reflection

Besides giving the reader insight into reflective writing for an assignment at the masters level, Susan's narrative informs regarding the nature of clinical supervision and its potential to enable supervisees to reflexively learn within the broader vision of the learning organisation. Note how Susan emphasises 'It would seem that contributing to the emergence of a Learning Organization from the current cultural stance poses a considerable challenge and requires real determination from the transformational health care practitioner/leader of today'. Her words reflect how the prevailing transactional organisation was not a learning organisation and indeed, might even resist such development. As she noted, a cultural revolution is needed. Yet the impact of her guidance with Sarah was profound in her transformation.

References

1. Senge, P. (1990) *The Fifth Discipline: The Art and Science of the Learning Organization.* Century Business, London.

2. National Health Service Management Executive (N.H.S.M.E.) (1993) *A Vision for The Future.* HMSO, London.

3. Halligan, A., Donaldson, L. J. (2001) Implementing clinical governance: turning vision into reality. *British Medical Journal* 322(7299), 1413–1417.

4. Donaldson, L. J. (2001) Safe high quality care: investing in tomorrow's leaders. *Quality in Health care*, 10, 8–12.

5. Department of Health. (1999) *Making A Difference.* HMSO, London.

6. Nursing and Midwifery Council (2002) *Midwives Rules and Standards.* Nursing and Midwifery Council, London.

7. Garside, P. (1999) The learning organization: a necessary setting for improving care? *Quality in Healthcare* 8, 211.

8. Hall, C. (2003) *Nurse Shortage in the NHS is Near to Crisis Point*. Daily telegraph 29th April.

9. Wall, T. D., Bolden, R. I., Borril, C. S. (1997) Minor psychiatric disturbance in NHS trust staff. *British Journal of Psychiatry* 171, 519–523.

10. Moss, F. (2001) Leadership and learning: building the environment for better safer healthcare. *Quality in Healthcare*, 10(supplement 2), 1–2.

11. Malby, R. (1996) The need for nursing leadership. *British Journal of Healthcare Management* 2(3), 18–19.

12. Rippon, S. (2001) Nurturing nurse leadership: how does your garden grow? *Nursing Management*, 8(7), 11–15.

13. Johns, C. (2022) A system to enable practitioners to develop personal mastery towards realising their vision of practice. In C. Johns [Ed.] *Becoming A Reflective Practitioner* (sixth edition). Wiley-Blackwell, Oxford, 245–258.

14. Cottrell, S. (1999) *Some Current Beliefs in the NHS and Some Consequences for Implementing Clinical Supervision*. Excerpt from conference address http://www.clinical-supervision.com.

15. Johns, C. (2001) Depending on the intent and emphasis of the supervisor, clinical supervision can be a very different experience. *Journal of Nursing Management* 9, 139–145.

16. Scanlon, C., Weir, W. (1997) Learning from practice? Mental health nurses' perceptions and experiences of clinical supervision. *Journal of Advanced Nursing* 26, 295–303.

17. Gilbert, T. (2001) Reflective practice and clinical supervision: meticulous rituals of the confession. *Journal of Advanced Nursing* 36, 199–205.

18. Bond, M., Holland, S. (1998) *Skills of Clinical Supervision for Nurses*. Open University Press, Buckingham.

19. Burrows, D. (1995) The nurse teacher's role in the promotion of reflective practice. *Nurse Education Today* 15, 346–350.

20. Lyle, D. (1998) Opinion: is clinical supervision the answer to quality care? *Nursing Management* 5(6), 3.

21. Goorapah, D. (1997) Clinical supervision. *Journal of Clinical Nursing*, 6(3), 173–178.

22. Ghaye, T. (2000a) Colleague centred care: the reframing of clinical supervision. In T. Ghaye, S. Lillyman [Eds.] *Effective Clinical Supervision*. Mark Allen Publishers, Dinton.

23. Ghaye, T. (2000b) The role of reflection in nurturing clinical conversations. In T. Ghaye, S. Lillyman [Eds.] *Effective Clinical Supervision*. Mark Allen Publishers, Dinton.

24. Power, S. (1999) *Nursing Supervision: A Guide for Clinical Practice*. Sage Publications, London.

25. Heath, H., Freshwater, D. (2000) Clinical supervision as an emancipatory experience: avoiding inappropriate intent. *Journal of Advanced Nursing* 32, 1298–1306.

26. Johns, C. (2003) Clinical supervision as a model for clinical leadership. *Journal of Nursing Management* 11, 25–34.

27. Wade, S. (1999) Promoting quality of care for older people: developing positive attitudes to working with older people. *Journal of Nursing Management* 7, 339–347.

28. Courtney, M., Tong, S., Walsh, A. (2000) Acute care nurses attitudes' towards older people: a literature review. *International Journal of Nursing Practice* 6, 62–69.

29. Schön, D. (1987) *Educating the Reflective Practitioner*. Jossey-Bass, San Francisco.

30. Smith, G. (2000) *Friendship within clinical supervision: a model for the NHS*? http://www. clinical-supervision.com.

31. Schuster, J. (1994) Transforming your leadership style. Leadership, 39–43.

Notes

i. Susan wrote her narrative as an assignment for the 'Ensuring quality' module within the MSc Leadership in Healthcare degree at the University of Bedfordshire.

ii. See Figure 8.5.

iii. See Figure 2.2.

PART 2

Transition into Formal Education

CHAPTER 14

The Person-centred Reflective Curriculum

Most reflective learning takes place within educational curriculum. It has become a key issue for curriculum development within nurse education (1) and for all healthcare professions. For example, the International Federation of Sports Physical Therapists (2) – quoting (3, p. 133) –

'Requires physiotherapist applying for their accreditation process to demonstrate a variety of reflective pieces relating to their devised sports physiotherapy competencies'.

The foundation of any healthcare curriculum is to enable students to realise a professional vision of their discipline. Design stems from that. For healthcare, and nursing in particular, its professional vision is indisputably person-centred practice (see Chapter 1). Ideally, the vision should not simply be imposed but be an initial point of dialogue between teachers and students, for students to reach the conclusion that realising person-centred practice is the aim and focus of their education. Students should be viewed from the outset not merely as vessels to be filled with knowledge but as intelligent persons with a background of experience. As Freire (4, p. 68) noted –

'The starting point for organizing the programme content of education must be the present, existential, concrete situation, reflecting the aspirations of the people. It is not our role to speak to the people about our own view, not to attempt to impose that view on them, but rather to dialogue with the people about their view and ours'.

Vision gives meaning and direction for the curriculum. The curriculum is then designed to enable students to develop the necessary knowing in practice to competently realise person-centred practice at the pint of registration.

Roots

Let me take a step back to my first engagement with guiding undergraduate nursing students in my role as a lecturer-practitioner at Burford Hospital. The role involved both supervising the students' practice and teaching for the rehabilitation and elderly care modules.

My initial approach was to construct the module as 10 × 2 hour weekly sessions over the placements. I constructed narratives characteristic of patients with conditions experienced at the hospital. This was akin to a 'Problem Based Learning' (PBL) approach.[i] On evaluating the impact of the first course, I questioned myself – 'Why construct PBL scenarios when the students have their own experiences?'

In response, the second time I taught the module, I shared and reflected on my own experience and contracted with the students to bring to each session reflections on their own experiences of working with patients at the hospital. This radically shifted the power differential within our teacher–student relationship by giving voice to the students' experiences. However, my authoritative voice could not be denied. Its presence was always there and yet I could quieten it to enable the students' voices to be heard. I was the servant-leader (see Chapter 8), servicing the dialogue in ways to ensure an effective learning experience. I 'fed in' relevant theory in context with the shared experiences so that theory became subjective and contextual rather than abstract. The students stated that learning was meaningful, intense, more responsible than other learning modes and enjoyable. Listening to their peer students' stories had a profound impact on their senses drawing them into dialogue and relating with their own experiences.

Woolf writes [5, p. 127] –

> 'One sees more intensely afterwards, the world seems bared of its covering and given an intense life. Learning should be memorable. As for the students, it was a learning experience I will never forget. I will keep trying to explore storytelling within the limiting confines of the system and perhaps ripples will become waves. Stories are empowering- we all leave the room richer for the experience'.

Surprisingly, I met little resistance from the students. I say surprisingly because, as Hooks [6, p. 142–3] writes –

> 'The urge to experiment with pedagogical practices may not be welcomed by students who often expect us to teach in the manner they are accustomed to'.

I had challenged myself – 'How will the students react if I teach through reflection on their experiences?' I imagined their lament – 'give us the facts'. Students know the lecture approach and learning outcomes – 'by the end of the session the student is able to ...' is the bread and butter of teaching. Writing modules at the University is prescribed in such a way. The logic being both the student and teacher know what to expect. Indeed, teachers often churn out the same lesson plan semester after semester. The university set the module outcomes. Teachers become chained to organising their teaching to meet these outcomes and yet the sessions at Buford evidence they could do that more easily through guided reflection than their previous learning experiences. More significantly, the classroom became 'active'. As I supervised the students' clinical practice, I knew the patients the students reflected on. This had the advantage of feeding in detail as appropriate and facilitating reflection in practice. Coherence between learning process and clinical practice outcome is a significant student motivator.

A number of factors facilitated my lecturer-practitioner role

- The school of nursing was dynamic in its approach to nurse training through the idea of appointing lecturer-practitioners to both deliver module content and supervise students' practice. I had license to interpret and deliver the module content as I deemed appropriate. Students knew I was an expert practitioner, which gave me credibility with teaching. I knew what I was talking about.
- The students were required to reflect on how they had met the module objectives [as set by the school]. As such, grounding their learning in reflection made meeting their module objectives more meaningful and useful.
- I was undertaking a doctoral study guiding practitioners to learn through reflection. As such, I was relatively skilled in reflective teaching.

- As clinical leader I had authority for determining practice.
- I had effective administrative support to enable me to maintain patient contact two days a week as an associate nurse, enabling me to be available to students in practice and demonstrate my clinical credibility.

Journal Entry 14.1

I gained insight into how reflective teaching was being taught in the university's technical rational undergraduate nursing degree curriculum when invited by a group of second-year nursing students to talk about reflection. They were frustrated with reflection. They said it felt like a chore with little value except to answer reflective type assignments that made them anxious. Could I help? We had two hours.

I asked about the way they had been taught reflection. As I suspected, they were given a model of reflection with little guidance as if the model was self-explanatory, and told to apply it to an experience. Their assignment was based on applying the model.

I shared my story concerning my experience with Violet [7]. It took about 20 minutes to narrate. When teaching reflection, I share a personal narrative especially if I expect students to write and tell their own stories. This role models what a narrative looks like and my risk in sharing it. I finish by inviting the students to dialogue with me, encouraging them to draw their own insights and share their own stories. I emphasise my experience as a contextual moment situated in history – a personal, social, cultural, professional, political, environmental, professional, gendered history. I say 'it's like peeling back an onion skin to reveal deeper contextual layers'. A bit deep for them, but I wanted them to think about that; that reflection had critical depth.

The students say the narrative was engaging. Two students, bold enough, related to the narrative with their own similar stories. A buzz about the place. I then invited them to write a description of a recent experience. I gave them 15 minutes. After an initial flurry of comment between them, the room went very quiet as pens raced across pages.

I then illuminated how the Model for Structured Reflection cues (Figure 5.2) could enable them to explore their experience, prompting the students to apply the cues to their own stories and draw out tentative insight. I then invited them to share their reflections, guiding them to reveal insight by asking 'What do you learn from this?' The two hours passed quickly. However, some students stayed on, wanting to talk more about reflective practice. Some said that they had no idea that reflection could be so creative and exciting. Some exclaim 'Why haven't we been taught reflection like this?'

I suggested it was a problem with accommodating reflection within a programme grounded in the school's dominant technical rational approach to learning and teaching. The students understood but were frustrated. I further explained that their reflective assignments were designed to measure their application of a reflective model supported by references [a pseudo-intellectual game] with no credit for aesthetic expression. I suggested that reflective assignments should be constructed around insights gained. The students said they played the game. 'What game is that?' I inquired. 'Guess what is in teacher's head – that way at least you pass'. What kind of education is that? 'If I had submitted my story as an assignment, would I pass?' 'No', was the general consensus, 'it doesn't tick the boxes'. Is education no more than ticking the boxes? If so, what a parlous approach to learning, and yet this scenario appears normal throughout nurse education. The students said their teachers don't share their own stories as I had done. It reinforced my belief that teachers need to be reflective practitioners and teach through their stories as exemplars of reflection. Then, reflection made sense to students. They could see themselves in their stories. It stimulated their interest in reflection and the learning embedded in them.

Some days later, their course teacher, who was also head of curriculum development for pre-registration nursing, approached me and fed back the students' enthusiastic response. The power of students' voices could not be discounted. She was convinced of a need for a new approach to reflection within the curriculum. She asked if I would lead a specialist sub-group for the curriculum revalidation for degree nurse training. I agreed but that's another story. Not a positive one. Perhaps I went about it the wrong way suggesting our existing curriculum needed to be radically revised around a reflective practicum. Resistance was grounded in the idea that the existing approach to reflective teaching was fit for purpose. People just couldn't imagine the radical shift. Resistance won the day. The result was more of the same just wrapped slightly differently and more frustration for second year nursing students.

My experience with these students revealed how reflective practice was bolted onto the curriculum as another technical rational approach whereby students were directed to reflect using a prescribed model of reflection and students were tested on their ability to apply the model. Clarke [1] emphasises that reflection should be an integral part of teaching and not perceived as something to add on. I assume that many of the teachers directing reflective learning have little or no experience of being a reflective practitioner. Teachers live out illusions that they know and teach reflective practice. As Bailey [8, p. 194] noted –

'I was largely resistant for many years to the conscious use of reflection in my personal and professional life. I perceived the reflective path to be one I had already walked, as though reflection has some definitive end point'.

As such, the beneficial impact of bolted-on reflective learning is minimal. Instead, the students were dissatisfied with their reflective learning became it was a task to do that many viewed as irrelevant or intrusive. The technical rational approach is based on imparting facts and students are primed to want to know the facts. Imagine the cry of the conditioned technical rational student 'give us the facts, not this navel gazing which is both uncomfortable and meaningless'! If students do not find reflective learning meaningful, they will not take it seriously. Then it is likely that only lip service is given to it. Indeed, many teachers imbued in a technical rational culture share this attitude reflecting a profound fear of change that threatens teacher identity. Teachers adopt 'piecemeal gestures' because they can be accommodated within the existing technical rational culture with minimal disturbance. In this way, they can confidently assert they have incorporated reflective learning within the curriculum. If a reflective curriculum is to be realised, then people involved have to realise the future is going to be different, that they must move beyond piecemeal gestures and begin to see the systems in which they are embedded. My experience with the students reminds me of Schön's words [9, p. 8] –

'What aspiring practitioners need most to learn, professional schools seem least able to teach' is to navigate the swamp effectively'.

The swamp is the messy, complex and indeterminate nature of everyday practice. This is more so with person-centred practice because of the practitioner's necessary personal involvement and acknowledged uniqueness of every situation.

Stemming from my experience with the second-year students, I surmised the existing curriculum was inadequate to enable students to become reflective practitioners for a number of reasons:

- Reflection was bolted onto the curriculum in a very limited way rather than integrated within the curriculum. Thus, there was no sense of continuity of learning through reflection or linked to specific curriculum aims resulting in failure to develop reflective skills.
- The sessions on reflective practice were focused on introducing a reflective model of nursing and setting some case study assignments where the student is asked to reflect on

an experience. This approach reflected the college's dominant technical rational approach whereby reflection was 'taught' from a more theoretical rather than practical perspective.

- The majority of nurse teachers did not practice nursing [at least in any meaningful way to be a credible nurse]. Neither were they reflective practitioners and thus not credible to teach reflective practice. Indeed many nurse teachers resist reflection because it threatens their credibility and control. As a consequence, both nursing and reflection are generally taught from a technical rational perspective.

- The existing curriculum was very teacher-centric. Teachers are comfortable with this approach.

- Reflection was 'forced' into the curriculum as a teaching technology. Its significance or application wasn't understood enough. Teachers assumed that reflection was simply thinking. These concerns are highlighted in the literature. Beauchamp [10, p. 126] quotes Russell [11] 'Has reflective practice done more harm than good in teacher education?' Beauchamp [10, p. 127] notes that Russell identified that –

  'Teacher educators have failed to provide adequate clarity on the meaning of reflection, have not necessarily modeled its practice themselves and have maintained their focus on it outside the realm of real action and experience'.

- The curriculum lacked a direct focus on developing the necessary knowing in practice to realise person-centred practice. As such, reflection had no depth or meaning.

A Potential Person-centred Reflective Curriculum Model

A potential person-centred reflective curriculum model is sketched in Figure 14.1. It is a 'whole systems' or 'system thinking' model, whereby all its parts are connected in which every action affects the whole system.[ii]

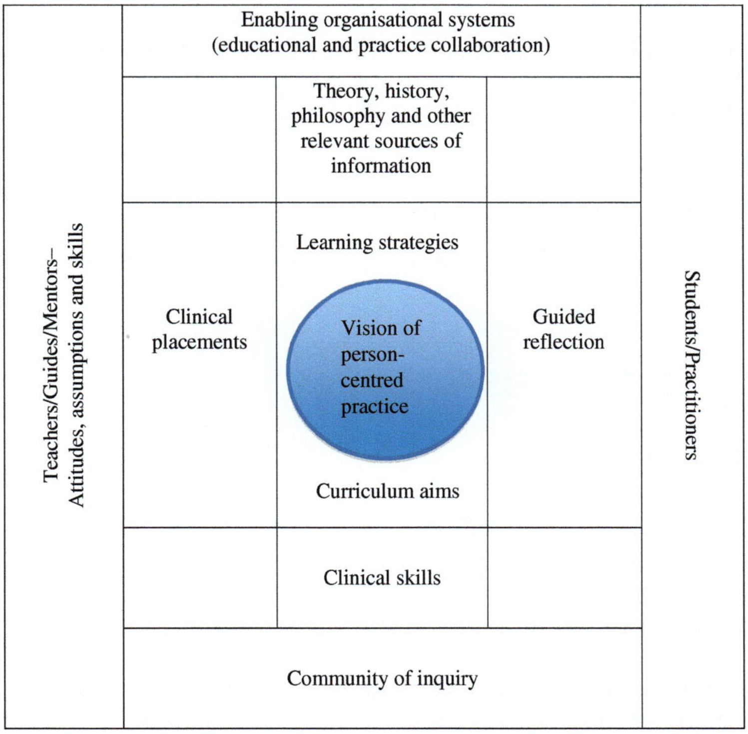

FIGURE 14.1 A template for the person-centred reflective curriculum.

Any curriculum has to respond to the demand of governing bodies, for example, the Nursing and Midwifery Council for approval of the nursing programme, where specific regulations and outcomes must be met. In addition, approval of programmes is determined by university validation events and the demand of NHS Trusts within the vagaries of tendering. NHS nurse education contracts are big money! As such, the reflective curriculum is not a blank canvass. It is a contested political canvass.

Curriculum Aims

Practitioners emerge from the programme with a strong sense of professional identity and professional artistry:

- They are competent in person-centred practice.
- They are adept reflective practitioners.
- They take co-responsibility for their learning.
- They speak with an informed, politically astute and assertive voice.
- They are leaders, adept in collaborative ways of working.
- They can articulate a strong professional vision and identity.
- They develop necessary mentorship skills to guide students in practice.
- They are poised and able to mitigate the possibility of 'reality shock'.

Co-centric Curriculum

The curriculum aim that students are co-responsible for their learning shifts the curriculum from being *teacher-centric* where teachers control the learning space to *co-centric*. In other words, it is collaboration between teachers and students working together to achieve the curriculum aims.

Research suggests that if students are permitted to make decisions about the focus of reflection and the process of reflection, more meaningful reflections are generated [10, 12]. It gives students the freedom to wander off the beaten paths and explore the surrounding areas. As such, each step along the journey becomes significant rather than looking at the outcomes. Each step is an event in itself not merely a means towards the end. This paying attention to experience creates the reflexive momentum. As Pirsig [13, p. 208] writes –

> 'To live only for some future goal is shallow. It's the sides of the mountain which sustains life, no the top. Here's where things grow'.

Learning Strategies

Guided Reflection

The core learning strategy is guided reflection. It brings together the other learning strategies to inform the students' development of knowing in practice.

I envisage that students would spend six hours each week in 2 × 3 hour guided reflection groups guided by a teacher over the whole programme. In practical terms, I suggest groups of eight students.

My experience with student nurses at Buford informed me that guided reflection is a viable learning approach within curriculum. It is a co-centric approach, whereby the students and guides co-create the students' insights or learning. This approach structured the post-registration 'Being and becoming a reflective and effective practitioner' programme delivered over two semesters. Hence, it has been tried and tested with positive impact (details set out later in this chapter).

I cannot assert enough the significance of extending guided reflection over time. My extensive experience of guiding practitioners informs that it takes about six months of intense guided reflection to grasp the nature of reflection and begin to reap its benefit in terms of internalising reflection and gaining insight. Practitioners talk about emerging into a clearing where suddenly learning becomes deeply meaningful.

Quoting Schön supports my assertion. He writes [9, p. 311] –

> 'A reflective curriculum demands intensity and duration far beyond the normal requirements of course … students no longer attend classes but live in them … nothing is indicative of student progress than the acquisition of artistry as the students' discovery of the time it takes – time to live through the initial shocks of confusion and mystery and unlearn initial expectations'.

Space within the curriculum for guided reflection is created with a reduction in traditional classroom teaching on topics that are better learnt within guided reflection: topics such as caring, relationships, ethics, knowing self, poise, communication skills and professional issues, such as leadership, guidance skills, conflict management, assertiveness and reality shock. This necessitates that teachers widen their theory base to be knowledgeable about these topics. An idea of this range is found in the exemplars of guiding reflection within the book.

Lectures

Lectures and internet programmes on more technical topics around disease and medical treatments can be picked up and related to practice within guided reflection. The approach to anatomy and physiology is more speculative. One approach is to structure the first year of the curriculum to gain a diploma in anatomy and physiology through specifically designed online courses supported by seminars and workshops to introduce basic clinical skills. One obvious risk with simulation teaching is that if you talk to a doll object long enough, that's the way you will be with patients and families.

Theory and Practice

The relationship between theory and practice is redefined. In a practice discipline, such as nursing, it is self-evident that we learn through doing. There are theories of how to do nursing but that doesn't mean we know what it is to nurse. As such, the conventional curriculum has blocks of theory and blocks of practice but that doesn't mean the twain shall meet. It is legend that nurses learn one thing in the classroom and another thing in clinical practice – what is historically described as the theory-practice gap.

The problem with theory prior to practice is that the student has nothing to hang the theory upon. As such, it is difficult to assimilate theory into personal knowing. It remains 'out there' as an abstract idea. The problem with theory after practice is to let students loose in practice with little idea about what they might be trying to achieve with patients. So, clearly students need to be informed before going into practice. However, within guided reflection, significant aspects of practice become a focus for attention yet are always set against the experience's context and wider theoretical and philosophical background. In other words, theory is introduced at a time when it is most meaningful and can be assimilated into personal knowing. The student has a hook to hang it on [14].

Link with Practice

Teachers (guides) need to become highly visible in clinical practice. Yet few teachers get meaningfully into practice. They would ideally spend one day a week in clinical practice to support both students and mentors in practice, to be more credible teachers and to collect personal experiences for role modelling reflection and illuminating the nature of person-centred practice. Teachers also reveal their vulnerability in sharing their experiences and, in doing so, opening themselves to dialogue and student inquiry. In doing so, students are encouraged to share and dialogue with their own experiences. It shows students that their guides can 'walk the talk'.

Mentors

The role of mentors is crucial, especially in the first few years of transition before the first cohort of students qualify and are prepared for mentorship. Mentors need to be reflective and person-centred practitioners, role modelling reflection as a way of being in their practice, offering a running commentary of their narrative practice, and ever mindful of the possibility of reality shock as noted as a curriculum aim. Supporting students in clinical practice is potentially problematic with the pressure on clinical staff in a stressed clinical environment due to less staff and a greater workload. Perhaps even more so with the government funding more nurse training places.[iii] Fewer qualified staff means less mentors. As such, teacher presence, at least once a week, will be vital to sustain and develop the clinical learning environment.

Thus, the curriculum planning team will need to look at mentor development and supporting association with practice partners. This can be linked to the NMC requirement for revalidation with its reflective practice requirement. It is noticeable that when I have taught clinical supervision to experienced healthcare professionals, professions that have seriously incorporated reflection into their curriculum are better equipped for supervisory roles than those professions, such as nursing, that have not. Thus, it is vital to get the clinical environment right.

Lecturer-Practitioners

Perhaps the best way to get the clinical environment right is appointing lecturer-practitioners. Vaughan's [14, p. 109] definition states that

> 'Lecturer practitioners have responsibility and authority for both practice and education within a defined clinical area with two broad but clearly defined aims: to identify and maintain the standards of practice and policies within a defined clinical area; to prepare and contribute to the educational programme of students in relation to the theory and practice of nursing in that unit'.

To guide students requires both reflective skills and clinical credibility. Lecturer-practitioners diffuse the educational organisation into communities of practice, giving greater autonomy to teachers and breaking up large cohorts of students into workable guided reflection groups within the practice setting. It also facilitates practice units as communities of inquiry. Fundamental to the role is direct patient contact [15]. My experience at Buford demonstrated (at least to me) the value of this role in enabling students to develop reflection and experience within a person-centred practice environment.

In the abstract to their paper, Driver and Campbell's [16, p. 292] note –

> 'The aim of this study was to determine if nursing diploma students recognized a difference in the nature of classroom teaching between lecturer practitioners and university-based senior lecturers in nursing. The study generated both qualitative and quantitative data from a sample of

117 student nurses completing an elderly care module. Analysis of the data suggested that the students associate lecturer practitioners with a realistic, evidence-based presentation of contemporary nursing practice, which they found both academically liberating, and efficacious to their practical training. Such associations were less apparent when analysing student responses to senior lecturer teaching. The study underlines the potential of lecturer practitioners to make a positive and far-reaching contribution to the future of nurse education'.

To Mitigate the Potential of Reality Shock

A significant value of lecturer-practitioners is to present a realistic presentation of practice whereby the tensions and contradictions between an idealised version and a realistic version are surfaced and explored. Rafferty et al. [17, p. 685] note –

> 'Such an approach has much to offer in helping students deal with reality shock and make sense of their experience as they confront the ambiguities, uncertainties and contradictions that characterize the stock-in-trade of professional life'.

Reality shock is the practitioner's dissonance between their expectations of practice and its reality and is a major reason why nurses quit nursing [18] creating a 'perfect storm' retention crisis.[iv] Yet reality shock can be mitigated through understanding its nature and developing the ability to counter it in collaboration with practice mentors.

Future Shock

The reflective/person-centred curriculum is in stark contrast with the predominant technical rational curriculum that the second-year students experienced. It is radical in terms of pedagogy and organisation. Envisaging such curriculum shift can be best described as a kind of 'future shock'.[v] It requires a significant shift in norms, assumptions, attitudes and learning strategies. It also requires a complementary shift within organisations to ensure person-centred practice where students are placed. Thus, organisational representatives need to be included in developing the reflective curriculum. It would create massive contradiction for nurses to be taught to become person-centred practitioners and then to practice where such practice is not reinforced. It requires education to work in harmony with organisations working together to realise a collective vision of person-centred practice.

The challenge is – How can it be realised given its radical difference when the teaching culture is rooted in technical rationality? How do assumptions and behaviours need to change?

Driving Change

The reflective curriculum is an ideal. Just because reflection and person-centred practice are mandated, it doesn't mean the conventional technical rational curriculum will change, embedded as it in tradition and authority. Therefore, it is necessary to consider how the transition can be understood and led.

Forum for Change

The first step is to establish a viable forum for change to direct the change comprising key representatives from education and practice. The key change agents from both education and practice are committed to the ideal.

Old norms to support the existing technical rational curriculum	New norms to support a reflective curriculum
Teachers control and are responsible for the educational environment (teacher-centric)	Teachers and students collaborate with contracted shared responsibility for the educational environment (co-centric)
The curriculum is predominantly theory led to prescribe practice.	The curriculum is practice led whereby theory informs rather than prescribes.
The curriculum aims are focused on the medical model and practitioners role to support.	The curriculum aims are focused on enabling practitioners to realise person-centred practice.
A focus on what nurses do.	A focus on who practitioners are (ontological shift)
The educational structure is transactional through hierarchy.	The educational structure is transformative through a community of inquiry.

FIGURE 14.2 Impression of movement of norms necessary to govern a reflective curriculum.

Change Process

Ottaway's [19] theory of change moving from one set of social norms to another set of social norms is useful to frame the change process by unearthing the norms or assumptions that govern the existing curriculum against a new set of norms or assumptions to govern the person-centred reflective curriculum. These new norms will not actually exist but can be assumed (see Figure 14.2).

Force Field Analysis

Lewin's force field analysis [20][vi] is a useful framework for considering the movement of norms to identify and map out both driving and resisting forces towards establishing the new 'status quo'. The status quo is a reflection of social norms. The fact is that teachers and students who have embodied an existing and particular way of thinking and acting cling to the 'status quo' of the existing model and resist attempts to disturb it if they feel they will be disadvantaged in some way. It is fundamentally a comfort issue irrespective of the rational for change, no matter how compelling the rationale. Resistors are very powerful to protect the 'status quo' and reflect how a rational approach to curriculum change won't work, especially if the envisaged change is disturbing.

The key to managing change is to focus on resisting forces when the temptation is to reinforce the driving forces. However, this is likely to reinforce resistance if the resisters feel they have not been involved in the change process.

Driving Forces for Change

The change process must generate *felt need* for the change. Both professional and governmental ideology emphasise person-centred practice and reflective practice that sets the foundation for change. Such emphasis is literally set in stone and cannot be rationally resisted. The bottom line for practice organisations is the curriculum results in competent person-centred practitioners.

This begs the question 'What is the evidence to support the envisaged curriculum will meet its curriculum aims?'

Professional bodies have made a link between reflective practice and competency. For example, the International Federation of Sports Physical Therapists, to quote Paterson and Chapman [3, p. 133], 'requires physiotherapist applying for their accreditation process to demonstrate a variety of reflective pieces relating to their devised sports physiotherapy competencies'. This needs to evidence professional development and its impact on an individual's practice increases pressure for physiotherapists to become competent reflective practitioners. However, as Paterson and Chapman [3, p. 33] note Mann et al.'s [21] observation that there is little direct evidence in the literature associating reflective practice and competency.

Clarke [1] notes –

'Reflection and reflective practice has become a key issue for curriculum development within nurse education. The Nursing and Midwifery Council has linked the demonstration of reflective skills to clinical competence to gain entrance onto the professional register. However, despite a significant volume of literature on reflection there is a paucity of research evidence regarding how nurse educators teach mental health nursing students to reflect and become effective reflective practitioners and, little research exploring experiences of staff and students engaged in reflection for teaching and learning purposes'.

Evidence to support the efficacy of the curriculum to realise its aims can be technical rational evidence (where it exists) and reflexive narratives (such as those included in this book). The most significant evidence that guided reflection 'works' is from practitioners' reflexive narratives because they clearly evidence the impact of guided reflection on enabling them towards realising their vision of practice as something lived [8, 22–28]. These narratives are all products of post-registration and post-graduate courses as outlined later in the chapter.

Evidence from narratives goes against the grain of the technical rational dominated university that will always give greater value to technical rational knowledge as indeed does health care generally waving its banner of 'evidence-based practice'. There are studies on teaching reflective practice that a curriculum group would naturally investigate, for example [29–33], amongst many others.

One study [34], involving 50 students from one cohort in their final year degree course in community health care nursing, sought to ascertain whether the students found reflection to be a meaningful activity, whether there are perceived benefits associated with reflective practice, and whether it is a valid process on which to access the outcomes of the course relating to the competencies of specialist practice. The data were collected via a web-based discussion board and focus group interview. The findings neither fully support nor refute the usefulness of reflective practice. It became apparent that the student's learning style was pertinent to his or her perception of the usefulness of reflection. However, it is not possible to draw any insight from this study because it paid no attention to the quality and exposure of the student's reflective experience, reflecting the limited value of technical rational studies to inform.

Other evidence is drawing on the experience of other educational organisations that have implemented a person-centred reflective curriculum, if these exist, or ideas about what the reflective curriculum could be like as set out in this chapter. Focus groups with students reflecting on their reflective learning would give feedback about students' perceptions.

Resistant Forces to the Reflective Curriculum

The resistors are powerful to protect the 'status quo' and reflect how a rational approach to curriculum change won't work, especially when the proposed change is radical. Resistance is a stimulus for dialogue within the planning team as a part of the change process to move towards consensus where resistance can be acknowledged with respect and patience.

Beau and Dracup [35] note that resistance is reduced when:

- Resisters perceive respected others supporting the change
- Their needs will be better met within a new status quo
- They feel involved in decision making or, put another way, are not victims of change
- When they have the opportunity to experience change with minimal threat

Both teachers and students are likely to resist a reflective curriculum.

Teacher Resistance

The biggest resistors will be teachers. Few teachers will appreciate being told that what you've been doing for years is no longer appropriate. Teachers have been socialised into a comfortable set of assumptions that support a traditional teacher led technical rational curriculum that makes it natural to resist such an envisaged radical shift despite any rational claim that a reflective curriculum focused on enabling students to realise person-centred practice could be better.

Imagine typical teachers' responses to resist the reflective curriculum (to name but a few):

- The existing curriculum works well. We teach reflective and person-centred practice satisfactorily despite Chris's experience with second-year nurses. They are just moaners, always complaining about something or another. So, there is no real need to change. Granted, our teaching approach is largely didactic but we do take account of the student's experiences. Dialogue is not our approach as it leads to too much chat when we need to get through the lesson's objectives.

Hooks [6, p. 148/151] writes –

'Focusing on experience allows students to claim a knowledge base from which they can speak. [However] many professors are critical of the inclusion of confessional narrative in the classroom, where students are doing a lot of the talking because they lack the skill needed to facilitate dialogue'.

- We have been socialised into a set of assumptions that support a traditional teacher-led technical rational curriculum. We are so rooted in a technical rational approach to learning/ reflective practice – How can we view the curriculum from such a radical reflective perspective? The technical rational is so embodied within us as individuals and within the university system that we naturally resist a shift.
- Democratising the classroom with its shift of power leading to a co-centric milieu will result in chaos and issues around 'who controls the learning environment'. Students simply are not responsible enough.

As Hooks [6, p. 152] writes –

'That's the difference education as the practice of freedom makes. The bottom-line assumption has to be that everyone in the classroom has to act responsibly. That has to be the starting point – that we are able to act responsibly together to create a learning environment. All too often we have been trained as professors to assume students are not capable of acting responsibly, that is we don't exert control over them, then there's just going to be mayhem'.

- We are comfortable in our current teaching roles although we accept there has been little demand for us to account for our teaching practice and demonstrate teaching development. It is probably true we churn out the same 'old stuff' yet we feel that is effective teaching.

- We are naturally reflective. You can't teach otherwise. It is absurd to suggest we are not and suggestion that we lack the ability to teach through reflection and dialogue is slanderous.
- We do not have the time to return to clinical practice as envisaged. We do not view our lack of practice credibility as significant because the students have mentors in practice. We know how to bridge the theory-practice gap.
- Our bottom line is that we like the 'status quo' and naturally resist any attempt to disturb this when we might be disadvantaged in some way. As it stands all we see is one big headache, disrupting things for the sake of a few zealots for change.

Hooks [6, p. 142–3] notes, shifting one's pedagogical practice is difficult –

'I want to reiterate that many teachers who do not have difficulty releasing old ideas, embracing new ways of thinking, may still be resolutely attached to old ways of *practicing teaching* as their more conservative colleagues. This is a crucial issue. Even those of us who are experimenting with progressive pedagogical practices are afraid to change. My point is that it takes fierce commitment, a will to struggle, to let our work as teachers reflect progressive pedagogical'.

Student Resistance

Journal Entry 14.2

Some time ago I met a district nurse at my local village fete. My partner mentioned that I was a bit of a guru in reflective practice. The district nurse recoiled and said she hated reflective practice, that she had had it shoved down her throat. No one liked it, it was a waste of time! I was left wondering why she had such a hostile attitude towards reflection.

I considered that students may resist a reflective curriculum because:

- They may feel threatened by the intense gaze particularly if they lack commitment to practice or study. It is less prescriptive and therefore more 'adult' and requires more responsibility and self-direction. It is not what they have been used to in schools.
- The shift from student passivity to student agency may feel threatening to the student if not frankly overwhelming. Quoting Hooks [6, p. 143] –

  'The difficulty getting students to take responsibility is that they have already learnt that they are not the ones with legitimate authority. Students have learnt the left brain approach and expect to be taught in the manner they are accustomed to'.

- They do not like or value reflection as experienced. They have an attitude – 'give us the facts necessary to pass assignments'. They have embodied a technical-rational learning style grounded in an evidence-based mentality. This is not surprising considering healthcare's demand that practice should be evidence-based.

Susan Brooks writes [36] –

'I commenced the course (MSc leadership in healthcare) as a die- hard, almost evangelistic, theorist. I had previously studied the four learning styles of Honey and Mumford [37] and recognised that my preference was always for logically sound theories that fitted into rational schemes. As a theorist I readily accepted, usually without question, basic assumptions, principles, theories and models and preferred rational objectivity rather than anything subjective or ambiguous [37]. I often rejected the other learning styles of activism, pragmatism and reflection and they were not really part of my psyche. I had paid scant attention to them in the past only where necessary to fulfil the requirements of academic courses attended. My theoretical stance was probably based on my strong adherence to the notion of evidence based practice, that is 'doing the right things right' - a belief so strongly felt that I was chair of the Evidence Based Practice Council for my organisation. Evidence based practice has arguably become the 'buzz word' of healthcare in recent years and has become somewhat hegemony in nursing. It had been a foremost element in the linguistic currency of my nurse training and is a pervasive element in the clinical governance agenda so widely espoused in my organisation'.

The UK government's drive to modernise health care includes a commitment to the provision of health services based on evidence and published strategies for nursing emphasise the need for a robust evidence base [38]. I saw this need for evidence as a basis for effective practice as paramount and, to me that meant adherence to objective and proven theory. I felt comfortable with this concept possibly because, as Craig and Smyth [39] note, evidence-based practice is a phrase that trips lightly off the tongue, engenders a reassuring glow that all is well and signifies that nurses merely need to implement the available evidence. As the course developed, I recognised that 'evidence based practice' is one of the most used but least understood adjectives in health care [39]. Nursing (and nurse leadership) does not always lend itself to the application of research evidence and technical rationality as I learned through Schön's [9] work on reflective practice, and I was exposed to the opportunity to consider a new way of thinking. This course was about to challenge and question my mode of (limited) thinking, radically alter my previous learning style and open doors into other ways of thinking and perception. This new way of thinking was particularly exciting to me and I am now acutely aware that such a strong and rigid adherence to the notion that evidence can provide all of the answers brings with it the danger of stifling creativity'.

Brooks' reveals how her learning style shifted through exposure to guided reflection. It was transformative.

- Students may have little sense of and value in 'owning their learning'. As a result, reflection is a learning style that some students will resist. Plazer et al. [40] noted that the nurses' previous educational experience made the self-directed approach associated with the adult-learning process difficult, as nurses had not been encouraged to think for themselves.
- Students may fear exposing themselves and their emotions, particularly students who lack confidence in themselves [40, 41] and where reflection is viewed as a type of surveillance, assessment and control [42]. This is understandable considering guided reflection is about 'who I am' where learning becomes personal. Main [41, p. 97] notes:

  'If reflection comes slowly to some people because they have little sense of involvement in their own learning, it comes unwillingly to others because they have little belief in its value for them'.

It follows that teachers and students must necessarily unlearn previous attitudes, assumptions and behaviours when they are comfortable doing what they have always done. Thus, the forum for change acts to ensure that [19]:

- All people involved have *ownership* of the curriculum to offset any sense of not being involved or it being imposed on them. The point is to encourage commitment rather than compliance to the curriculum resulting in passive resistance.
- The curriculum is *tailor made* to suit the local circumstances rather than a model taken of the shelf to give a sense of ownership.
- Necessary staff *development* to ensure the success of the curriculum are identified and established.
- To establish a *pilot site* to test and evaluate the new curriculum.
- To establish feedback loops, for example, the use of the 'classroom critical incident questionnaire' (Appendix 1) to facilitate student responsibility for their learning, involvement and feedback.

Leap of Faith

At the end of the planning forum's dialogue, there needs to be a leap of faith when the forces for the change out weight the forces against it – termed the critical mass. This can be mitigated through a pilot curriculum where processes and outcomes can be monitored and evaluated and the curriculum adjusted in response.

Thus, the involvement of resisters in the forum for change is essential to give voice to their concerns and involve them in planning the change. Through dialogue, old and new norms are revealed revealing the creative tension as the focus for change. Wheatley [43, p. 130] notes

> 'Behaviours don't change by announcing new values. We move only gradually into being able to act congruently with those values. To do this, we have to develop much greater awareness of now we're acting: we have to become for more self-reflective than normal. And we help one another notice when we fall back into old behaviours. We will all slop back into the past – that is unavoidable – but when this happens, we agree to counsel one another with generous spirit. Little by little, tested by events and crises, we learn how to enact these new values. We develop different patterns of behaviour. We slowly become who we said we wanted to be'.

This long quote reflects the necessary spirit, pace, tolerance and culture of change, acknowledging the radical shift requires a dialogical community of practitioners working patiently together.

Staff Development

The transitional success to realising the person-centred reflective curriculum will depend on enabling all involved to shift their assumptions and develop new skills.

1. Establishing teacher guided reflection groups for all staff, both educational and administrative, led by person either within or outside the organisation with acknowledged reflective skills. After six sessions, the group can become peer-led with an expert guide shadowing. After 12 sessions, the teacher guided reflection groups are rolled out to be self-sustaining.
2. Establishing mentor-guided reflection groups in a similar format as above. Developing mentors' reflective capacity links into the Nursing and Midwifery Council for the UK's requirement for revalidation with its reflective practice requirement.[vii] As noted in the curriculum aims, student practitioners become mentors – a 'grow your own' approach.
3. The development of lecturer-practitioners. This can be linked to developing nursing development units as pilot sites for the development of person-centred reflective curriculum and become centres of expertise for other units.

Community of Inquiry

The planning team will morph to become a community of inquiry or learning organisation. Wheatley and Kellner-Rogers [44, p. 70] state –

> 'A system [such as the curriculum] is fluid relationships that we observe as a rigid structure. If we look past these structures, we see that systems spring to life from agreements among individuals [us] on how best to live [and work] together. From this multitude of individual explorations, a system may suddenly appear [that] individuals didn't know they were creating'.

The community of inquiry is a creative space where student practitioners, teachers and practice staff *collaborate* to ensure the new programme works effectively based on the premise that every individual takes responsibility for their own performance and for the functioning of the group as a whole. Without mutual responsibility, the group will fail. Peers offer an invaluable resource to each other as they relate to each other's experiences. Wheatley and Keller-Rogers [44, p. 53] write –

> 'When we link up with others, we open ourselves to yet another paradox. While surrendering some of our freedom, we open ourselves to even more creative forms of expression. This stage of being has been described as communion, because we are preserved as our selves but are shorn of our separateness or aloneness. What we bring to others remains our self-expression. Yet the meaning of who we are changes through our communion with them. We are identifiable as our selves. But we have discovered new meaning and different contributions, and we are no longer the same'.

A community of inquiry dialogue to learn positively from conflict and mistakes towards consensus to further develop the person-centred curriculum. It does not blame and shame. Obviously, conflicts arise but are viewed as opportunities for learning. Such a community is extensive governed by a council of representatives (the hub of a wheel) in collaboration with splinter groups (the spokes of the wheel). A wheel is round reflecting dialogue and collaboration with no pinnacle of authority. People may consider the person-centred reflective curriculum as utopian. Of course it is not. There is a 'real world' where life simply isn't like that. But it is a vision to strive towards and with vision, commitment and determination it can be realised.

Post Registration Education

Moving from Buford into the university setting opened an opportunity for me to develop reflection within curriculum notably at post-registration and graduate level.

Becoming a Reflective and Effective Practitioner

Based on my 'roots' experience at Buford in teaching undergraduate nursing students through guided reflection, I designed the 'Becoming a reflective and effective practitioner' programme within a BSc Nursing Studies degree for post-registration practitioners. The programme was originally designed as a double module delivered over one semester (12 weeks). However, it became evident that students were just beginning to grasp reflective learning by this stage. Thus, the programme was extended into two double modules over two semesters to enable students to embody reflection and reap its full benefit in terms of realising their visions of practice (30 weeks including holiday breaks). The programme recruited 16 practitioners divided into two guided reflection groups that met weekly comprising 30 × 4 hourly study days.

Twenty-four days were designated guided reflection sessions and six comprised workshops that focused on journaling, reflective theory, standards of care, art workshop, narrative construction, evaluation.

The students undertook three assignments:

1. To write a reflective narrative based on an experience shared within guided reflection revealing tentative insights gained.
2. To construct a personal theory of reflection based on their initial exposure to guided reflection in dialogue with an informing literature.
3. To construct a reflexive narrative of insights gained evidenced by at least three experiences.

Students were given leeway to interpret these assignments in creative ways. Exemplars are shown in Chapters 18, 21–23, evidencing the efficacy of the programme alongside other publications as previously noted. 'The proof was in the pudding' to coin a phrase, meaning that the value, quality, or truth of something must be judged based on direct experience with it – or on its results.[viii]

MSc Leadership in Healthcare

The becoming a reflective and effective practitioner course proved the efficacy of guided reflection towards enabling practitioners to realise their visions of practice, visions that had been constrained for whatever reason. Based on this 'knowing' I set about establishing a MSc Leadership in Healthcare. I knew from my experience as clinical leader at Buford hospital that facilitating person-centred practice at Buford required a certain type of leadership. In my opinion, the best fit was servant-leadership [45, 46], the qualities of which I set out in Chapter 8. The programme ran for 12 years until my early retirement, during which more than a 100 leadership students participated from diverse professions and roles.

The programme was designed as community of inquiry. It met for a whole day every two weeks to share and reflect on their experiences of becoming a leader guided by myself. The student leaders' backgrounds were not significant representing a diverse range of nurses from staff nurses to directors of nursing. Diversity of health care disciplines added a rich mix to the community.

The curriculum was constructed as a series of modules (Figure 14.3) that covered the spectrum of leadership activities, arranged to inform the core dissertation module of 'Becoming a leader' presented as a reflexive narrative.

The Modules[ix]

- 'Visions of leadership' was designed to enable the 'leaders' to construct a tentative vision of leadership. In response to setting out leadership theories, all the students aspired towards a transformational type or servant leadership in sharp contrast with the transactional organisations in which they worked. This immediately set up the creative tension between transformational/servant-leadership and transactional management that became the focus for understanding and resolving throughout the programme.

Year 1 Semester 1		Year 1 Semester 2		
Visions of leadership	Conflict management	Managing change project		
Dissertation – 'Being and becoming a leader'				
Developing quality project		Alternative perspectives on leadership	Leading in a chaotic world	Dissertation support [June–October]
Year 2 Semester 1		Year 2 Semester 2		Extension of year 2 until submission of dissertation end of October

FIGURE 14.3 MSc leadership in health care programme.

- Managing conflict module focused the leaders to reflect on how they managed conflict situations in tension with how they would ideally manage conflict in tune with their emerging vision of leadership.
- The change and quality modules were designed as projects that involved student presentations at conferences organised by themselves.
- The leading in a chaotic world module was designed to enable the leaders to explore how practice is structured through strange attractors governed by meaning and self-organisation rather than through command and control. This module was a pivotal moment within the programme where the leaders had a much greater sense of themselves as leaders within practice and had become adept at reflection.
- The alternative perspectives module involves shadowing a 'leader' within the student's organisation and 'measuring' them against their own vision of leadership. It also involves giving feedback to that leader and contrasting this feedback with an appraisal of their emerging leadership.
- The dissertation module commenced at the beginning of the programme as a continuous core throughout the whole programme. After completion of the last 'taught' module, the student-leaders had five months of intensive guided reflection sessions focused on developing their reflexive narratives.

Structuring the Reflexive Narrative Dissertation

The reflexive narrative dissertation was structured of five chapters:[x]

1. Background
2. Methodology and method (research process)
3. The reflexive narrative
4. Discussion of insights
5. Reflection on the process of self-inquiry

The background chapter is necessary for the reader to position the student within the narrative due to its subjective and contextual nature. It sets the scene. To structure background, I adapted Heidegger's notion of Fore-structure to structure background [47, p. 198–9]. It sets out three levels of prior reflection, all of which are influential in interpreting their experiences through self-inquiry:

- Fore-having – where interpretation is set against the student's understanding of prior relevant experience. This includes upbringing, education, experience of leadership, role and suchlike. It sets out 'where the practitioner is coming from'.
- Fore-sight – where interpretation is an understanding as to how to approach becoming a leader from an understanding of their current role within the organisation set against a tentative vision of leadership. It sets out 'where the practitioner is now'.
- Fore-conception – where interpretation is set within the student's expectations of self-inquiry realising its achievement as a reality rather than an idealistic understanding. It sets out 'where the practitioner is heading to'.

Methodology and Method

Reflexive narratives written as formal research at all academic levels require an appreciation of self-inquiry through guided reflection as a methodology. The students were introduced to the reflexive narrative bricolage (Figure 1.2) that sets out philosophical and theoretical influences on reflexive narrative offering various pathways of exploration and presentation. The two constructs of methodology and method are combined because methodology is only of relevance to inform the process of constructing a reflexive narrative rather than prescribing its form. Thus, the student references any methodological idea in relation to their learning experience.

Discussion of Insights

In this chapter, the practitioner pulls out from their reflexive narrative significant insights in becoming a leader to explore with a deeper immersion and dialogue with informing theoretical sources. At this level, new 'knowing in practice' is expounded.

Reflection on the Process of Self-inquiry

The final chapter asks the practitioner to reflect on the process of constructing their reflexive narrative revealing the influence of guided reflection. It invites an evaluation of the process adding to the understanding of reflexive narrative as a formal research process. Excerpts from this chapter are offered in the book and in Chapter 26.

Collaborative Inquiry

The programme was established as a collaborative inquiry into becoming a leader whereby students agreed for me using their assignments and dissertations for analysis, edit as necessary, and publish. In total, more than 100 reflexive narrative dissertations became available guided by myself and which I meta-analysed resulting in the book 'Mindful leadership' [46] evidenced by four student narratives. This analysis revealed and illuminated the creative tension between the student leaders' vision of transformational leadership and the realities of everyday practice that constrained its realisation, and how these constraints were understood and overcome to varying degrees of success. The book illustrates how reflexive narratives can generate theory through systematic self-inquiry and the transformational power of guided reflection to enable leadership.

Conclusion

If we truly desire reflective practitioners, then we require compatible educational and clinical environments. If not, then we will always be scratching at the surface of what being a reflective practitioner might mean. Scratching that becomes painful to the point whereby even bothering is just a waste of effort. Reflective learning cannot simply be bolted on to an existing technical rational curriculum without it being perceived as itself a technical rational perspective. I couldn't agree more with

Coleman and Willis's [48, p. 910] comment –

> 'If students are to truly maximise the benefits of reflection and reflective writing there needs to be a paradigm shift in nursing pedagogy away from traditional models of reflective writing and assessment'.

References

1. Clarke, N. M. (2014) A person-centred enquiry into the teaching and learning experiences of reflection and reflective practice – Part one. *Nurse Education Today* 34, 1219–1224.

2. Bulley, C., Donaghy, M., Coppoolse, M., Bizzini, M. (2005) *Sports physiotherapy competencies and standards.* www.sportsphysiotherapyfor all.org/publications [accessed August 18th 2015].

3. Paterson, C., Chapman, J. (2013) Enhancing skills of critical reflection to evidence learning in professional practice. *Physical Therapy in Sport* 14, 133–138.

4. Freire, P. (1970) *The Pedagogy of the Oppressed.* Penguin, Harmondsworth.

5. Woolf, V. (1945) *A Room of One's Own.* Penguin Books, London.

6. Hooks, B. (1994) *Teaching to Transgress: Education As the Practice of Freedom.* Routledge, New York.

7. Johns, C. (2014) An enquiry into the spiritual. *International Practice Development Journal* 3(2), [9].

8. Bailey, J. (1998) The supervisor's story: from expert to novice. In C. Johns, D. Freshwater [Eds.] *Transforming Nursing Through Reflective Practice.* Blackwell Science, 194–205.

9. Schön, D. (1987) *Educating the Reflective Practitioner.* Jossey-Bass, San Francisco.

10. Beauchamp, C. (2015) Reflection in teacher education: issues emerging from a review of current literature. *Reflective Practice* 16(1), 123–141.

11. Russell, T. (2013) Has reflective practice done more harm than good in teacher education? *Phronesis* 2, 80–88.

12. Ramsey, S. (2010) Making thinking public: reflection in elementary teacher education. *Reflective Practice* 11(2), 205–216.

13. Pirsig, R. (1989) *Zen and the Art of Motorcycle Maintenance.* Vintage, London.

14. Ausubel, D. (1967) *Learning Theory and Classroom Practice.* Ontario Institute for Studies in Education, Toronto.

15. Vaughan B. (1990) Knowing that and knowing how: the role of the lecturer practitioner. In B. Kershaw, J. Salvage [Eds.] *Models for Nursing 2.* Scutari Press, Harrow, 103–113.

16. Elcock, K. (1998) Lecturer-practitioner: a concept analysis. *Journal of Advanced Nursing* 28(5), 1092–1098.

17. Driver, J., Campbell, J. (2013) An evaluation of the impact of lecturer practitioners on learning. *British Journal of Nursing* 9(5), 292–300.

18. Rafferty, A. M., Allcock, N., Lathlean, J. (1996) The theory/practice 'gap': taking issue with the issue. *Journal of Advanced Nursing* 23(4), 685–691.

19. Kramer, M. (1974) *Reality Shock: Why Nurses Leave Nursing.* C. V. Mosby, New York.

20. Ottaway, R. (1978) A change strategy to implement new norms, new styles and new environment in the work organization. *Personnel Review* 5(1), 13–18.

21. Lewin, K. (1951) *Field Theory in Social Science.* Harper & Row, New York.

22. Mann, K., Gordon, J., Macleaod, A. (2009) Reflection and reflective practice in health professions education: a systematic review. *Advances in Health Science Education* 14, 595–621.

23. Davis, M. (1998) The rocky road to reflection. In C. Johns, D. Freshwater [Eds.] *Transforming Nursing Through Reflective Practice.* Blackwell Science, 206–213.

24. Latchford, Y. (2002) Finding a new way in health visiting. In C. Johns [Ed.] *Guided Reflection; Advancing Practice.* Blackwell Publishing, 144–165.

25. Madden, I. (2002) Working with women following traumatic childbirth. In C. Johns [Ed.] *Guided Reflection; Advancing Practice.* Blackwell Publishing, 187–212.

26. Jarrett, L., Johns, C. (2005) Constructing the reflexive narrative. In C. Johns, D. Freshwater [Eds.] *Transforming Nursing Through Reflective Practice* (second edition). Blackwell Publishing, Oxford, 162–179.

27. Lee, S. (2009) Reflection on caring. In C. Johns [Ed.] *Becoming A Reflective Practitioner* (third edition). Wiley-Blackwell, 164–171.

28. Priest, J.-M., Johns, C. (2010) More than eggs for breakfast. In C. Johns [Ed.] *Guided Reflection; A Narrative Approach to Advancing Professional Practice* (second edition). Wiley-Blackwell, Oxford, 195–214.

29. Fordham, M. (2010) Falling through the net and the spider's web; two metaphoric moments along my journey. In C. Johns [Ed.] *Guided Reflection: A Narrative Approach to Advancing Professional Practice.* Wiley-Blackwell, 145–163.

30. O'Connor, A., Hyde, A., Treacey, M. (2003) Nurse teachers' constructions of reflection and reflective practice. (Qualitative research into tutors'

perceptions and experiences of using reflection with diploma nursing students in Ireland.) *Reflective Practice* 4(2), 107–119.

31. McGrath, D., Higgins, A. (2006). Implementing and evaluating reflective practice group sessions. *Nurse Education in Practice* 6(3), 175–181.

32. O'Donovan, M. (2007). Implementing reflection: insights from pre-registration mental health students. *Nurse Education Today* 27(6), 515–664.

33. Mann, K., Gordon, J., MacLeod, A. (2009) Reflection and reflective practice in health professions education: a systematic review. *Advances in Health Sciences Education* 14, 595–621.

34. McCarthy. J., Cassidy, I., Tuohy, D. (2013) Lecturers' experiences of facilitating guided group reflection with pre-registration BSc Nursing students. *Nurse Education Today* 33, 36–40.

35. Smith, A., Jack, K. (2005) Reflective: a meaningful task for students. *Nursing Standard* 19(26), 33–34.

36. Beau, C., Dracup, K. (1976) Implementing nursing research in a critical care setting. *Journal of Nursing Administration* 6(10), 14–17.

37. Brooks, S. (2004) *Becoming A Transformational Leader*. Unpublished MSC Leadership in healthcare dissertation, University of Bedfordshire.

38. Honey, P., Mumford, A. (1989) *The Manual of Learning Styles* (second edition). Peter Honey Publications.

39. Department of Health. (1997) *The Evidence Base of the Public Health Contribution of Nurses and Midwives*. HMSO.

40. Craig, J. V., Smyth, R. L. (2002). *The Evidence-Based Practice Manual for Nurses*. Churchill Livingstone, Edinburgh, Scotland.

41. Platzer, H., Blake, D., Ashford, D. (2000) Barriers to learning from reflection; a study of the use of group work with post-registration nurses. *Journal of Advanced Nursing* 31(5), 1001–1008.

42. Main, A. (1985) Reflection and the development of learning skills. In D. Boud, R. Keogh, D. Walker [Eds.] *Reflection: Turning Experience into Learning*. Kogan Page, London/Nichols Publishing Company, New York, 91–99.

43. Cotton, A. (2001) Private thoughts in public spheres: issues in reflection and reflective practices in nursing. *Journal of Advanced Nursing* 36(4), 512–519.

44. Wheatley, M. (1999) *Leadership and the New Science*. Berrett-Koehler.

45. Wheatley, M., Kellner-Rogers, M. (1996) *A Simpler Way*. Berrett-Koehler, San Francisco.

46. Greenleaf, R. (1977/2002) *Servant Leadership: A Journey into the Nature of Legitimate Power and Greatness*. Paulist Press, New York.

47. Johns, C. (2016) *Mindful Leadership: A Guide for the Healthcare Professions*. Palgrave, London.

48. Dreyfus, H. (1993) *Being–in-the-World: A Commentary on Heidegger's Being and Time, Division 1*. The MIT Press, Cambridge MA.

49. Coleman, D., Willis, D. S. (2015) Reflective writing; the student nurse's perspective on reflective writing and poetry writing. *Nurse Education Today* 35(7), 906–911.

50. Yew, E., Goh, K. (2016) Problem-based learning: an overview of the process and impact on learning. *Health Professions Education* 2(2), 75–79.

51. McCormack, B., McCance, T. (2021). The person-centred nursing framework. In: J. Dewing, B. McCormack, T. McCance [Eds.] *Person-Centred Nursing Research: Methodology, Methods and Outcomes*. Springer, Cham.

52. Toffler, A. (1984) *Future Shock*. Pan Books, London.

53. Johns, C. (2021) *Reflexive Narrative; Self-Inquiry Toward Self-Realization and Its Performance*. Sage, Thousand Oaks.

Notes

i. Google problem based learning to locate a plethora of articles. One example is Yew & Goh, [49].

ii. A pertinent exemplar of systems thinking is 'The Person-centred nursing framework' [50]. This framework offers a potential template for appreciating the 'whole' structure of person-centred practice to inform curriculum.

iii. NHS Forward Review 2015. https://www.england.nhs.uk/wp-content/uploads/2014/10/5yfv-web.pdf.

iv. The Royal College of Nursing analysed the latest Nursing and Midwifery Council (NMC) data of UK-educated nursing staff leaving the register in England. Between 2021 and 2024, the numbers leaving within 10 years of registering increased by 43%, whilst those leaving within five years rose a staggering 67%. According to the NMC's leavers survey, nursing staff cite poor physical and mental health, burnout or exhaustion, and changes in personal circumstances as key reasons for leaving nursing outside of retirement. https://www.rcn.org.uk/news-and-events/Press-Releases/huge-increase-in-nurses-quitting-early-in-perfect-storm-for-patientcare#:~:text=According%20to%20the%20NMC's%20leavers,leaving%20nursing%20outside%20of%20retirement. (November 11th, 2024).

v.   Future Shock is a book written by the futurist Alvin Toffler [51]. In the book, Toffler defines the term "future shock" as a certain psychological state of individuals and entire societies. His shortest definition for the term is a personal perception of "too much change in too short a period of time". https://en.wikipedia.org/wiki/Future_Shock.

vi. Force Field Analysis offers an effective reflective framework in change management for looking at forces for driving or resisting change in relation to the status quo. The theory suggests that change agents should focus primarily on minimising resisting forces as strengthening driving forces would lead to strengthening resistance.

vii. http://www.nmc.org.uk/standards/revalidation/provisional-revalidation-requirements/ [accessed 18th August 2015].

viii. https://www.dictionary.com/e/slang/the-proof-is-in-the-pudding/.

ix. A detailed content of the modules is published in Mindful leadership [46].

x.   This blueprint for constructing the reflexive narrative was further developed into a doctoral programme structured within the community of inquiry resulting in the publication of 'Reflexive narrative' [52]. At the time I termed this 'reflexive narrative' research. However it is more accurately termed 'Guided reflection' research as stated in Figure 1.2, presented as a reflexive narrative.

CHAPTER 15

The Tale of Two Teachers

Introduction

How might teaching from a reflective perspective differ from a conventional technical rational approach? Janet and John are two nurse teachers who have a remit to teach stroke management to second-year degree students. The students will be on medical ward placements where stroke patients reside.

Janet believes strongly in a reflective practice approach to teaching, whereas John is oriented towards a conventional technical rational approach. The students in both institutions have been introduced to reflective practice earlier in their nursing education.

John

John sets out his teaching plan with aims and measurable objectives.

At the end of this session, the students will:

1. Understand the aetiology of cerebral vascular accident.
2. Recognise its common symptoms.
3. Know the range of investigations to establish diagnosis.
4. Have gained a critical understanding of nursing care alongside other professionals.
5. Appreciate the social and psychological impact on the patient and family.

John prepares a power-point presentation to enable him to move smoothly between the objectives supported by references. He has two hours to deliver. All in all, a solid lecture with some discussion time built in for students to express any thoughts they might have, acknowledging that some students may have previous experience of caring for stroke patients.

For the assignment John writes – 'A case study reflecting the essential aspects of treating a stroke patient. It is expected the assignment will show evidence of knowledge of stroke aetiology and symptoms, investigations, and nursing care'.

Janet

Janet sits at her computer wondering how best to deliver this session. She considers her range of options. First, a solid lecture based around a series of objectives. She senses many students would like this approach, as it fits with their normal approach to teaching. She is mindful that she is 'out on a limb' regarding teaching from a reflective paradigm despite the curriculum expectation to teach reflection. She knows that many of her peers teach reflective practice purely from a technical rational perspective that only gives lip service to its learning potential. She decides to deliver the session from a reflective perspective using performance.

She drafts her lesson plan. The objective is – 'to understand the needs of the stroke patient and the family and the response of the health care team to meeting these needs'.

She muses – 'How best to deliver this session?'

The first need is to prime the students by talking through the teaching approach. Then share a brief narrative of caring for a stroke patient and relatives to develop the idea of how to construct a narrative. In doing so, she will make herself vulnerable by sharing. Taking a risk. She knows that students will appreciate this. It brings her closer to the students, more working with them rather than talking at them. Diffusing the power differential between them.

Collecting the story should be relatively easy as she works one day a week on a number of medical wards supporting students in practice and staff who mentor them. She can arrange to meet stroke patients and their families and the health professionals involved in their care. She can even arrange to give care herself.

For the assignment, she writes 'Insights gained from appreciating patients' and relatives' experiences and needs of suffering stroke and the nurses' response in collaboration with other health professionals'.

Janet considers the students should now be adept with the idea of gaining insight from reflections in their second year of training. She phones Peter, one of the few teachers she feels she has a philosophical rapport. He can see the bigger picture and the competing assumptions that govern it. She talks through her session idea with him.

Peter is supportive. 'Go for it! Janet. Create some ripples and stir up the pond'.

'Thank you. I need that. Just knowing that at least one other person can see the bigger picture and the options is helpful. In a practice discipline such as nursing, we must focus on practice rather than theory as the primary source of learning. I know it goes against the grain that most of my colleagues will reject this claim but I think their resistance comes from an ignorance because they are not reflective about their own work, so how can they teach reflective practice except from a technical perspective?'

'That's very true Janet! You inspire me to consider reflective practice beyond the technical rational'.

Janet puts down the phone more resolute in her intention.

Next morning, she puts on her clinical dress and goes in search.

She also arranges to meet April, a teacher from performing arts who has expressed an interest in reflective practice, over lunch to explore how performance might work.

Basically, April will introduce some movement exercises to counter inhibition and some breath and voice projection exercises. She will then take a couple of scenarios from Janet's narrative to involve the group. She suggests I read around 'Performance studies' by Richard Schechner [1].

Two weeks later Janet and April enter the classroom. Janet introduces April as a teacher from school of performing arts is joining our session to help prep performance. She commences by 'bringing the mind home' to help the group focus on the task. Just three minutes and the group are quieter, more present.

Janet outlines her plan:

- First hour – explore her narrative of caring for stroke patients.
- Second hour – prepare for the follow-up study day in four-week time.

Key components:

- This will be organised in groups of six students.
- Go out onto wards and talk with stroke patients, their relatives and health professionals – what are the significant care factors, what investigations have been carried out, what is the resultant aetiology?

- Use the Model for structured reflection (see Figure 2.2) as a framework to consider the experiences of different people involved in stroke care [patients, relatives, health professionals]. In particular consider how people felt and reasons for that. Consider – 'Do the actions of health professionals really meet needs of patients and relatives?' Be critical – if needs not met – then why? How might real needs be known and met?
- Identify and critique a list of key texts to explore these issues from a theoretical perspective to critically inform your insights.
- Reflect on your findings and construct a 'performance' of findings to illuminate stroke care together with written commentary based on two 10-minute scenarios around insights gained for when we meet at our study day in four-week time. In total, each group has 20 minutes. Choose a narrator who can link the experiences with relevant sources of information.
- Janet and April will be available for consultation as necessary.

The group buzz with novel excitement, seemingly not fazed by the task. Indeed, they seem to relish the creative responsibility. Janet then shares her narrative. Posing questions to engage the group, drawing on their previous nursing experiences, linking with stroke theory and research. She explicitly uses cues from the MSR to illuminate their value in gaining insight. An hour quickly passes. April takes over and the group play with performance ideas using Janet's narrative as an example of how narrative can be acted out.

John Reflects on his Session

'It went fine as usual. I was in control and moved through the objectives seamlessly. We had only a brief time for discussion of previous experience. However, that was useful. It added a learning flavour to the session. Maybe more time would help. Generally the assignments were descriptive Not very reflective but then that's to be expected from students. However the students showed a reasonable understanding of stroke and its nursing care'.

Janet Reflects on her Session

'No time to fit it all in. However we were available for ongoing support. Performance is complex and may need more prep time. However they got the gist of it and will learn through the experience of doing it. I checked which wards had stroke patients and were willing to talk with the students'.

'The performances were brilliant. I never expected them to rise to the challenge so well. The performance students would like to be involved next time we do something similar. The assignments were so reflective- really highlighted the core issues especially around emotional and psychological issues, challenging whether stroke care was empathic enough. Will definitely approach other "conditions" in this way. It goes to prove that if you give students responsibility they rise to the challenge. Mind you it is not without some trepidation. I felt very anxious about the "performance" part, knowing little about performance as learning. Without expert help I do not think I would have contemplated it. I would have been exposed as an imposter and looked foolish in front of the students. But I did say – "this is learning for me as well" dropping any pretence of knowing. Risky stuff – Does such confession undermine students' confidence especially with something that goes against the grain taking us all out of our comfort zones? I had to trust the students and my own instinct that this approach made good pedagogical sense'.

I asked the students to evaluate the session – What would they do differently given the experience again? Is there anything more I [as teacher] could have done to support them. All reflective teaching, by its very nature, needs a critical evaluation rather than take it for granted. I find 'The classroom critical incident questionnaire' enables this [2] (see Appendix 2).

I suggested the students also give me anonymous written feedback for me to consider and discuss with them before we do further performance learning. It's quite emotional – I feel closer to the students as if we have bridged a gap between us. I no longer teach at them but teach with them. Rather like the way we value working with patients rather than nursing at them. Shift from teacher-centric to student-centric.

Feedback from Alan – 'I asked the group about the session. The feedback was positive despite one or two dissenting students who felt "lost" in the task'.

I responded – 'fancy teaching with me next time? I think it will work better with more than one teacher'. He responded – 'Perhaps we can set up a performance workshop to explore the milieu more deeply with our performance colleagues?' I know he was hedging his bets, wanting to be open to the idea but cautious. Always a fear of incompetence or peer criticism holds us back, making us fall back on known approaches within our collective comfort zone.

I sense a pressure on me to conform as if using a performance approach threatens the status quo. An older colleague who always seems to put others down sarcastically remarked at a team meeting if I was hoping for an Oscar? It caught me off-guard. I tried to explain my reflective approach. With withering scorn, she suggested I focus on my real role as a teacher and stop using the school as a playground. Teaching is serious stuff and teachers must control the classroom or anarchy would ensue. I must admit it knocked my confidence being slated in public like that.

Nursing is a practice discipline. As such practice must be at the core of any curriculum. Theory and research exist to inform practice. It cannot predict practice because nursing is essentially unpredictable and complex because of its human nature. Therefore, nursing is always interpreted at the point of contact. As such practitioners require necessary knowing in practice to navigate the seemingly indeterminate nature of practice towards realising person-centred practice.

References

1. Schechner, R. (2002) *Performance Studies: An Introduction* (second edition). Routledge, New York.

2. Brookfield, S (1996) *Becoming A Critically Reflective Teacher*. Jossey-Bass, San Francisco.

CHAPTER 16

Guiding First-year Nursing Students

Introduction

In the person-centred reflective curriculum group, guidance is the primary teaching mode. In the first guided reflection session, the guide contracts with the students so that they understand and accept their respective responsibilities to ensure the group's effectiveness. The ideas of reflection, the curriculum aim of person-centred practice, keeping a reflective journal to record reflections on experiences, especially those experiences felt as significant in some way and those they are willing to disclose and dialogue as the mode of communication, notably to listen carefully to their peer's experience with openness, curiosity and respect have all been explored (as explored in Chapters 8 and 9).

Guiding Reflection with First-year Nursing Students

In the following scenario, the students have been learning for eight months. They are on a surgical ward placement. Lucy, their lecturer-practitioner has organised delivering the module through guided reflection sessions twice weekly for two hours. Their guide is Lucy. Today is Michelle's turn to share an experience.

Michelle's Experience[i]

Lucy [to the whole group] 'As you listen to Michelle's experience note issues you feel are significant especially in context of your own experiences. Also think about the MSR cues'.

Michelle reads from her journal: 'Mrs Morris was admitted for a breast biopsy. She had been a nurse, a fact that made me feel slightly on edge wondering if she would judge me. But not to worry, she was a pleasant lady. The next morning I was doing the drugs with Katie, a senior staff nurse who is also my practice mentor. Katie can be rather brusque when anxious and that morning we were hectic chasing the clock. It became a task to rush through which I know is not good practice when it concerns patients' medications'.

Michelle paused as if waiting for comment. She looked at Lucy for permission to continue. Lucy simply smiled and nodded.

'When we got to Mrs Morris I asked her whether she had any pain?' She was written up for some paracetamol as required. She was due to go home later that afternoon after the consultant had reviewed her results and explored treatment options. She said 'No .... oh I feel weepy' and then she burst into tears. I said 'what's up Mrs Morris?' She said 'My friends were saying how scared they would be if it was them having a breast biopsy. I hadn't appreciated these feelings until now. Oh my husband and my children!'

It made me think – she's a nurse and she's so vulnerable. I just stood there not knowing what to do. What to say that would help? I looked at Katie uncertain what to do but she had moved on with the medicine trolley and I knew she expected me to rejoin her. I said to Katie 'hold on a moment'. I said 'I'm sorry you feel so weepy'. I passed her a tissue. I said I'll come back later if you like'. Mrs Morris said – 'yes, I know you're busy'. I expect she'd been watching us. I told Katie what had happened. She said it must be awful for Mrs Morris and that she would go back later and talk with her. I felt so sad for her. She could have been my mum. We have quite a few women undergoing breast biopsy. I get the impression nurses are not as sensitive to these women as we should be. They look jolly and jovial outside but inside it's like a bombshell!'

Lucy: 'Finding an upset patient whilst doing the medicine round is a common occurrence on hospital wards. It's often one of the few times patients get direct attention especially for short stay patients like Mrs Morris having a biopsy. Put yourself in her shoes. You spent just a few minutes with her. Why did you respond as you did?'

Michelle: 'To help her. I mean to respond to her distress. I couldn't have walked by. I had to do something. Maybe Katie could have closed the cart for a few minutes and come over. I thought it was insensitive of her. I know she was anxious about time. It's difficult to balance things. Blow the pills, no-one will come to any harm. It made me feel so vulnerable- what do you say?'

Lucy: 'Did you have to say anything?'

Michelle: 'Silence is difficult. It's keeping quiet I find the hardest. Did we give her the opportunity to chat? Did we keep away because she was a nurse? Are we frightened of being patronising? Should she be treated any differently?'

Lucy: 'Can you answer your own questions?'

Michelle: 'I don't know. I was afraid of making things worse'.

Lucy: 'I understand that. It's not easy. For example, Kopp [1] suggests that nurses aren't very good at sitting and listening. I'll post that paper on the intranet'.

Anita: 'I can really relate to your story Michelle. I can see why we need counselling skills. I would also be at a loss to know what to say to her- worrying if I'm helping or hindering'.

Other students then shared brief descriptions of situations where they had felt clumsy talking to patients who were angry or emotional in some way.

Patricia: 'It makes you want to avoid them. The other day in shift report, this staff nurse labelled one patient 'a real pain'. The charge nurse sympathised with her and said we know 'she can be difficult' but it's not her fault, so let's be positive about helping her. Staff can be so judgmental and loose compassion for patients. It's like turning your head away and pretending not to see them. It's almost you can't afford to care because it takes time!'

Lucy: 'Well spoken Pat. It is a sobering thought to consider how many women suffer in silence and how nurses might be ill equipped to respond to suffering and as a consequence avoid it. Did you use ethical mapping in preparing to share this experience today?'

Michelle: 'Actually I did! It was the first time I really tried to apply it. It made so much sense. I've put it on a power point. I'll talk through it (Figure 16.1)'

Rona: 'It's so easy to glibly reassure people. I hope I don't but like Michelle has said – 'what do you say to patients like Mrs Morris'? Perhaps letting Katie respond would have been better if we feel we lack skills rather than make a mess of it?'

Michelle: 'Yes, but she said it to me not to Katie – I felt I had to respond – I would have felt stupid if I just asked Katie to help!'

Patient's / family's perspective:	What ethical principles inform this situation?:	Michelle's perspective
Mrs Morris was visibly upset and needed care at that moment. Other patients were probably watching. I sensed they expected me to comfort her but also knew I was busy with the meds. Maybe they expected us to give them their meds first and then return to Mrs Morris. I don't know.	I needed to weigh up the needs for Mrs Morris against the needs of others to have their meds. That is the utilitarianism perspective. I don't think the other patients would have come to any harm if they waited a few minutes more for their meds. This is the non-malevolence perspective. I did wonder if I had the autonomy to act on my initiative and comfort Mrs Morris. Somehow my sense of integrity said I should.	I was anxious if I stopped to comfort Mrs Morris, the staff nurse, Katie, would criticise me as she wanted the meds finished. We were running a bit behind as it was. I was a little fearful if I could actually help Mrs Morris. Did I have the skills? It was a new situation for me. What do you say in that situation?
How can any conflict of perspectives and principles be best resolved?	Did I/we act ethically?	Consider the power relationships that determined action
Other health care workers' perspectives: Katie indicated she wanted me to continue the meds with her. I guess the doctors would want patients to received meds on time. We could always tell Mrs Morris we will see her afterwards. Makes her seen like a task to do!	How can a similar situation be responded to most ethically? 'I remain uncertain. It depends on the situation- every situation is different and needs weighing up. What is important is remaining available to Mrs Morris, showing my concern for her, so she knows I would go back if unable to stay with her in that moment'.	The organization's perspective: Not sure about what they would say. I guess they would sympathise with my dilemma. At least I hope so. What do others think?

FIGURE 16.1   Michelle's application of 'ethical mapping'.

Lucy: 'Michelle's exposition of ethical mapping really highlights tension in acting for the best. The utilitarian idea of needs of the individual versus needs of the many and its impact on the way we manage time and set priorities seems significant?'

Roy: 'It also highlights Michelle's uncertainty in being able to make her own decisions as a junior student nurse'.

Lucy: 'Indeed. I appreciate claiming autonomy to decide and act can seem impossible for students but learning to read the politics of ward culture is useful. Seeing things for what they are even if our hands feel tied. Let's consider `Katie's position more carefully – her dilemma that if she stopped then other patients might suffer by having their medication delayed?'

Michelle: 'Gosh, I hadn't seen Katie's perspective clouded by Mrs Morris's upset'.

Connie: 'She just wants to get the task done. You see that all the time. It's quite upsetting to think about it'.

Lucy: 'Picking up the Organization's perspective. I know we've only touched upon the nature of organizations in any depth, but it's worth considering the way the organization would view an event like Michelle's. I suggest a good place to start is the book 'Mindful Leadership' [2]. It explores the struggle of nurses to realize leadership within transactional organizations, which are more concerned with their own smooth running than the patient's experience'.

Roy: 'By its own smooth running do you mean the organization is more concerned with itself than with Mrs Morris getting effective care? Like getting the work done on time?'

Lucy: 'Sounds about right. What do others think?'

Michelle: 'Yes, that's how I think as well. I know its wrong but I feel care for patients is a secondary concern to getting the work done as Roy suggests'.

Roy: 'It's such a contradiction between the idea of caring and its reality'.

Lucy: 'That is why you need to understand this and appreciate the ethics involved even at your early stage of training. We'll pick up organizational issues as they emerge through our reflections'.

Lucy: 'Michelle, did you use the MSR anticipatory cues?'

Michelle: 'I did think about that but my mind went blank. I think I was too caught up in the emotion of it I couldn't see another way. I think it's more difficult when you do not know the patient. It's not easy when patients have such a quick turnover'.

Connie: 'Maybe we set our relational expectations too high?'

Roy: 'But then how do you help someone like Mrs Morris when caught on the hop?'

Lucy: 'OK. Let's consider - if you were in Michelle's shoes how you would have liked to respond and the likely consequences. Make a note of these responses and then we can feedback to Michelle and let her choose what response if any would have helped her'.

(The group spend about 10 minutes writing).
Responses included:

- 'Ask Katie to get someone to take over the medication round with her. That's about making a stand. It becomes an ethical thing – about how to set priorities and use time although Katie might be put out as a consequence. I mean Katie's priorities were different to Katie's and Katie has the power. She could make it difficult for Michelle if she resisted her?'
- 'Tell Katie you need to spend some time with Mrs Morris. That's what you did anyway, so I'm agreeing with you'.
- 'Have definitely gone back to talk with her no matter what Katie had said. You would have felt better for doing that and Mrs Morris would have more trust in us a consequence'.

Michelle: 'Thanks guys. I agree with going back to talk with her later rather than disrupt the medicine round but in the moment it's tough to walk away. It is so important for my own integrity that she knows that I am available to support her'.

Lucy: 'Let's pick up on the idea of being available and remind you of the being available template as a framing device for person-centred practice. Michelle's experience is a good opportunity to look again at this template because it sets out a whole theory of caring based on the idea that, from a person-centred perspective, the nurse's role is to be available to the person/patient- to enable that person to find meaning in their experience, in this experience Mrs Morris having a biopsy for a breast lump, and enabling her firstly, to make best decisions about her health needs and secondly, to assist her as necessary and skilfully to meet those needs. Can anyone remember what the determining influences on being available are?'

After some debate, these are identified as holding a vision, concern for the person, knowing the person, responding with skilled action, poise and creating an environment where it is possible to be available (see Figure 5.3).

Michelle: 'This is such a useful framework. I can really look at my response. It reminds me of the importance of knowing Mrs Morris and having concern'.

Lilly: 'It's so easy to take people like Mrs Morris for granted, especially as they are only in for the day. Just treating them like objects- I see that all the time even in my short experience'.

Michelle: 'Tell me about it! I don't like to criticize but I felt the staff nurse was like that. I felt I wasn't poised and very uncertain of my how best to respond. So much to learn!'

Lucy: 'Our responses are very much focused on the event itself- finding Mrs Morris tearful. Could staff have done something earlier in the day to support Mrs Morris?'

Michelle: 'We could have been more available to her pre-operatively and more empathic of what the biopsy meant to her. I know I couldn't have made it better for her, change what was wrong. I don't think the pre-operative planning is very good at psychological care. It's all rather processed. Another one on the conveyor belt!'

Lilly: 'As if she is an object Maybe it's easier for staff not to see the person. That's shocking saying that!'

Lucy: 'You can't take concern and empathy for granted with the excuse of being busy. You said Michelle that it had been a busy morning?'

Lilly jumps in: 'Maybe when you do the same thing day after day you get into a routine and not pay attention to how the person is feeling?'

Michelle: 'Yes I can see your point although I wouldn't like to say Katie or other staff are like that. I like to think that if Katie had not put pressure on me to continue the drugs I wouldn't have left her but I wouldn't have been so calm. I'd have been thinking more about other work that needed to be done; premeds, eye drops, and things, thinking I wish you'd hurry up. That's really wrong- how do we get over that?'

Lucy: 'That's what our learning is about. Perhaps as practitioners we need to be more prepared to defend our actions'.

Michelle: 'Its true I am worried what others think of me being relatively new to the ward. I don't like conflict so conform to expectations on me. But this experience challenges that- I would have felt guilty if I hadn't responded to Mrs Morris in the moment. I felt better having spent just a few minutes with her'.

Lucy: 'I think it is an opportune time to explore more about communication skills. We have noted Heron's "Six Category Intervention Analysis" [3] as a way to develop communication skills. Can anyone remember?'

Colin: 'I think so because I actually played with them in my own reflection. Heron split them into two categories; authoritarian and facilitative'.

Colin marked them out on the whiteboard (Figure 16.2).

Lucy: 'That's correct Colin. Each communication skill is significant dependent on the situation'.

Gaylor: 'Can you remind us of confrontation?'

Lucy: 'It is challenging someone's viewpoint if you think it is not helpful. You can see how that would work within ethical mapping when faced with conflicting perspectives. Catalytic

Authoritarian	Facilitative
Giving information	Catalytic
Giving advice	Cathartic
Confrontation	Supportive

FIGURE 16.2 Six-factor intervention analysis.
Source: Adapted from [3].

skill is enabling someone to talk through an issue. Cathartic skill is enabling someone's expression of emotion especially if they were bottling it up. OK. Can you apply each of these six skills for use with Mrs Morris?'

Annie: 'I can see that cathartic and catalytic skills were vital – *"How are you feeling now Mrs Morris?" "I'm here if you want to talk about it."* Lucy, I remember you saying something about glib reassurance - how it is used to make us feel more comfortable but unhelpful to the patient'.

Lucy: 'Yes like saying something like- *"Come along Mrs Morris, don't worry, its not so bad"'*.

Michelle: 'That's probably what I would have said!'

Lucy: 'And probably most nurses. It's as if we say it to ease ourselves rather than the patient because the patient's suffering makes us uncomfortable and we do not know better ways to respond. This came up in our last session. So I did some research. - In his story of Alice, Johns [4, p. 200] notes that Alice was told not to worry about her blood stained sputum. I'll read from his book that I conveniently have with me –

> *'But she does. She sits and worries' He asks 'why do health staff who work with people suffering from cancer offer such glib reassurance – 'don't worry'. Do they merely try and reassure themselves or get the patient off their back?'*

Lucy pauses to gauge reaction. 'He goes on to say *'Perhaps a bit of both, but either way it is unskilful because it does the opposite, it feeds rather than melts anxiety'.*

Peter: 'Just listening to that I can sense how Mrs Morris sits and worries. It's good Lucy the way you feed theory into these sessions, especially stories. It makes the issues feel more real because it's linked to a real situation and illustrates the power of reflection'.

Roy: 'Also information skills- about who Mrs Morris could talk with from a more authoritative perspective. I don't see any value in giving advice or confrontation- just imagine saying *"stop crying. It doesn't help"* or something like that. How perverse would that have been?!'

Martha: 'And supportive skills like eye contact is vital in order to communicate one's concern. Perhaps touch might also be helpful?'

Michelle: 'I did put my hand on her arm when she apologised for crying. Not knowing her well enough stopped me from holding her hand. I love the story of touch by Jill Jarvis in 'Becoming a reflective practitioner' [5] (see Chapter 20) but touch is not yet something I really appreciate or feel comfortable with'.

Mark: 'I haven't read that but it reminds me of the experience I shared a few sessions back when I touched a distressed young female patient on the shoulder and she recoiled. Ouch! I recoiled back. It made me realise just how sensitive I need to be when using touch especially being a male nurse. I reflected ion the experience and checked out some relevant research Lucy had listed for us about the use of touch. It seems to be potentially problematic for male nurses. Is it Ok to read this passage from Evans's paper [6, p. 446]?'

Lucy: 'Go ahead'.

Mark read:

> *'The gendered nature of men nurses' caring interactions reveals the ways in which gender stereotypes create contradictory and complex situations of acceptance, rejection and suspicion of men as nurturers and caregivers. Here the stereotype of men as sexual aggressors creates suspicion that men are at the bedside for reasons other than a genuine desire to help others. When this stereotype is compounded by the stereotype of men as gay, the caring practices of men nurses are viewed with suspicion in situations where there is intimate touching, not only of women patients, but of men and children as well. In each of these patient situations, men nurses are caught up in complex and contradictory gender relations that situate them in stigmatizing roles vulnerable to accusations of inappropriate touch'.*

Roy: 'Blimey Mark. That's food for thought! Better leave my tights at home'.

Lucy: 'Good idea Roy. It suggests how we can take nothing for granted. We've had several experiences concerning touch. It's recurring theme to explore. Ok, where are we with alternative options?'

Clare: 'Did you go back and see Mrs Morris later as you suggested you would?'

Michelle: 'I said to Katie 'shall I go and talk with her? I felt I needed permission after Katie had suggested she would have a word with her. Katie affirmed she would when it was quieter so I didn't. I did go to say goodbye when she went home. I don't know if Katie had a word with her or not. I feel a bit awkward about that now. Bit guilty that I let her down. If it happened again I would certainly go back and talk with her irrespective of Katie'.

Lucy: 'To clarify- given the situation again you would go back to Mrs Morris after the medicine round had been completed despite Katie saying she would. It is something I need to see through using facilitative communication skills. Is that correct Michelle?'

Michelle: 'Yes. Good intention but could I actually do it?'

Lucy: 'The MSR guides us to consider whether we can act differently (see Figure 2.2) – *"Am I able to respond as envisaged?"* To help with this cue the MSR asks:

Am I skilful and knowledgeable enough to respond differently?
Am I powerful enough to respond differently?
Do I have the right attitude?
Am I poised enough to respond differently?

Michelle: 'My communication skills are really weak. Part of it is lack of confidence and fear of saying the wrong thing. However I do feel exploring Heron has totally expanded my frame for viewing communication with Mrs Morris. I actually feel confident I could use these, especially catalytic and cathartic skills. I know it's not easy for me to cope with someone's distress but now we've reflected on it I feel I can be more poised rather than be a wobbling mess. If Katie said "I'll go and see her" I don't know what I would do. Could I assert my right to do it? I don't know? What do the rest of the group feel?'

(They felt much the same as Michelle.)

Lucy: 'Do you felt that working through the ethics informs you and strengthens your voice?'

Michelle: 'Definitely. I feel it does give me power to voice my perspective. It makes being involved in decisions easier. It's hard to refute what the best thing to do is'.

Lucy: 'Did you find any literature that might have informed you?'

Michelle: 'I did a literature search around breast biopsy and found an informative paper by Woodward and Webb [7, p. 30]'. I wrote this down in my journal –

'The quality of life a woman experiences during the process of investigation and treatment for breast disorders is linked with the communication and support provided by others, and includes family members, friends and clinic personnel'.

Another paper by Knopf [8] recommends that nurses working with breast cancer develop strategies to help patients clarify, interpret and process information. They say that greater attention should be given to the emotional experiences of all women during the diagnostic phase of breast disease that breast biopsy is not a benign experience – citing Northouse et al. [9]'.

Roy: 'Wow that is so impressive Michelle- can you give us those references?'

Lucy: 'Let's summarise – Michelle what's been insightful?'

Michelle: 'Without doubt reflecting on ethics and using Heron's work especially the cathartic and catalytic skills. I can really see how I could have used them with Mrs Morris. Reflecting on my own emotional response has also been good. It links with previous shared experiences by people – that it's more difficult to be available to people who are emotional if we are not poised'.

Lucy: 'What have others learnt?'

The other members of the group then summarised what insights they had gained.

Roy: 'The significance of knowing the person is so evident within Michelle's experience. It really makes me think to the extent I know patients and relatives and the extent I need to know them. That's such food for thought. I am also really hooked on the Black Lives Matter movement. It has really made me look at myself as a white guy and practice in a new light as if I just hadn't seen it as an issue before'.

Alice: 'As a black woman I heartily endorse your sentiments. I feel the Black Lives Matter movement helps to liberate me to express myself. I feel I can hold my head higher, not that I have overtly experienced racism at work yet I feel it is always there under the surface or built into the woodwork. On another point, Michelle seemed so concerned for Mrs Morris and yet it made her feel vulnerable. I guess that's poise? Being able to manage ourselves so we are not overwhelmed yet are available to the patient?'

Michelle: 'That has got me thinking. Would I have responded to Mrs Morris differently if she had been black? I've really got to think about that'.

Lucy: 'Google "cultural safety" and consider this as a background for experiences to bring next session'.

Anita: 'On top of that, having the autonomy to respond for the best. I guess that will take some practice! As first years' our voices are so fragile being shaped by authority figures. Just understanding that is so helpful'.

Lucy: 'All the points such as poise that have been raised are attributes of the Being Available template that offers a framework for framing your insights. It is based on person-centred nursing as we have discussed that we ideally aspire to realise. Try using it. How do you feel now Michelle?'

Michelle: 'So much better. I know I've got to be more confident with my communication skills. I shouldn't be so anxious about messing it up. Maybe I shouldn't have judged Katie so harshly saying she was insensitive. I hope she did go back and have a word with her. I can ask her tomorrow. We don't find time to talk much'.

Lucy: 'Yes, it's good to follow up events and discuss more with your ward mentors. They are there to support you although as you say, they also need support. Perhaps the school could do more? I'll raise that again in my next team meeting. We can pick up your feedback with Katie when we meet next Friday. Mark- I believe it is your turn to next share an experience?'

Lucy's Reflection

Lucy shared this session within her own guided reflection group of peer teachers who meet once a month for two hours.

Lucy: 'I've drawn a number of insights from this session'.

- I used the MSR to structure the session. The cues flowed well. The student had prepared as contracted with a good description. She used dialogue, raised questions and expressed her feelings, all of which gave the description a vivid richness. Other students easily identified with it and drew some useful insights.
- I am convinced that all the attributes of using the 'Being Available Template' to help the students view themselves were evident in Michelle's concern and poise with 'being available' to Mrs Morris. All the template's attributes are relevant within every situation and emerge as a vital aspect of developing knowing in practice and can be meaningfully developed through guided reflection.
- Ethical mapping proved to be a useful tool to facilitate teaching of ethics. Ethics can seem such a dry topic for students but when linked to actual experience it becomes intensely relevant and meaningful.

- I used Heron's Six Category Intervention Analysis as a way to help the students develop communication skills. It reminded me of the way I try to use facilitative skills in de-emphasising my authority as 'teacher'. Using facilitative skills role models them for the students – what Johns terms as 'parallel process framing' (see Figure 5.2). I thought I would be giving more advice or confronting actions that I felt weren't appropriate, but it hasn't generally been necessary. Using Heron's communication skills planted seeds in their minds to germinate in future situations.
- Theoretical mapping is such a useful approach to introduce relevant theory into the session that both informs and challenges the students' insights notably when students themselves have done the homework. Theories on touch, gender and breast biopsy were researched and fed in by the students.
- The technique 'of being in the other's shoes' creates options that are essentially confrontational but in a safe and non-authoritative way. It illustrates how giving advice from peers offers multiple perspectives on the situation that is helpful and non-threatening.
- The above points convince me that the key element of what we do in guided reflection groups is to facilitate student growth. I take the idea of growth from Mayeroff [10, p. 1] who notes –

> 'To care for another person, in the most significant sense, is to help him grow and actualise himself'.

That growth is a reciprocal thing – I also felt myself grow through dialogue with the students. It's a development curve for all of us. I don't set myself up as 'expert'.

- My vision as a teacher is aspiring to be a 'servant-leader' [11], notably being of service to the students and to my peers. It reflects a shift from 'teaching at them' to 'learning with them' within a community. The students have become more responsible for their learning even in the short time the group has been together. In fact, I'm surprised at just how much the group works together. I know some of the students are quiet and others talk a lot. Peter, for example, tends to dominate and be quite opinionated. But he's changing. I don't tend to interfere or censure because I sense the group will find its synergy. Also, the structures we use – students taking it in turns and 'being in the others shoes' facilitate participation from quieter members.
- The whole issue of authority is challenging. We, as teachers, are so used to being in authority with students that it's difficult for us to shift and yet it is vital. As Bohm stated [12, p. 42] –

> 'The school is a very authoritative structure. It has it's value but it is a structure within which it might be difficult to get dialogue going ... there is no place in the dialogue for the principle of authority and hierarchy'.

I replaced 'family' in Bohm's text with 'school'. This is the fundamental assumption that has to change – that if we are going to work through dialogue, then we must adopt the assumption that our role is to serve students to grow, and that requires a radical shift in our relationships with students. More adult-adult and less maternal – using a TA perspective [13]. I know this is contentious because of the resistance some teachers have to such a shift, especially a maternal attitude towards first years. I've often heard it said that students are irresponsible children, but perhaps that's because we don't give them enough responsibility?

- This leads on to the idea of 'community' – that what is nurtured in group guided reflection is a community of inquiry. It develops from moving from an individual consciousness to a group consciousness or coherence where the whole is greater than the sum of the parts. Bohm [12] suggests that coherence has a very high creative energy that we put to work through reflection and dialogue.

- At times I wanted to assert my own perspective as I knew the person involved but I bit my tongue to enable the students to take responsibility and work things out for themselves to really good effect.
- Using the 'classroom critical incident questionnaire' gave really helpful feedback (Appendix 1). What surprised the students most was how liberating and enjoyable the task was once they got into the groove. It was a new approach to learning for them. A few students feedback the task initially seemed daunting but more positive group members were very supportive.

Summary

Lucy's reflection on her session with the first-year students draws out her insights to share within her peer group. Such groups are vital within the reflective curriculum, for as Lucy highlights – it is a learning curve for guides as well as students. The guide's approach may be informed with theory or ideas (Chapters 8 and 9) but it can only be developed through doing it – what Beck [14] described as 'running in place' (Chapter 1). In Chapter 17 I offer a contrasting illustration of guiding third-year nursing students.

References

1. Kopp, P. (2000) Overcoming difficulties in communicating with other professionals. *Nursing Times* 96(28), 47–49.

2. Johns, C. (2016) *Mindful Leadership: A Guide for the Health Care Professions*. Palgrave Macmillan, London.

3. Heron, J. (1975) *Six-Category Intervention Analysis*. Human Potential Resource Group, University of Surrey, Guildford.

4. Johns, C. (2004) *Being Mindful, Easing Suffering*. Jessica Kingsley Publishing, London.

5. Johns, C. (2022) Grading reflective assignments. In C. Johns [Ed.] *Becoming A Reflective Practitioner* (sixth edition). Wiley Blackwell, Oxford.

6. Evans, J. (2002) Cautious caregivers: gender stereotypes and the sexualisation of men nurses' touch. *Journal of Advanced Nursing* 40(4), 441–448.

7. Woodward, V., Webb, C. (2001) Women's anxieties surrounding breast disorders: a systematic review of the literature. *Journal of Advanced Nursing* 33(1), 29–41.

8. Knopf, M. (1994) Treatment options for early stage breast cancer. *MEDSURG Nursing* 3, 249–257.

9. Northouse, I., Jeffs, M., Cracchilo-Caraway, A., Lampman, L., Dorris, G. (1995) Emotional distress reported by women and husbands prior to breast biopsy. *Nursing Research* 44, 196–201.

10. Mayeroff, M. (1971) *On Caring*. Harper Perennial, New York.

11. Greenleaf, R. (1975/2002) *Servant-Leadership*. Paulist Press, New York.

12. Bohm, D. (1996) In L. Nichol (Ed.) *On Dialogue*. Routledge, London.

13. Stewart, I., Joines, V. (1987) *TA Today: A New Introduction to Transactional Analysis*. Russell Press, Nottingham.

14. Beck, C. Y. (1989) *Everyday Zen*. Thorsons, London.

Note

i. This experience was originally shared by Janet Graham from guiding a student nurse on a surgical ward. Janet was the ward manager.

CHAPTER 17

Guiding Third-year Nursing Students

Introduction

As you might expect, the tone and depth of a guided reflection session with third-year students will differ in contrast with guiding first-year students (Chapter 16). The following narrative illustrates guiding third-year nursing students undertaking the professional placement module. They have met twice weekly for three hours in guided reflection sessions since commencing the curriculum.

The guide is Gary. It is Karen's turn to share. She practices on an elderly care unit, where she has been provisionally accepted for a staff nurse position. The ward has established mentorship whereby Toni, the ward sister, mentors Karen.

Karen's Experience[i]

Karen [reading from her journal]: 'One night last week Hank, one of the patients, complained to me about the actions of one of the night care assistants. He said she was very rude when he asked for help. She told him curtly that he would have to wait, that he wasn't the only patient on the ward. He was very angry and distressed about it. I felt awful for him. Somewhat impetuously I wrote about his complaint in the notes. I did this because I felt angry on his behalf but also to cover my own back because if something had happened because of that, if he had got worked up and had a heart attack or he made a formal complaint. I didn't state who was involved or the nature of the incident. Christine, the staff nurse on duty that night, picked up what I had written in the notes and told me that she felt 'very sad that I had to write that, that some things were better said, not written'. She didn't deny the incident happened but criticised my documenting it'.

(Karen pauses, clearly upset recounting the situation.)

Gary: 'I can see you are upset by the event. Is that because of the way you handled it or because you still feel angry on Hank's behalf or both?'

Tom interjected: 'I'd feel angry if I had been in your shoes'.

Pauline: 'Me too! Some of these care assistants shouldn't be allowed loose!'

Karen: 'Thanks guys. I was anxious about Christine's remarks as if it was me who was the villain. I re-read my notes of the incident because I had written them in a hurry. You know, in the heat of the moment. I realised I had used a word that could have been replaced by a better one'.

Gary: 'An antagonistic word?'

Karen: 'Yes. I made a further comment and replaced my initial note to make it clearer to people reading it. What got me was Christine criticising me about my way of documenting it when The Nursing Times and the Government bang on about "whistle blowing" and how complaints should be documented. I felt she was trying to cover for the person involved though she did acknowledge the event had happened'

Gary: 'And now?'

Karen: 'I pointed it out to Leslie as he was the staff nurse on duty that morning looking after Hank. He was working a long day and said he would have a word with the person involved when she came on for the night shift. I went home and worried about it all day, worried how she would take it, what she would say'.

Gary: 'You were worried about comeback that somehow you had broken an unwritten rule about being loyal to colleagues in spite of the patient's best interests? Let's cut to the anticipatory cue and consider what you would do differently if you found yourself in the same situation again? It might be helpful if the whole group considered what they would do if in your shoes'.

(After a few minutes pause)

Karen: 'This is a hard one. The only thing I could have done differently would have been to ring her and ask her to explain from her point of view'.

Louise: 'What response might you have got?'

Karen: 'From my perspective, if it was me I would have appreciated it'.

Gary: 'And knowing the person involved?'

Karen: 'I can't say. She could nearly be my grandmother'.

Tom: 'How do you normally get on with her?'

Karen: 'I see her in the evenings and nights when she works but I don't have much to do with her. I suppose my relationship with her is superficial'.

Gary: 'Do you think this action against Hank was out of character for her?'

Karen: 'I think it was an exaggeration of her normal character'.

Gary: 'You think?'

Karen: 'I don't work with her. It's difficult to know how she is with other patients. The event itself was quite trivial, its Hank's anger that got to me'.

Lil: 'Do you think Hank's anger was reasonable? I mean is he always giving staff grief?'

Karen: 'If it had been me on the receiving end then I would have been upset and angry. She was inflicting her values on him, not respecting him'.

Gary: 'I sense you feel you didn't handle Hank's complaint in the best way. Have you shared this in your practice mentoring?'

Karen: 'No, not yet. It's helpful to work it through here first'.

Gary: 'Do you think writing a complaint in the notes was the best way of reporting patient distress?'

Karen: 'I'm not sure. Do you think it was the wrong approach?'

Gary: 'Let's open that up'.

Pauline: 'I guess that altering the notes might be construed as unprofessional. Perhaps other staff should have picked that up. I know you were trying to dampen down the conflict'.

Karen: 'Yes I was. What would you have done?'

Pauline: 'Umm, tricky. I know you were emotional because of Hank and the hostile feedback. Maybe discuss the situation at shift report would have been better? Reporting the incident to the staff nurse sounds good. It's not unreasonable to expect him to deal with it'.

Karen: 'He's a conflict avoider! He would have conveniently forgot about it and brushed it under the carpet. That would have made it worse. I can imagine them saying I went running to mother and got them into trouble'.

Gary: 'What other options do you have? Think about what would have been the "right" response- use ethical mapping?' (see Figure 4.2)

Karen: 'OK. Clearly Mandy, that's the care assistant, was in the wrong – she abused a patient and that cannot be tolerated. She has no defence for this except to play down the incident or accuse Hank of lying. I know I should have been more mindful of the consequences of writing as I did in the notes. It wasn't the best way of reporting this. Altering the notes was not a good response as it looked as if I was trying to cover up my 'mistake'. I'm fearful of conflict but I do need to talk this through with Mandy either face to face or phone her at home'.

Lyn: 'What would Hank want you to do?'

Karen: 'That's a good point to consider his perspective. I could have asked him if he wanted me to report the situation. I've rather taken that for granted. I have a moral duty to care and expose situations of abuse'.

Ann: 'Yeah, so many experiences we reflect on involves conflict and yet it seems we are not good at dealing with it.

Karen: 'I know. I put myself into the Thomas-Kilmann conflict mode instrument [1]. I know I am a conflict avoider or at best accommodate conflict'.

Peter: 'Where do you want to be?'

Karen: 'Collaboration of course. It is the ideal but everyday situations seem like a barrier towards achieving that. Maybe, it's because I'm a student and anxious about confronting more experienced staff. To confess, I know I avoid conflict. However I can voice my ideas, for example in looking at what is the best, but usually only when asked. I always give way or accommodate those with authority. Compromise is partly assertive/cooperative, finding a way to move through the conflict. Competition is around the struggle to see who wins and looses! I feel I am in this position with Hank's complaint. Unwilling to back down fuelled by my outrage. Collaboration is where I would like to be. But I am not skilled or poised enough am I?'

Gary: 'Maybe not yet. You're not alone. Cavanagh [2] indicated that nurses and nurse managers most used avoidance, then accommodation, then compromise, then collaboration and then competition. But we can see how the framework helps us understand where we are at and where we want to be. The constant challenge through reflection on conflict experiences is to find the collaborative way that begs the question- can you be collaborative? If not, what prevents you?'

Pauline: 'Yes, that's reflected in your earlier comment about Leslie brushing it under the carpet. That relates to the 'harmonious team' [3] whereby staff are more loyal to their colleagues than to their patients and as such sacrifice the patient's best interests in favour of avoiding conflict with their colleagues to maintain a harmonious façade. From this perspective Karen becomes the problem not the care assistant because she broke this "rule"'.

Karen: 'That's true but really uncomfortable. How do we overcome this and achieve collaboration? I sense we have to shed the fear of sanction or consequences and that's exactly what I fear to the extent I sense that I wouldn't report the complaint again especially as I'm going to work on the ward as a staff nurse'.

Gary: 'But then you do not act for the best and sacrifice your integrity'.

Lil: 'Ouch. That's tough but true'.

Karen: 'Any tips for speaking with the care assistant?'

Gary: 'Let's imagine I am the care assistant. The key factor is to keep the situation grounded in the situation rather than it becoming a secondary situation of interpersonal conflict, as indeed it threatens to become. Remember the maxim- 'tough on the issues, soft on the person'. See taking action as an act of personal integrity as fearful as you are of its potential consequences of ostracism'.

Sophia: 'I'm thinking about using confrontation, one of Heron's six-factor intervention analysis skills [4]. How to do that non-threateningly?'

Karen: 'Give me a clue?'

Sophia: 'Hi Mandy. Its Karen. I wanted to speak with you and clear up any misunderstanding between us about Hank's complaint. I know I should have spoken with you directly rather than write it in the notes. That was naïve of me. However Hank was really upset, which made me upset on his behalf. We really do need to respect all our patients'.

Karen: 'Wow. That sounds good'.

Gary: 'Managing conflict has clearly emerged as a significant professional issue. Can I suggest you read up on Cavnagh's paper [2]. I will also post Valentine's paper [5] on the intranet. Its titled – "Management of conflict: do nurses/women handle it differently?" These references are rather dated so do some searching to find other relevant papers'.

Next Session

Gary: 'Ok guys. Let's just focus on our breath a moment to quieten our thoughts and bring ourselves fully present to this moment'.

Mo: 'I've been using that with engaging with patients and colleagues. It makes me feel so much more focused, confident and present'.

(General agreement amongst the group)

Gary: 'Any pick up from the conflict literature?'

Pauline: 'It just reinforced what we discussed about avoidance and the difficulty with competition … how and why nurses generally respond to conflict'.

Tom: 'Yes, it gives conflict management a reassuring theoretical edge'.

Gary: 'Karen?'

Karen: 'Well, I went home and phoned her!'

Lil: 'Good for you. How did you feel when you picked up the receiver?'

Karen: 'Terrified! She was angry but she didn't get as angry as she possibly could have done. I think she was feeling guilty'.

Wilson: 'Her anger was you breaking the rules of the harmonious team?' [3]

Karen: 'I don't know. I'm really dejected and yet I can sense it's vital that I am not intimidated. If we can't raise issues because of fear of conflict then we all go about as if wearing masks. I can't simply sweep this under the carpet'.

Peter: 'You haven't – you did phone her and refused to play the harmonious team game. When is your next mentoring session?'

Karen: 'Tomorrow! I feel like a chicken at the prospect of talking about this situation but I must. I must be assertive and not a coward. Why did Hank wait to see me!? He was probably just thinking about it when he saw me'.

Lil: 'Perhaps he trusted you?'

Karen: 'I like to think so. It is important that patients can trust nurses to act for them as necessary'.

Lil: 'How do you think the care assistant might be feeling now?'

Karen: 'I hope she thinks I had the courage to ring her'.

Gary: 'So be positive about this- your phone call to Mandy was an act of integrity. Her anger was her guilt. You enabled her to release that energy, yet she was also confronted with the fact that she did not act appropriately towards Hank. You can rationalise her anger in this way. It's imperative that you do not see yourself in the wrong. It's easier with the charge nurse because that's what mentoring is about- a non-judgmental space to reflect on and learn through experience'.

Karen: 'I hear what you say but it's not easy. I'm not assertive'.

Gary: 'So let's talk about assertiveness. It links well with conflict management. What do we know about it?'

Peter: 'Well, we've explored the 'Assertiveness action ladder' in a previous session. It offers a practical approach to reflecting on the self being assertive and where we might get stuck on the way up. Shall we use that to position ourselves up the ladder?'

(The group agreed)

Gary: 'Peter, talk us through it'.

Peter looks it up in his tatty copy of becoming a reflective practitioner and talks through the 10 rungs (Figure 17.1).

Karen: 'Well, on the bottom run I certainly felt the need to assert myself. Working through the ethics I know I am in the right to assert myself although perhaps I needed to have asked Hank if he was Ok with taking action on his behalf. Respecting his autonomy. I get stuck at rung 3 'authority to assert self'. Being a student and not wanting to upset the apple cart. However, on rung 4, I've got a good argument and, on rung 5, mentoring is the optimum opportunity to express it. I appreciate the challenge of rung 6 - JDI! That's another block! I realise I need to be able to jump that rung!'

Gary: 'Consider rungs 7 to 10 on the ladder. On rung 7, the idea of "being heard" is significant. We might have something to say but will the other person hear you? It suggests that being assertive is being heard. Remember we considered confrontation in our last session with Karen anticipating phoning the care assistant'.

Ann: 'I like the idea of giving the charge nurse information that Hank complained and how Karen dealt with it. Then, depending on how she responds, to be confrontational- "what is she going to do about it?" There seems little room to use the more facilitative skills of catharsis or catalytic although I imagine if she is any good at mentorship she can respond with those techniques'.

Peter: 'If I was the charge nurse I would want to intercede and confront the care assistant's and the night staff nurses' behaviour'.

Gary: 'Rung eight 'staying in adult mode' is the default pattern of communication to realise person-centred practice. This is such a recurring theme in your reflections. Let's revisit TA theory we looked at some time back. You can use this framework to position yourself in

10	Treading the fine line between pushing and yielding	
9	Playing the power game	
8	Staying in adult mode	
7	Being communicatively skilful	
6	'Just do it!' [JDI]	
5	Creating the optimum conditions to assert self	
4	Making a good argument	
3	Authority to assert self	
2	Ethically right to assert self	
1	Feeing the need to assert self	

FIGURE 17.1 The assertiveness action ladder.

relation with others to explore and understand why you are in your respective ego modes, and how to move to a compatible adult-adult mode to realise person-centred practice'.

(Gary digs into his satchel for the TA handout that the students had previously engaged – Figure 17.2).

As we can see on the handout, when people get anxious, they can flip into either learnt parent or child mode. When the situation is with someone in authority and anxious – for example, the charge nurse is anxious about the complaint or altering the notes, then they are more likely to flip into critical parent mode. That creates anxiety for Karen who is then likely to respond by flipping into child mode. In this way, the pattern of communication is reciprocated and doesn't breakdown.

Cues:

- Is the actual pattern therapeutic?
- What factors influence both self and other into this pattern of interaction?
- Is this a repetitive pattern?
- What pattern is desirable ? [plot]
- What do you need to do to move to this new pattern?

Karen: 'As a student it is so easy to fall into 'child mode'. Indeed, I think some staff view students as children and naturally respond in parental mode. Hence, if we speak up and voice our views as adults their response is condescending pushing us back into child mode reminding us of our place within the ward hierarchy. Rather than being seen as a naughty child I am submissive to avoid conflict and be seen as a "good child"'.

Gary: 'You've expressed that very well Karen. It becomes learnt behaviour unless we can break the pattern'.

Karen: 'It is a repetitive pattern but that's going to change! That's my insight- to see beyond my own ego to something far greater if I am going to be an effective person-centred practitioner. TA theory is so helpful! I can really see myself within these modes! It just shows how easy it is to flip into parent or child mode even though you know it is not therapeutic.

Parent: Nurturing Critical Tolerant	P	Fear of: Losing control; Losing self-respect; Losing respect of others.	P	Parent: Nurturing Critical Tolerant
Give yourself permission to stay with your uncertainties; Accept your emotions as energies rather than anxieties or symptoms to be locked away; Witness your responses rather than indulge or swamp yourself in them.	A		A	Allow yourself to make mistakes; Share your insights, observations, feelings with others; Avoid win-lose situations; Don't defend your views, just share your evidence; Stay aware off your defences and work towards giving them up.
Child Rebellious Conforming Hurt	C	Fear of: persecution; Rejection; Being overwhelmed	C	Child: Rebellious Conforming Hurt
	self		Other	

FIGURE 17.2 Transactional analysis template.

Even if you could resist the pull into child mode I'm not sure if I could help the charge nurse also stay in adult mode?'

Peter: 'I can dig that. Yet it would be the only way you can have a mutually responsible 'adult' conversation. Staying in adult mode and enabling the other to respond in adult mode is the power game – rung 9 on the assertiveness ladder'.

Dirk: 'And that just leaves rung 10. I sense that's mindful of the power game as it's being played. Sensing that fine line between pushing the issue and yielding because we know we can't win'.

Pauline: 'And yet we know we've got our message across. We've made the argument. We've been heard. We live to fight another day'.

Lil: 'And most significantly we have asserted ourselves and not failed'.

Karen: 'Food for thought'.

Gary: 'Time is getting on. Karen and the group - can you summarise what insights you have gained'.

Karen: 'Reflection has reinforced my patient centred values – the importance of listening to and working with patients like Hank. It involves a moral responsibility. I realise I do care about patients. I'm not good at conflict and felt intimidated – I need to develop a greater sense of poise so I am not so easily rattled by such issues. As a result I feel I have grown through this experience – more grown up, more adult, less like a frightened panicky child. It has exposed the myth of collaborative relationships. The idea of the harmonious team is compelling – I can see it. My assertive, conflict management and communication skills all need developing- and yet I do feel more assertive. I will talk to the charge nurse tomorrow, shed my fear of "telling tales" and keep us both in adult mode!'

Lil: 'No pressure then!'

Gary: 'Before we go, any further thoughts on the Valentine paper if you had the chance to read and reflect on it?'

Lil: 'I was struck by the notion that women may respond differently to conflict then men. It made me rethink the idea of 'finding voice' and the difficulty women might have in having a voice in a generally patriarchal culture. Why do women always want to avoid issues or compromise! I think it's a form of peacekeeping. Not very assertive'.

Karen: 'Linking that to my experience I definitely agree. I hate the idea of competition. I would much rather avoid the situation but as my experience showed you can't avoid or compromise if it's important in terms of realising care'.

Peter: 'As a man I can empathize what Lil and Karen have said. The paper made me more aware and sensitive to gender issues'.

Gary: 'Good stuff. See you next session'.

Next Session

Gary asked Karen for feedback.

Karen: 'Yes I did talk to Toni the ward manager. I knocked on her door. I took a deep breath to bring my mind home and relax myself. I told her about Hank's complaint and my response to it. She asked "What do you want me to do about it?" Initially I was flummoxed. I said something like "I want you to deal with it. I'm sorry I changed the notes, that was so unprofessional. It won't happen again". She said it wasn't very clever of me to change the notes but she understood why I did it. She said it couldn't have been easy confronting Mandy. She isn't easy. She said that Mandy had been on the ward a long time working nights and admitted I had actually done her a favour. She will have a word with Christine and remind her that any abuse of patients will not be tolerated and that perhaps then she will be more mindful of her own responsibility and take action with Mandy if she's abusive to patients. I said I was so anxious coming to see her today. Anxious that she would be angry at me and not want me on the ward as a staff nurse. Conflict is so hard and yet it shouldn't be if we were all responsible for our actions and working towards the same values? She said "my door is always open but from next month you won't be a student but a staff nurse". She was really receptive. I tried to be in adult-adult mode although I could easily have slipped into child mode if she had not been so receptive. It shows how easily I'm intimated by senior staff'.

Lil: 'I think we would all agree with that but why?'

Gary: 'Why do you think?'

Lil: 'I suspect as a fairly newly promoted charge nurse she's anxious and critical of every little thing. She needs to be in control of things to feel secure. I think Karen's honesty and openness enabled her to respond to Karen in adult-mode'.

Karen: 'Yes, as if she could let go with me and trust me. I really felt different about her after that – like empathy, knowing how she was feeling and how tough it was for her dealing with people like Mandy. She didn't want to appear as if she wasn't coping so hence her tough parental front'.

Peter: 'I've noticed that with charge nurses and sisters I've worked with. They are like critical parents always at you for little things. You're right – it is as if they are anxious and flip into this parental role. It's hard not to respond as a child especially when you rely on them for good reports'.

Gary: 'There is so much pressure on organisations to perform. It is as if the whole organisation is anxious and this gets transmitted down the hierarchy into every member of staff at every level. So no doubt Toni gets treated like a child from her modern matron and all the way to the boardroom. It's like an anxiety transmission that is very hard to breakthrough. It requires a massive transformational shift throughout the organisation where the blame shame culture is put to rest. Can we see how this fits within French and Raven's power typology? [6] (Anyone remember it?)'

Jeanne: 'Yes. French and Raven set out six sources of social power that are either authoritative or facilitative. Authoritative sources are positional, coercive and extrinsic reward for example promotion. In contrast, facilitative sources are relational, expert and intrinsic reward for example helping someone and being thanked'.

Gary: 'Thanks Jeanne. Karen's experience suggests that most managers are authoritarian relying on position and sanction power with rewards for "good children." A transformational organizational shift requires leaders who emphasise facilitative sources of power notably expert and relational sources of power. Or framed within TA, who communicate from adult-adult ego mode all the way down the system'.

Pauline: 'It must be hard to resist the threat of sanction. Yet how can staff grow into adults when their superiors flipping into parental mode?'

Lil: 'I have an experience to share that relates to Karen's. It is about me pushing an issue and getting slapped down when I told the senior nurse I couldn't do as she requested as I was talking with a patient. She told me to stop that and do as she requested. I said no. She shouted at me in front of the patient to do as I was told – she had certainly flipped into critical parent. I felt humiliated. I apologised to my patient trying to stay in adult mode and did as she requested. The patient seemed to understand ward politics and gave me a smile so I didn't feel I had failed her'.

Ann: 'Pushing the fine line- step ten of the assertiveness ladder. You didn't know when to yield! Ouch'.

Lil: 'Yes it did hurt but I felt outraged. She could see I was with a patient talking about discharge. She said I could do that later as if talking was some low level task'.

Gary: 'And if it happened again?'

Lil: 'Good question. I know I must keep my cool, be poised and not get outraged. Perhaps play the power game knowing she is such a tyrant with student nurses but be mindful I am yielding so that I don't feel such a failure'.

Ann: 'Yielding. Pushing the fine line – treading careful not to overstep the mark and get punished. That's quite some skill, to be that mindful. It's a form of retreat from a situation you can't win to preserve your integrity. Hands up – I yield!'

Peter: 'Surviving to fight another day!'

Gary: 'Thanks Ann. Knowing when to yield is an important professional skill. As Ann says it is about maintaining one's integrity. This sense of outrage – is that healthy or professional?'

Lil: 'No! Some days stress eats me alive!'

Ann: 'Yeah some days I could do with a suit of armour as protection'.

Gary: 'Managing our stress is clearly a vital aspect of professional practice because it consumes vital energy and hence makes us less available to our patients and colleagues. Poise is an element within the "Being available template" as we have constantly referred to throughout the whole programme (Figure 5.3). It is similar in nature to emotional intelligence' [7].

Lil: 'I probably let stress build up in me until it explodes. Obviously I didn't explode with the senior staff nurse. Subdued by her authority over me. Later Jenny, a second year nurse asked me something silly and I exploded at her. I later apologised'.

Peter: 'Is that horizontal violence? Feels like bullying to me?'

Ann: 'Yes, one thing that bothers me about Karen's experience we haven't really touched upon is the notion that she felt bullied by the night staff nurse. Bullying is an insidious and debilitating experience for its victim. It is difficult to resist, possibly the reason why the 'bully' has picked on that person. Both bully and victim get caught up in a pattern of behaviour from which neither can easily break free. As I read it, Karen threatens her control and thus becomes a target as if a naughty child being scolded by a critical parent. I wonder- does the staff nurse realise she is a bully?'

Gary: 'This is such an important point. Picking up Peter's point, horizontal violence occurs when someone is unable, for whatever reason, to turn their outrage against its proper target. The staff nurse lashed out at Karen because she is a softer target than the care assistant. Hence she becomes a bully'.

Peter: 'Well, it shouldn't be tolerated and yet recognising its endemic nature makes it difficult to tackle'.

Ann: 'I was inspired by Otter's storyboard of nurse bully and the sheep [8]. It showed me how we can fight back against bullying although, as Otter implied, it isn't easy. Has anybody read that?'

Lil: 'Yes I did. I agree it was inspiring. Mentioning it now it makes me want to use storyboard as a creative approach to reflection and narrative especially linked to an informing literature that suggests bullying is to quote (turning to the sixth edition of Becoming a reflective practitioner, [8, p. 146] one of the biggest untalked about problems in the delivery of good care to patients caused by the NHS's hierarchical culture and occurred across all staff groups. Maybe we could have a session on taking care of ourselves using storyboard?'

Gary: 'That's a good idea. I hadn't thought of using storyboard myself. Shall I arrange that?'

(unanimous group agreement)

Gary: 'One approach to reflecting on stress is using "the feeling fluffy, feeling drained scale." We can locate it in 'Becoming a reflective practitioner'.

Gary: 'Let me elucidate. The scale is a visual analogue scale 10cm long. You mark along the scale the extent you feel either "fluffy" or "drained" at the end of your shift. The scale poses three questions:

- What factors contribute to your sense of feeling drained?
- What factors contribute to your sense of feeling light and fluffy?
- What can you do to go home feeling more fluffy and less drained?

So think about your recent practice placement and answer these questions'.
[group spend about 15 minutes applying this task]
Gary: 'Karen would you like to apply the scale to your experience?'
Karen: 'I reckon my average stress score is about 4. I've scored it as 2 after my experience with Hank. I've listed factors to each question (Figure 17.3) (talked through)'.

Other group members including Gary talked through their own lists.

Karen: 'Having talked with Toni, my mentor and ward manager I felt my stress melt away. I felt understood and vindicated. It made me feel positive to work on the ward despite Mandy. Yes, I felt empowered! It made me feel more adult and more responsible. I hope I can keep it up'.
Lil: 'Looking at Karen's example – it was a bad day at the office for her! I can identify with her experience – dealing with angry staff scares me and yet it is such an important part of practice. I know we must take responsibility and put our hands up if we are wrong but it's tough when we do our best and still get shit'.
Pauline: 'Yes, I agree. I notice Karen scored 2. I get stressed over the smallest thing because nursing is such a responsibility especially as you get more senior. All that stress accumulating until I want to explode like you Lil!'
Lil: 'Maybe. But I can see how the scale works, that by becoming more mindful of our stress we can begin to work out ways of dealing with it – for example – next time we are faced with angry relatives we are more likely to handle it better. That in itself is rewarding and stress breaking. Give ourselves positive feedback. Sharing here in the group is really helpful. As Karen said "empowering"! Like draining the stress butt before it gets too full and using that energy to stop the butt filling in the first place'.
Peter: 'The water butt theory of stress. (see Chapter 4) I like the way we introduce theory to fit with the experiences we share and then use those theories to develop our reflections as per the MSR cue – "what knowledge did or should have informed our actions"'.

I go home feeling light and fluffy	0 / 10	I go home feeling totally drained
	2	
What factors contribute to my sense of feeling drained?	• Situations of conflict with patients, relatives and staff. • Being blamed. • Witnessing other nurses' poor practice. • Not feeling supported.	
What factors contribute to my sense of feeling light and fluffy?	• Having time to practice as I feel I should. • Being acknowledged by patients or staff for doing a good job – positive feedback. • Having support from colleagues and being able to talk through things.	
What can I realistically do to go home feeling more fluffy and less drained?	• Get the support I need to talk through the stressful situation – using my mentor if she's on duty. • Saying goodbye to the patients I have been caring for.	

FIGURE 17.3 Feeling drained, feeling fluffy scale applied to Karen's experience.

Ann: 'I feel I am just beginning to learn how to be a nurse. You can learn all the technical stuff easy but these professional issues are really tough. The ward is certainly a political and social cauldron'.

Gary: 'The scale is a good example of a practical reflective tool in which to view yourself. Try keeping the scale over the next few weeks and see if we can reduce our stress scores and understand why stress occurs and what factors emerge as significant in dealing with it. As Karen identified, genuine support from clinical colleagues seems vital whereby staff are available to each other. Perhaps only then can you be available to patients – a reciprocal relationship in creating a clinical environment to support person-centred practice. Check out the Being Available Template (Figure 5.3). I say genuine rather than glib reassurance or false harmony. Is everyone feeling good after such dialogue?'

(Group affirm)

Gary: 'I'll dig out some theory on horizontal violence for the intranet'.

Gary posted a footnote

Karen's experience reveals the phenomena of horizontal violence [3, 9–11] as a toxic form of dealing with stress. The idea of horizontal stems from bureaucratic – hierarchical systems, whereby the subordinate person [the nurse] is unable to project her anger or frustration at her more powerful oppressors. She can only fire at her those on her own level or below her. Yet, even on her own level, this violence is muted within the harmonious team, perhaps because people are motivated to be partially invisible, to keep their heads down to avoid criticism and conflict [12]. Hence, 'the harmonious team' is a collusive strategy to contain the team's unresolved conflict, brushed under the carpet to fester.

Reflection

The guided reflection dialogue followed its chaotic path around Karen's reflection of her experience with Hank. And yet, within the apparent chaos order emerges because Gary enables the dialogue to flow guided in a less directive fashion than with first year nurses. The third-year students have now become relatively experienced reflective practitioners. They know the ropes and can almost guide themselves. Gary has a pivotal role in drawing out and focusing key issues of professional practice and feeding in relevant theory as visual reflective frameworks to enable the students to position themselves within it. Insights tumble out. A wealth of professional practice issues is covered, threads picked up from previous sessions, seeds laid for future sessions. It is dynamic, fecund. It reflects that most aspects of knowing in practice are not possible to teach from a technical rational approach. They can only be appreciated through experience and developed through guided reflection.

References

1. Thomas, K., Kilmann, R. (1974) *Thomas Kilmann Conflict Mode Instrument*. Xicom, Toledo.

2. Cavanagh, S. (1991) The conflict management style of staff nurses and nurse managers. *Journal of Advanced Nursing* 16, 1254–1260.

3. Johns, C. (1992) Ownership and the harmonious team: barriers to developing the therapeutic nursing team in primary nursing. *Journal of Clinical Nursing* 1, 89–94.

4. Heron, J. (1975) *Six-category Intervention Analysis*. Human Potential Research Group, University of Surrey.

5. Valentine, P. E. B. (1995) Management of conflict: do nurses/women handle it differently? *Journal of Advanced Nursing* 22(1), 142–149.

6. French, J., Raven, B. (1968) The bases of social power. In D. Cartwright, A. Zander [Eds.] *Group Dynamics*. Row Peterson, Evanston, IL, 150–267.

7. Goleman, D., Boyatzis, R., Mckee, A. (2008) *The New Leaders, Transforming the Art of Leadership into the Science of Results*. Sphere, London.

8. Johns, C., Rose, O. (2022) Narrative art and storyboard. In C. Johns [Ed.] *Becoming A Reflective Practitioner* (sixth edition). Wiley Blackwell, Oxford, 143–150.

9. Duffy, E. (1995, April) Horizontal violence: a conundrum for nursing. Collegian. *Journal of the Royal College of Nursing Australia* 2(2), 5–17.

10. McKenna, B., Smith, N., Poole, S., Coverdale, J. (2003) Horizontal violence: experiences of registered nurses in their first year of practice. *Journal of Advanced Nursing* 42(1), 90–96.

11. Hutchinson, M., Vickers, M., Jackson, D., Wilkes, L. (2006) Workplace bullying in nursing: towards a more critical organisational perspective. *Nursing Inquiry* 13(2), 118–126.

12. Street, A. (1992) *Inside Nursing: A Critical Ethnography of Clinical Nursing*. State University of New York Press, Albany.

Note

i. This experience was originally shared by Kate Butcher, an associate nurse at Buford Hospital, in guided reflection with myself.

CHAPTER 18

Weaving the Reflexive Narrative: The Fifth Dialogical Movement

Introduction

In previous chapters, I set out the first four dialogical movements. These movements are fluid and interwoven towards enabling the practitioner to develop tentative insights to inform and develop the necessary knowing in practice towards realising their vision of practice. In the fifth dialogical movement, the practitioner weaves a reflexive narrative to communicate the extent they have realised their vision with the purpose of presenting the narrative to an audience. Most often, practitioners write a reflexive narrative as an academic assignment or research dissertation, as shown through exemplars in this book.

Narrative Plot

The plot of all reflexive narratives is to communicate the practitioner's journey of self-inquiry towards realising their vision of practice. Mattingly [1, p. 813] notes –

> 'It is the plot that makes individual events understandable as part of a coherent whole, one which leads compellingly towards a particular ending. Any particular event gains its meanings by place within this narrative configuration, as a contribution to the plot'.

The narrative has a beginning and end determined by linear time. At the end, it leaves a trail for the practitioner to pick up and continue. I make this point to encourage practitioners not to simply view reflective practice as a means of completing an academic requirement but to view reflection as a life-long commitment whereby one's practice becomes a 'lived' narrative as a reflective practitioner. This has a practical spin-of whereby maintaining a reflective journal can morph into a compelling professional portfolio necessary for re-registration purposes.

Weaving the Narrative

Let me be clear at the outset – there are no firm guidelines as to how to weave a reflexive narrative. It is both a creative act and logical exposition. Some structure is necessary from the perspective of illustrating reflexivity as a dynamic movement through the narrative. Reflexivity is 'looking back' to self-emerging through a sequence of experiences marked by insights or moments of transition that form the threads that are woven together to create the pattern of the whole narrative.

Chase [2, p. 656] notes, weaving is

'Organizing events and objects into a meaningful whole, and of connecting and seeing the consequences of actions and events over time'.

Events are the practitioner's experiences. This may simply be one or two experiences or a chain of experiences, usually depending on the reflective time span. The number of experiences drawn on to support insights over time is clearly significant, as it is difficult to demonstrate reflexive development over a short period of time or grounded in just one experience, whereby the practitioner anticipates responding differently. However, where a narrative consists of just one experience, it must include a follow-up, revealing the consequences of taking action or taking non-action.

Dewey gives clarity to this process [3, p. 4/5].

'The successive portions of reflective thought grow out of one another and support one another; they do not come and go in medley. Each phase is a step from something to something. Technically speaking, it is a term of thought. Each term leaves a deposit that is utilised in the next term. The stream or flow becomes a train or chain. There are in any reflective thought definite units that are linked together so that there is sustained movement to a common end'.

The 'deposits' Dewey refers to are recorded in the practitioner's reflective journal. When 'linked together' these deposits, consisting of insights supported by experiences form the reflexive narrative. For longer reflexive narratives associated with masters or doctoral research stemming over two or three years, the practitioner can periodically to step back to review and summarise this linkage as a platform for continuation.

Dewey suggests a logical flow from one experience to the next suggesting a linear flow. However, in weaving the narrative, the practitioner may consider commencing the narrative with its ending and then weaving how that was realised through a succession of experiences. Films often use this mode. The narrative 'More than eggs for breakfast' [4] used this approach.

Shifting through perhaps dozens of collected experiences, the practitioner must decide what to put into the narrative and what to leave out. They are all meaningful in their own right, yet some will stand out as being particularly meaningful that mark a turning or transformative point towards realising their vision of practice.

At first, experiences may seem like a jumble as the practitioner seeks to make linkage between them and identify the threads to weave. The practitioner needs to stand back to see the whole picture to begin to see an emerging pattern within the whole. As Wheatley notes [5, p. 126] –

'To see patterns, we have to step back from the problem [text] and gain perspective. Shapes are not discerned from close range. They require distance and time to show themselves. Pattern recognition requires that we sit together reflectively and patiently. I say patiently not just because patterns take time to form, but because we are trying to see the world differently and there are many years of blindness to overcome'.

It may not be easy to weave the narrative pattern. The mind is not trained to see reflexive patterns. Yet there is always connection between experiences, however random they may appear. The pattern is likely to be intuitively appreciated rather than rationally forced. Tuffnell and Crickmay [6, p. 41] note –

'Creating becomes a conversation when we enter into a *dialogue* with whatever we are doing. In this conversing we are drawn along the in the moment-by-moment flow of sensation, interchange and choice, rather than following a predetermined intention or idea. Conversations grow as we listen and explore – a constantly shifting process of discovery that changes in momentum, rhythm, clarity or chaos as we work'.

Journal Entry 18.1

As if by serendipity I open Margaret Wheatley ad Myron Kellner-Rogers' book 'A simpler way' and they write about tinkering – 'this world of exploration is one which tinkers itself into existence' [7, p. 17]. 'Tinkering is making small changes to something, especially in an attempt to repair or improve it'.[i] It is playing with the narrative to make it work better or as Wheatley and Kellner-Rogers add 'it tinkers towards order [7, p. 17]. The writer's search for pattern is sensed in moments of revelation by dwelling within the whole messy fabric of words that may be scattered randomly throughout the journal. The linkage between words, events and feelings are not necessarily found as a neat analytical process, but deeply complex that defy simply reduction into an orderly pattern and representation. Again quoting Wheatley and Kellner-Rogers [7, p. 17] – 'but how it gets there violates all of our rules of good process: life is not neat, parsimonious, logical, not elegant. Life seeks order in a disorderly way. Life uses processes we find hard to tolerate and hard to believe in- mess upon mess until something workable emerges'. I must believe in this for myself when my aching logical mind screams for order. My students also ache and scream at me when they write and write again, and, slowly find form that works, emerges, until the sense of creation and its beauty astounds them. Creation is a relentless process. It is surrender to deeper intuitive forces beyond the grasping rational and analytical mind that always seeks to censor and impose order. Order is found from within, not from outside. It writes from the senses, from the body. Hence, we must find a place where we can dwell with our words and ideas, to push aside the rational mind, where we can reveal to ourselves the art of holding creative tension. A place where the cubic centimetre of possibility becomes a wide open space. It is about creating our own world rather than being confined to a world created by others. It commences in our journals and continues within our communities of inquiry. I am drunk with reading. I need to walk and let the ideas ripple through and play with them. Reading crowds my mind. At first, it excites me, and then it over-whelms me. Reading in short bursts is helpful with a pencil in hand to mark the serendipity. Only then do I really listen, opening myself up to the possibilities of what the text has to say. In guiding students, I cannot rush them into a creative space. First, they must come to realise that their learnt processes are no longer adequate to guide who they desire to be. That their learnt processes have been forged on the Newtonian anvil that constrains their creative becoming. Hence, on the surface of things, we pull at the order of things, exposing paradoxes, ruffling feathers, making it messy, slowly opening ourselves to the possibilities of different shapes and forms to represent the mystery of our journeys towards becoming who we strive to become.

Metaphor

Metaphors hold meaning and give the narrative rich description. Thus, the narrative is more creative to weave and more engaging. In her leadership narrative, James [8] marks her narrative journey with the metaphoric theme of observing crab apples from her office window. She writes –

> 'I joined my new organization today. My window looks over a wild garden. The crab apple trees are covered in small yellow apples the size of large marbles. Apparently there is a lunar eclipse followed by a full moon, a time of new beginnings, and that's how it feels' (p. 35).
>
> 'The birds are pecking at the small yellow apples on the trees outside my window, taking full advantage of autumn's bounty ... it is the fourth week in my new post' (p. 38).

'The crab apples are now bereft of leaves. Only a few small apples cling to the branches. The cold kiss of frost has withered and discoloured them but they stay attached to the tree defying both birds and weather' (p. 43).

'I look at my window and imagine the crab apples decked with lights as Christmas approaches' (p. 44).

'The trees outside my window have never looked so forlorn, and only the grey mists and short days shroud their vulnerability. It is as if they are suspended, waiting, waiting for the signal to emerge again. This is how I am feeling' (p. 47).

'The cold winter wind has finally changed direction and eased. I can see tight buds ion the crab apple trees ready to unfurl and bring fresh growth' (p. 59).

'The garden outside my window is transformed. The crab apples are green and the long grass revived' (p. 59).

James's imagery of crab apples reflects her transformation as a leader, moving through a sense of desolation to new growth and abundance that marked her emergence as a transformational leader after a seemingly long winter where it seemed nothing would grow, or that all might perish. It creates a vivid sense of her narrative journey. Such playful imagery spins the transformational story. The imagery helps its audience visualise her journey, drawing them into her journey. It binds the narrative. The narrative vibrates with energy.

In weaving a narrative, I suggest to the practitioner to visualise the impact of your words upon an audience. What words to emphasise, plant questions for the audience to consider, dramatise the turning points, using imagery or poems, journal extracts, dialogue from practice and guided reflection; all creative ploys to lift the text beyond the prosaic to engage its audience in dialogical play.

Show or Tell

Weaving the narrative, the practitioner reveals their insights. These can be spelt out directly – 'these are my insights' perhaps woven into a developmental framework. Telling the audience is like reading a report as a fact. Alternatively, the practitioner may weave a story of their journey where their insights are shown or pointed to less directly to be discerned by the audience, inviting the audience to draw their own insights. Thus, the audience are active. Indeed, reflexive narrative always intends to inform others towards social action – what I term the sixth dialogical movement.

As Okri notes [9, p. 41] –

'The writer does one half of the work but the reader does the other. The reader's mind becomes the screen, the place, the era. To a large extent, readers create the world from words, they invent the reality they read. Reading is therefore a co-creation between writer and reader'.

Showing is more creative and engaging than telling. It is also more risky from a traditional technical rational perspective. Teachers might insist that insights are spelt out rather than being interpreted from the text. As such, the practitioner may feel forced to lean towards telling rather than showing. That, of course, doesn't prevent the reader from drawing their own insights. Validity of an insight can be gauged by the description of experience to support it. Thus, the reader must appreciate the nature of reflexive narrative and those who might grade it guided by appropriate grading criteria (see Chapter 20).

I always advocate the practitioner invites its reader to dialogue with the narrative text with an open mind as to what the narrative has to say rather than just passively reading it. Gadamer [10] asks the reader not to take offence at the text, especially if the text says something the reader disagrees with. As such, the invitation to dialogue should ask the reader to be aware of and suspend their assumptions and prejudices, yet read with a sceptical mind. The audience can read between lines, pick up clues, use their imagination and pursue them. This is the posture of the reflective reader: to be open, curious and sceptical as to what the text has to say.

Ruth Morgan [11] wrote –

'The construction of my autobiographical narrative has taken many twists and turns demonstrating the complex and changing scenes of my daily practice. The penetrative process of unravelling my own thinking and committing reflections to paper has itself altered my perceptions and created change. I have discovered that challenge is not to be feared, life need not be static and mountains can occasionally move. I invite my readers to ride in tandem with me viewing and moving the scenery through the filter of their own experience and applying it to their own lives. I depend on you, the reader, to move the narrative beyond an articulation of personal experience into the realm of wider interpretation and social relevance [12]. It is from you that the text gains its validity and movement. Stories can infect perceptions, invade complacency, amplify conscience and change lives. As Okri [9, p. 44] writes – "stories are living things; and their real life begins when they start to live in you". They are not dead scrolls. They pulse with the writer's experiences. There is always more to tell'.

As Morgan suggests, the narrative is both a window for the reader to view the lives of those within the narratives and a window to their own mind. Narratives are compelling because they capture the complexity of everyday practice without fragmenting it. They give testament to uncertainty. She invites her reader to dialogue. In her case, her audience was her academic marker. To engage a wider audience, reflexive narratives need to be published rather than left to gather dust on shelves where no dialogue beyond the examination of the dissertation can take place.

The narrative is not authoritative. It doesn't spell out facts. It is both contextual and subjective – 'this is how it was, and this is my understanding of it' although its subjectivity has been mediated through guidance. Feedback from academic marking should be with dialogical intent to enable the practitioner another level of dialogue through raising insights the reader has gained. The reader reads with the intent – 'What do I learn from reading this narrative?' Gadamer [10, p. 210] terms dialogue as the 'fusion of horizons' expanding and deepening the horizons for both reader and author.

Coherence

The practitioner is mindful of narrative coherence, the notion of weaving the narrative pattern into a coherent whole. Coherence is when the narrative holds together as a whole. The parts flow together towards the conclusion. The only criterion to judge coherence is its reflexivity. This is because every reflexive narrative is a unique self-inquiry that reflects a meaningful personal journey. Virginia Woolf [13, p. 105] notes –

'So long as you write what you wish to write that is all that matters; and whether it matters for ages or only for hours, nobody can say. But to sacrifice a hair of the head of your vision, a shade of its colour, in deference to some professor with a measuring rod up his sleeve if the most abject treachery'.

Madden reflects Wool's words with her dilemma in writing her dissertation between writing what she wishes to write against the prospect of the measuring rod [14, pp. 25–26].

'In a simple way, my feminist finds expression in my dissatisfactions and frustrations as a practicing midwife. This research is an exploration of those frustrations – teasing out the elements of constraint upon me to practice in ways congruent with my beliefs and ideals. I have already said that the writing of this project is its creation, but I am concerned that I find it so difficult to mould this dissertation into a compact, recognisable, academic piece of work. I search for the freedom to let it develop devoid of predetermined chapters and sections, finding it difficult or think in terms of self-contained, clearly demarcated issues and arguments. I tell myself this is laziness, that what results must be logical, and complete: beginning, middle, end. I worry about assessment and the need to gain accreditation. But Cixous an Clément [15] challenged me to write my femininity, "it is the whole that makes sense," and for a while I worry less about the fear of fragmentation. Cixous and Clément objects to what she sees as masculine writing, because it is cast in oppositions – it relies on reason and logic for its validity. She identifies women's writing as much more fluid, "marking, scratching, scribbling, jotting down," and argues that it is the flexibility that makes feminine writing potentially subversive and transformative. I am after all wring a story about myself here, surely that is not too difficult? But I am ever worried about the validity of the exercise, how can I make this academic? How can I turn this into knowledge that is "worth" something? Just as I seek the discourse of resistance ion women's narratives, so I resist the patriarchal, rational discourse of academic writing at the same time as attempting to gain from it? How can I reconcile these tensions, or live with them?'

Madden argues from a feminist perspective yet anxious about being judged against 'normative' academic writing. Madden is herself an academic and 'scribbles' to free herself from her own embodied dilemma. And yet she has been informed that she can write 'from the body' [1, p. 97], as Cixous and Clément [15, p. 97] note in a similar vein to Woolf [13] – 'Write yourself: your body must make itself heard. Then the huge resources of the unconscious will burst out'.

Madden's words were 'bursting out'.

'Rings True'

Because of their guided subjective and contextual nature, it is difficult to construct an inauthentic narrative. Thus, the reader will sense the extent the narrative 'rings true'. The audience should feel its authenticity. That it is compelling. That it is the practitioner's truth. Winterson [16, p. 18] notes –

> 'Truth for anyone is a very complex thing. For a writer, what you leave out says as much as those things you include. What lies beyond the margin of the text? When we tell a story we exercise control but in such a way as to leave a gap, an opening. It is a version, but never the final one. And perhaps we hope that the silences will be heard by someone else, and the story can continue, can be retold. When we write we offer the silence as much as the story. Words are part of the silence that can be spoken'.

So, play and converse with ideas and see where they lead. You can't force creativity but must let it flow. This may sound absurd to the practitioner writing a reflective assignment due next day mindful only of getting a pass grade. You might say 'that is the real world'. It behoves an educational culture that fosters creativity, otherwise reflexive narratives will be dry and stifled rather than brimming with life and meaning.

'Life Begins at 40' Introduction

'Life begins at 40' reveals what a reflexive narrative can look like. Clare, a psychiatric nurse, wove it as a final assignment undertaking the 'Becoming a reflective and effective practitioner' course (see Chapter 14). I invite you, the reader to dialogue with her narrative to draw out your own insights considering how they might inform your own practice.

Life Begins at 40

It was Pitkin W B [17], who coined the phrase life begins at 40, and how right he was. The first day I attended the course also happened to be my 40th birthday and where my life as a reflective practitioner was to begin, although at that point in time, I could not have envisaged the significant impact and influence the course would have on me. What follows is the story of how my practice developed as result and an analysis of factors that constrained my development. This will be illustrated through a series of experiences I wrote in my reflective journal, which, when viewed alone are perhaps not of great significance. However, like a children's dot-to-dot picture, it is only when the dots are joined together that a tangible picture becomes clear.

At the beginning of the course, I recorded my feelings and thoughts at the end of the day on a separate piece of paper in my journal. I felt I was reflecting. This made me question why I needed to be on an eight-month course to do this. Initially I was silent within the group, rather like a passive resister. It was only when I began to share my experiences within the group did I realise that all I was doing was stating what had happened and how I had felt. It was when I was challenged and forced to examine my feelings and view the situation from different perspectives that I started to learn from my experiences. However, it still took some weeks and a comment from the group's guide who informed me that, 'an effective practitioner is an informed practitioner', for me to ashamedly acknowledge to myself that knowledge acquisition does not happen magically but does in fact require a degree of effort on my part. It wasn't until the fifth session that I took the risk to seriously participate. Before then my participation had been zilch. I had been a passenger. I said something like 'I have something to share'....

Within my current practice one of my clinical responsibilities is to perform electrocardiographs (ECG) for all the inpatient units of the hospital. Initially I found this interesting. However, once the novelty had worn off, I viewed it as a task that had to be done. My lack of enthusiasm was quite evident in my journal entries until one day following an attempt to perform an ECG my journal entry was very different:

> 'When I arrived on the ward I was shown in to the ladies bedroom I introduced myself and started to explain the procedure the nurse interrupted me stating that I was wasting my time, "she doesn't understand a word you are saying, she has dementia". My anger levels rose but I carried on trying not to let my feelings show, the lady looked at me with watery pale blue eyes and speaking in a language of her own was trying to tell me something but I was unable to understand her, she kept tugging at my arm getting more frustrated with tears falling down her cheeks. I reassured her that I would not be performing the ECG and left the ward. The image of her eyes stayed with me, had they once been sparkling deep blue, full of life and what had those eyes seen in their 82 years of existence. I felt disgust with the nurse for treating her with disparagement and disrespect but I also had to acknowledge the uncomfortable feelings within myself about my view of performing an ECG as a tedious task and had appreciating the privilege of entering into this intimate relationship ...'

I would have liked to confront the nurse but I let it go. Swallowed my disgust but it left a nasty taste. I must admit I am a conflict avoider but then I guess most nurses are. The impact this experience had on me was immense; it enforced me to examine my attitudes, beliefs and focus my thoughts upon the nurse–patient relationship, especially the challenges faced when the patients' ability to communicate is compromised.

I asked myself – What sense do I make of this? Morse [18] states that the nurse–patient relationship is established as 'the result of interplay or covert negotiations until a mutually satisfying relationship is reached'. She discusses the types of relationships that exists and divides them into two categories, mutual or unilateral. The latter she describes as being asynchronous with one person unwilling or unable to develop the relationship to the desired level of the other. Morse [18] provides an example of why mutual involvement is not possible, that is when a patient is unconscious or in a psychotic state. Due to the fact that the lady with blue eyes was suffering from dementia automatically forced her into a unilateral relationship.

Rao [19] believes the act of communication comprises all of the ways that people send and receive messages. However, Miller [20] draws to our attention that most people do not think about the way they communicate on a day-to-day basis and are often unaware of how they relate to others yet communication is essential to our development as social beings and it is the ability to communicate that enables the development of short and long-term relationships. What happens then if the ability to communicate becomes impaired? Bush [21] suggests that people who cannot communicate, or who communicate inappropriately are often marginalised by society and run the risk of social alienation and diminished function and that as a result of the frustration of being unable to make needs and feelings understood by others challenging behaviour and behavioural disturbances can occur. It has been proposed by Lliffe and Drennan [22] that communication with the patient suffering from dementia may be the key to understanding and resolving behaviour disturbances. One method of communicating with people with dementia is validation therapy; this was developed by Feil [23] and attempts to help the person deal with their feelings by validating them, subsequently helping them to move from their inner world to the shared reality of the present. It is claimed that validation therapy promotes communication with the severely confused older person on their own terms, on subjects and issues that are chosen and are important to them, assuming that all the words and actions of a person with dementia have a real sense of purpose and value.

Picking up the story: as a consequence of confronting and examining my feelings, my attitude towards performing ECGs altered. I no longer viewed it just as a task that had to be done as quickly as possible but recognised that although only brief, I was engaging in a relationship with another person which should be given time and respect. Having shifted my viewpoint, I found that I once again found performing ECGs a positive experience. I was mindful of this when I received an ECG request from one of the wards that specialise in treating elderly people who are more severely confused, suffering from dementia or other organic brain disorders. The name on the ECG request seemed vaguely familiar; however, I was not prepared for the shock when I was introduced to the lady. Sitting slumped to one side with saliva dribbling out of the corner of her mouth was a lady with whom I had contact about a year ago when she received a course of ECT to which she responded well. My last memory of her was of a bright, smiling physically fit lady in her 50s who was able to return back to her work, which incidentally was as a healthcare assistant on one of the other elderly wards. This is an extract from my journal entry for that day.

> 'When I first saw her the shock was immense like a jolt of electricity had surged through my body causing my skin to prickle and take a sharp intake of breath, it took me a moment to recover. What message had my face portrayed and had she seen it? How lonely must it be to be trapped inside a body unable to communicate verbally and how must it feel to be reliant upon nurses, with whom you had once worked along side with, to feed, wash and dress you ... what is it about this situation that I find so uncomfortable I perform ECGs on other patients who are unable to communicate verbally and do not feel the same. Perhaps the sadness I feel is that she is too young to be treated on an elderly mental health ward and that her own profession has in some way let her down ...'

I remembered the group's guide had recommended an article about silent advocacy (Gadow [24]) and I set about finding it. However, it was then that I started to question my motives for doing this. Was it that if by being more informed about a situation helps me to become a more effective practitioner, or was it to help me resolve my uncomfortable feelings and feel better in myself?

It was this conflict that I shared with the group at the next session. I began by sharing the experience and discussing the conflicts I faced, which was helpful; the focus of the discussion wandered slightly with issues around communicating with patients with communication difficulties examined. One of the group members made a comment about how some nurses, without realising it, treated people as an object and lost sight of the person. That resonated within me. In response I was defensive and categorically stated that within the ECT department people were treated with respect, dignity and as individuals.

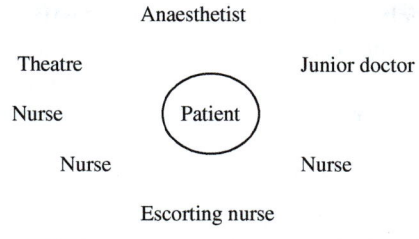

FIGURE 18.1 People in the treatment room.

But this comment niggled away at me. During the next two ECT sessions, I metaphorically took a step back and observed with more critical eyes how we regarded and treated the patients receiving ECT. I was reassured that the mental health nursing team did show respect for the patient, taking time to explain procedures and provide reassurance, although once the patient was asleep the focus of them as a person was lost. One thing that struck me was the amount of people that are present during treatment; on that day seven people, including the patient were in the present in the treatment room (Figure 18.1). Conversations took place that excluded the patient.

At the next clinical team meeting, I shared this experience and my observations, to generate discussion I posed some questions. 'How would you like to be treated if you were to receive ECT, what aspects of our practice are positive and what areas could we improve upon?'

To gain a better understanding, I suggested we recreate the scenario as fully as possible to experience first hand of being on the trolley with people attaching various monitoring equipment to you. Benner [25] highlights that good nursing practice requires ongoing clinical knowledge development through experiential learning. However, it is not automatic and requires openness, attentiveness and responsible engaged learning on the part of the practitioner. One of the team members was not a willing participant at first but did join in and, at the end of the session, commented that she had never thought about it from the patient's point of view.

We discussed this exercise in the next team meeting; we all felt it was worthwhile and that it gave us a better understanding of how the patient feels before they are anaesthetised. What struck us all was how vulnerable and intimidating it felt lying on the trolley with so many people surrounding you. From this, we considered ways we could improve our practice, limiting the amount of people surrounding the patient until they are asleep, encouraging the doctors to have discussions about treatment regimes out of earshot of the patients, and instead of having the radio on, play more soothing and related music. This exercise was only carried out with the mental health nursing staff, who felt it would be beneficial for the whole treatment team to undergo this, particularly with the theatre nurse and the anaesthetist, who by the nature of their work, spend the majority of the time with unconscious patients.

Morse [18] highlights nurses working in operating rooms use a strategy of depersonalisation, which includes transforming not only the person into a patient but also the patient into a case. According to Sisson [26] hearing is the last sense to go when a person becomes unconscious. Studies of patients' memories of their unconscious state indicate that they heard and understood various conversations that took place while they were unconscious [27–29]. It is imperative, as Leigh [30] points out, that health professionals evaluate the way in which they communicate with unconscious patients. Russell's [31] study concludes that hospitals are often noisy, which can make the patient anxious, whereas reassurance and explanations by nurses help them to feel safe, secure and feel less vulnerable. This study also found that where nurses became over involved with technical equipment and the physical aspects of care reduced the level of communication with the patient. While Podurgiel [28] and Green [32] both recommend that personalised care should be given through the use of effective communication strategies, such as speaking directly to the patient and using touch to enhance communication and express emotional support. Dyer [33] cautions that touch is a two-way process, and permission should be sought before a nurse invades a patient's personal space.

At the end of an ECT session, I shared our experiential experience with the theatre nurse, hoping that she would be receptive to the idea of participating in a similar exercise with the anaesthetist. 'Whatever did you want to do a thing like that for?' was her cynical reply. I attempted to explain that I felt it was important to view the care we gave from the patients' perspective. She ridiculed such an idea – *'What a load of poppycock, how do they know what they need, we are the anaesthesiology specialists not them, so how can they possibly know what they need and I certainly do not need to lay on a theatre trolley to know how to do my job'.*

She left the department with very ruffled feathers and I felt irritated and disappointed as this extract from my journal entry shows.

> 'My emotions are all in a muddle like a big ball of spaghetti lying heavy and uncomfortably in the pit of my stomach. I have experienced these feelings before, when I was a child in primary school there was one particular teacher who no matter how hard I tried to please and gain her approval she all ways knocked me back leaving me feeling angry and frustrated and confused. Only now I am not a schoolgirl I am a professional practitioner and believe in what I am trying to achieve. Why do I always let her get to me? Why do I feel intimidated by her and unable to assert myself with her when I can with other people? ...'

When I read this extract in the guided reflection group, Chris [the guide] in his ubiquitous coaxing manner simply asked – 'so why do I let her get to me?' A silence descended over the group as I contemplated this question. Was it a simple identification with a teacher from primary school? How could I know that? I connected this experience to another experience that concerned a junior doctor who was constantly late and on one occasion did not show up at all. I had no hesitation in letting the doctor know my feelings.

Chris asked 'How can you change things?'

I replied 'I can't imagine how I can'.

He suggested the other group members put themselves in my shoes to imagine how they would like to respond and what might stop them. Like me the group were uncertain. They could feel the conflict.

Chris suggested I use transactional analysis [34] to examine the pattern of communication between myself and the theatre nurse. The gist of this theory is that people communicate from learnt ego states – either parent, adult or child. Ideally, we should use adult–adult interaction as befits collaborative and responsible professionals. Effective communication is when lines of communication are not crossed – for example, adult–adult or parent–child. However, when someone gets anxious, they often revert to 'type' and move into either parent or child ego states.

Understanding this theory, I discovered the root of the breakdown. The theatre nurse's response was not the adult response I had invited. Instead, it was a cynical dismissive response I linked with the primary school teacher [critical parent]. It conjured up similar feelings that left me seething. I became the 'hurt child'. I had spoken to her as an adult, she responded as a critical parent. Stewart and Joines [35] describe this as a 'crossed transaction'. Cross is an apt description of how I felt! Looking again at how I communicate with the theatre nurse it became evident that I often revert into 'child mode' in response to her 'critical parent mode'.

Chris then talked through TA theory based on parent–adult–child interactions.

'So how can you stop reverting to a hurt child mode?'

I confessed 'I don't know'.

Chris asked 'Imagine the situation again – how might you respond differently?'

I mused 'he's using the MSR cues'. It reminded me of star wars and using the force. Uncanny. I smiled 'smack her in the teeth!' The group laughed. The spell was broken.

One of the groups suggested I might have said 'you sound just like my primary school teacher' and walk away. A subtle confrontation that keeps my integrity.

Applying the transactional analysis framework was most helpful using the labels of critical parent and hurt child – it enabled me to visualise the relationship between myself and the theatre nurse, and, perhaps most significantly engendered the feelings associated with those labels. It was illuminating and challenging and prompted me to examine my patterns of communication with other members of the team towards promoting more effective collaborative working.

Deepening Insight

The point of reflection is gaining insight. Whilst these are laced within the above description, I have been starkly reminded of my vision to realise person-centred nursing. I had become complacent! Practice had become routinised as if I was on auto-pilot most of the time. What a wake-up call! My concern for patients was relit. I learnt something about myself and improving my communication skills. Perhaps, most significantly, I acted to create a more therapeutic environment. Checking out insights is significant, because it helps to solidify learning.

One of the biggest factors that hindered my development was myself. At the beginning, my attitude was arrogant and the reasons for attending the course were influenced by the educational credits that could be obtained. Although I consistently kept a reflective journal my entries were descriptive, inexpressive and once written, were not returned to. I am not sure when exactly my transformation happened as it was a gradual process. However, I remember feeling uncomfortable when other members of the group shared their journal entries. The words of a teacher who taught spelling came back to me, he said, 'If you cheat you are only deceiving yourself and it will be you who has to face the consequences'. I felt like an impostor and my atheism would be exposed at any minute. Writing my journal was finding my voice. The emphasis on rich description focused me to pay attention, notably those things I had taken for granted, that had become part of the wallpaper. Perhaps that was why I had initially nothing to say. My lack of voice rendered me silent. Finding voice gave vent to thoughts and feelings, opening my mind to ideas, – what Belenky et al. [36] describe as the subjective voice – 'the quest for self'. Then I could explore, critique and juxtapose a literature to inform my emerging insights – the synthesis of what Belenky et al. [36] term the separate and connected procedural voices. This synthesis moulds the constructed voice. It made sense. It was empowering and led to action. The world became a better place for myself and for patients.

Finding my voice in my journal empowered me to find my voice in practice to question and challenge. I felt I had shed some dark fear lurking in me, implanted aeons ago during my childhood, schooling and nurse training – 'be a good girl – good girls are seen but not heard'. No longer will I be silent or silenced. It is an insult to my integrity to act for the good.

This journey has been lonely at times, but having undergone a complete transformation of my attitude and realised the power that reflection has to change and improve practice, I wanted to share this enlightenment and sought after converting my colleagues to my newfound faith. However, in my passionate and over zealous approach, what I in fact achieved was to alienate my colleagues, not bring them on board. I realised that in order for me to have any influence, a drastic modification of my approach was needed. Put another way, it's no good having a voice if it isn't heard!

There were times on this journey that I became exhausted and on occasions I wished I could remove my reflective lenses and view things through my old eyes. Reflecting daily on my practice constantly highlighted areas that need modification or change. Like a rolling stone gathering moss.

For me one of the immense values of this course was that the process of reflection was guided. Being in the reflective group helped me to remain focused and motivated me to continue on my journey. If my reflective journey had not have been guided, then I feel it may well have been more of a magical mystery tour.

Has attending this course helped me to become an effective practitioner? The answer is unequivocally yes. Although I am a novice in the world of reflection, I realise the potential reflective practice has on shaping the future of our profession whereby we can begin to value our practical expertise as a profession [37].

Commentary

Reading Clare's narrative and other narratives in this book, it is easy to feel their creativity, energy and transgression. She does not utilise a developmental framework or spell out her insights. Instead, she weaves her insights into the narrative fabric. As such, there is creative and dramatic flow running through the narrative that engages the reader. The reader wants to know what happens next.

The narrative is revealing and disturbing into ECT practice – as if the person being treated is some object, merely a task to do – the very antithesis of person-centred practice. She goes deep into the background of practice to reveal the assumptions, norms and relationships that govern existing practice and her efforts to shift these norms if a better, more satisfactory state of affairs is to be established. The narrative's transgression is palpable.

Turning Points

Clare's narrative can be viewed through pivotal *turning points* [38]. Turning points are the highest moments of tension within the narrative, the most revealing and possibly dramatic points within the narrative. They also mark insights.

One turning point is the revelation that ECT is not humane. Clare's shocking revelation – '*Swallowed my disgust but it left a nasty taste*'. It went right across the grain of her vision for person-centred practice. The emotional and creative tension woke her up that person-centred practice mattered, confronting her routine approach to practice. From that point, guided reflection also mattered, giving her voice and humbling her arrogance. Indeed, she emphasises this in concluding her narrative.

Another turning point is her interaction with the theatre nurse again triggered by strong emotion. The theatre nurse resisted her, mocked her, as Clare tried to apply her insights into the broader field of practice. It showed how deeply personal reflection becomes when practitioners are vision driven. Clare's use of journal reflections gives these turning points a strong sense of drama. This enables the reader to really feel Clare's experience, perhaps triggering their own emotions and reflections.

The use of reflective questions immediately engages the reader, helping the reader put herself in Clare's shoes – '*why do I always let her get at me?*' I am sure many readers can identify with this sentiment. Clare's use of description lifted from her reflective journal gives her narrative richness and adds to its authenticity. Its richness is reflected in her evocative use of language – '*the lady looked at me with watery pale blue eyes and. Speaking in a language of her own, was trying to tell me something ...*' And later in the same passage – '*the image of those eyes stayed with me: had they once been sparkling and deep blue, full of life, and what had those eyes seen in their 82 years of existence?*' Again in the same passage –'*I felt disgust with the nurse for treating her with disparagement and disrespect but I had to acknowledge the uncomfortable feelings within myself*'. In this passage, I sense the cathartic and creative impact of writing. Shaping words into images to enchant and disturb the reader.

Clare's use of metaphor holds meaning and create drama – '*When I first saw her the shock was immense like a jolt of electricity had surged through my body to prickle*'. She links the electricity shock to the patient to describe her feelings. Another example *'my emotions are all in a muddle like a big ball of spaghetti lying heavy and uncomfortable in the pit of my stomach.* The use of spoken words between herself and the theatre nurse also creates a vivid image and gives voice to the nurse, enabling the reader 'to walk in her shoes' to sense the feelings of anger behind her word and question shy this nurse was so threatened by Clare's proposal.

Clare repeats herself from time to time. It is intuitive as words unfold. By repeating, the narrative's messages are reinforced for readers to take notice. When Eva Hesse [39, p. 11] was asked 'repetition is very prevalent in your work. Why do you repeat a form over and over?' She replied 'Because it exaggerates. If something is meaningful, maybe it's more meaningful said ten times. It's not just an aesthetic choice. If something is absurd, it's more greatly exaggerated, absurd, if it's repeated'.

Clare explores the significance of guidance in enabling her to confront and change organisational practice against the barriers that manifest.

Summary

Constructing narrative is like following a stream and seeing where it flows. It seeks to capture the drama of the unfolding journey of becoming who one seeks to become within the context of realising one's vision of practice. Like experience itself, narrative is not formulaic even though we constantly seek to impose order on our practice.

Be soft in your practice
Think of the method as a fine silvery stream, not a raging waterfall.
Follow the stream
Have faith in its course.

It will go its own way,
Meandering here, trickling there.
It will find grooves, the cracks, the crevices.
Just follow it.
Never let it out of your sight.
It will take you.

Sheng-yen [40, p. 69]

References

1. Mattingly, C. (1994) The concept of therapeutic 'emplotment'. *Social Sciences and Medicine* 38(6), 811–822.

2. Chase, S. E. (2005) Narrative inquiry: multiple lenses, approaches and voices. In N. K. Denzin, Y. S. Lincoln [Eds.] *The Sage Handbook of Qualitative Research* (Third edition). Sage Publications, Thousand Oaks, 651–679.

3. Dewey, J. (1933) *How We Think*. J. C. Heath, Boston.

4. Priest, J-M., Johns, C. (2010) More than eggs for breakfast. In C. Johns [Ed.] *Guided Reflection: A Narrative Approach to Advancing Professional Practice*. Wiley-Blackwell, Oxford, 195–214.

5. Wheatley, M. J. (1999) *Leadership and the New Science. Discovering Order in a Chaotic World.* Berrett-Koehler, San Francisco.

6. Tuffnell, M., Crickmay, C. (2004) *A Widening Field.* Dance Books, Alton.

7. Wheatley, M. J., Kellner-Rogers, M. (1998) *A Simpler Way*. Berrett-Koehler publications, San Francisco.

8. James, P. (2006) *Being and Becoming an Effective Clinical Leader*. Unpublished MSc Leadership in Healthcare Dissertation, University of Bedfordshire.

9. Okri, B. (1997) *A Way of Being Free*. Phoenix House, London.

10. Gadamer, H.-G. (1960) *Truth and Method*. In G. Barden, J. Cumming [Eds.] Seabury Press, New York.

11. Morgan, R. (2004) *Realising Transformational Leadership*. Unpublished MSc Leadership in Healthcare Dissertation, University of Bedfordshire.

12. Pinar, W. (1981) 'Whole, bright, deep with understanding': issues in qualitative research and autobiographical method. *Journal of Curriculum Studies* 13(3), 173–188.

13. Woolf, V. (1945) *A Room of One's Own*. Penguin Books, London.

14. Madden, B. (2002) *Working with Women Following Traumatic Childbirth*. Unpublished MSc Dissertation, University of Bedfordshire.

15. Cixous, H., Clément, C. (1996) *The Newly Born Woman*. I. B. Tauris Publishers, London.

16. Winterson, J. (2011) *Why Be Happy When You Can Be Normal?* Jonathan Cape, London.

17. Pitkin, W. B. (1932) *Life Begins at Forty*. McGraw-Hill Book, New York.

18. Morse, J. (1991) Negotiating commitment and involvement in the nurse-patient relationship. *Journal of Advanced Nursing* 16, 552–558.

19. Rao, M. T. (1993) *Coping with Communication Challenges in Alzheimer's Disease*. Singular Publishing, San Diego.

20. Miller, L. (2002) Effective communication with older people. *Nursing Standard* 17(9), 45–50, 53, 55.

21. Bush, T. (2003) Communicating with patients who have dementia. *Nursing Times* 99(48), 42–45.

22. Lliffe, S., Drennan, V. (2001) *Primary Care and Dementia*. Jessica Kingsley, London.

23. Feil, N. (1993) *The Validation Breakthrough: Simple Techniques for Communicating with People with 'Alzheimer's-type Dementia*. Health Profession's Press, Baltimore.

24. Gadow, S. (1980) Existential advocacy. In S. Spickler, S. Gadow [Eds.] *Nursing: Image and Ideals*. Springer, New York, 79–101.

25. Benner, P. (2003) Clinical reasoning: articulating experiential learning in nursing practice. In O. Slevin, L. Basford [Eds.] *Theory and Practice of Nursing* (second edition). Nelson Thornes, London, 176–186.

26. Sisson, R. (1990) Effects of auditory stimuli on comatose patients with head injury. *Heart and Lung* 4, 373–378.

27. Tosch, P. (1988) Patients' recollections of their post-traumatic coma. *Journal of Neuroscience Nursing* 20(4), 223–228.

28. Podurgiel, M. (1990) The unconscious experience: a pilot study. *Journal of Neuroscience Nursing* 22(1), 52–53.

29. Lawrence, M. (1995) The unconscious experience. *American Journal of Critical Care* 4(3), 227–232.

30. Leigh, K. (2001) Communicating with unconscious patients. *Nursing Times* 97(48), 35–36.

31. Russell, F. (1999) An exploratory study of patient perception, memories and experiences of an intensive care unit. *Journal of Advanced Nursing* 29(4), 783–791.

32. Green, A. (1996) An explorative study of patients' memory of their stay in an acute intensive therapy unit. *Intensive and Critical Care Nursing* 12(3), 131–137.

33. Dyer, I. (1995) Preventing the ITU syndrome or how not to torture an ITU patient (part 2). *Intensive and Critical Care Nursing* 11(4), 223–232.

34. Berne, E. (1961) *Transactional Analysis in Psychotherapy. The Classic Guide to its Principles*. Grove Press, New York.

35. Stewart, I., Joines, V. (1987) *TA Today: A New Introduction to Transactional Analysis*. Russell Press, Nottingham.

36. Belenky, M. F., Clinchy, B. M., Goldberger, N. R., Tarule J. M. (1986) *Women's Ways of Knowing: The Development of Self, Voice, and Mind*. Basic Books, New York.

37. Bulman, C. (2004) An introduction to reflection. In C. Bulman, S. Schultz [Eds.] *Reflective Practice in Nursing* (third edition). Blackwell Publishing, Oxford.

38. Carson, J. (2008) *Spider Speculations: A Physics and Biophysics of Storytelling*. Theatre Communications Group, New York.

39. Hesse, E. (2002) *Eva Hesse*. In M. Nixon [Ed.]. MIT, Cambridge, MA.

40. Levering, M. (2000) *Zen*. Duncan Baird Publishers, London.

Note

i. https://dictionary.cambridge.org/us/dictionary/english/tinkering.

CHAPTER 19

Narrative as Poetry and Art

Weaving the reflexive narrative opens up a space to explore creative ways for representation of insights. Whilst most practitioners have a natural leaning towards a verbal prose mode of expression, others may lean towards more artistic modes of expression, such as poetry and visual art.

Loori (1, p. 84) highlights the significance of art as a learning milieu –

'Through our art we bring into existence something that previously did not exist'. What we bring into existence are our stories of everyday practice and what we have learnt from them, rich fuel for others to reflect on and learn through. As such, narrative art is active, open to interpretation, full of meaning both shown and told, dynamic in dialogue with others. Art forms fuel both the artist's and their audience's imagination'.

Wagner (2) interviewed 18 nurses for their reflections of family impact on the dying experience. She reduced these experiences into a set of categories using fragments of the nurses' reflections to justify each category. In doing so, I felt she lost the meaning in these nurses' stories. However, she then re-interpreted the nurses' words into poetry – 'as a way of knowing subjectively and inter-subjectively the fullest meaning of the data' (p. 21). Her poetry reflects a deeper level of interpretation beyond cognition; in my mind, it heals the story and makes it possible to connect with the experience because it is whole. Coleman and Willis (3, p. 906) facilitated nursing students, consisting of two focus groups of ten students, to use poetry as reflective writing. They concluded that –

'Poetry writing give students the opportunity for freedom of expression, personal satisfaction and a closer connection with their patients which the more formal approach of reflective writing did not offer'.

Prose Poetry

Prose poetry is a mode of aesthetic expression that balances the more cognitive approaches to reflection, a more holistic approach to tap the deep pool of tacit knowing [4]. Everyone is a poet although you, the reader, may not realise that potential. Remember, limits exist only in the mind. Some of us have had our imaginations so trimmed that we believe poetic endeavour is beyond us.

As Paramananda [5, p. 71] writes –

> 'Of course, the sad thing, the tragic thing, is that many of us do get trimmed. We all start off with real heads full of space and imagination, but slowly, somewhere along the path that we call growing up, our heads get trimmed. We become caught up in the doings of this world, the realities of adult life, and we get down to size ... without imagination the world loses its mystery and sense of depth in which we can find meaning'.

We lose touch with the imagination. Instead we are caught up in the demand to be rational that seems to govern much of professional life.

And yet, practice is performance – watch the practitioner dance as she moves through her practice. The greatest assets are perception, imagination, intuition, creativity, all assets generally denigrated and stunted. Art as reflection enables the practitioner to value and develop these qualities. In doing so, the practitioner begins to use her whole brain again, recovering the wilted right side where these qualities are generally considered to reside. And at the end of art workshops built into the reflective curriculum, smiles are broad, fears dispelled and a real sense of recovery and achievement generally expressed.

When given the opportunity to write poetry, practitioners often say that they do not know where their poetic words have come from. Many are astonished that they can write poetry, as if it is some untapped, latent potential within us all. Yet the latent artist lives within each of us. It just needs to be woken up and injected with some spirit. On a one-day workshop, I could have you writing poetry you would never believe possible. Let go of anxiety and the rational mind and let the creative juices flow, although this might be easier said then done when one's creative juices have dried up in the left brain world. Moving into poetic mode, we engage the right brain to unleash creativity. It is a sense of writing from the body, an altogether more intuitive representation of one's experience.

Tufnell and Crickmay [6, p. 63] capture this sense –

> 'By allowing words and images to spread out in response, we open up an imaginative field that plays upon and around what has occurred, writing as we might write a poem in order to touch the deeper currents felt within the moving'.

Roger, a primary nurse at Buford, shared a poem with me in one guided reflection session that reflect his feelings about a patient's death.

Remembering MA
Walking on a high wire above the trees
Below me is a broad river over-ripe with death.
From holding death's hand,
Looking death in the eye,
Washing and dressing death,
Laying death out,
And wrapping death in a sheet, yet
There is no understanding.

Dry, flaking skin stretched over bones
Sticking together in a creaking frame,
So frail it seems crushable.
Holding hands with life,
Feeling life fade away with last labour asps
Death creeps in.

I have heard the scream of love
And gathered the tears.

This bundle of dead cells is not the one we knew
Who once cried in her mother's arms,
Walked her first step.
Whose laugh and early words lit her parents' eyes.
This bundle of dead cells is not the lover once
Caressed and hugged close, nor
Yet a wife, a mother, a friend.
She has gone
And lives in the mind only, and
Caught in photographs.
Her friend told the nurse
'Nobody else understood her.
Nobody else knew her as I did'
There is no understanding.

I asked Roger why he had shared the poem with me. He was at a lost to know. I suggested it reflected his vulnerability as a person-centred practitioner. He says that in writing the poem he worked out his feelings. In doing so, he honours MA and himself. Perhaps only a poem was an adequate expression of his reflection.

Single Lines and Scrolling Down

My approach to writing prose poetry is to break the reflective text into single lines and then scroll down pausing at the end of each line as if to read between the lines. In scrolling down, imagine pulling away the veneer of normal practice to see self from a new, less familiar, perspectives, an approach inspired by Jeannette Winterson [7, p. 103][i] –

'There are so many lives packed into one. The one life we think we know is only the window that is open on the screen. The big window full of detail, where the meaning is often lost among the facts.

If we can close that window, on purpose or by chance, what we find is another view. This window is emptier. The cross references are cryptic. As we scroll down it, looking for something familiar, we seem to be scrolling into another self- one we recognize but cannot place. The co-ordinates are missing, or the co-ordinates pinpoint us outside the limits of our existence.

If we move further back, through a smaller window that is really a gateway, there is less and less to measure ourselves by. We are coming into a dark region. A single word might appear. An icon'.

You may find that as you break the text into single lines and scroll down, it takes you deeper into yourself, into regions you have not been aware of to find the icon or insight. Breaking the text into single lines rewrites the text into a poetic narrative form, rearranging words and adding new lines as new ideas emerge. You have created a prose poem! There is no need to make lines rhyme, although most poems have a metre noticeable in the length of the lines that becomes evident when the poem is recited.

'What Is Therapy?'

'What is therapy?' is my narrative based on my experiences with patients who had resisted or declined my offer of a 'hands-on' therapy in my work as a holistic therapist working in hospice. The genesis of these poems was written in my reflective journal as notes. I was the sense of pathos I felt for my experience of meeting the people involved in each poem. Looking back over these poems, I reflexively realised they all concerned experiences when I had not given a 'hands on' therapy, opening my inquiry – 'what is therapy?'

Thus, I returned to the texts and expanded them as a narrative.

The poems evoke the complex relationship between suffering and therapy. My plot is my vision of practice to ease suffering that provides a broad canvass against which to read these poems. The poems are presented in a linear time. The reader can scroll down the poems, and perhaps, reading between the lines, will discern their own icons or insights in relation to their own experiences. Without doubt, human suffering and dying have deep regions.

'What is therapy?': a narrative of my reflections on patients to whom I do not give a physical therapy to

Alfie Boundary

Despair ripples through him like a harsh wind,
It blows and distorts his counternance.
His face crumples to the inquiry;
Heart failure has reduced him, taken his vitality.
He is in the hands of others now.
His wife at her brother's funeral;
'I should be there' he cries.
Tears fall,
He has fallen.
I move a chair close to his bed
sit, move closer, as if moving into his suffering
whereas before, standing, I was on the margin.
Anxiety spills about going home,
'How will she cope?
She doesn't know yet ....?'
Words that drift off,
Other words spoken in silence.
Can suffering be eased with words?
In the silence we dwell
He declines a therapy.
Not in the right frame of mind
as if healing needs a particular frame.
My presence a pressure?
I conclude that sitting and listening is itself therapy with one's own concerns set aside
O'Donohue [8, p. 101] writes
> *Sometimes we listen to things, but we never hear them*
> *True listening brings us in touch*
> *Even with that which is unsaid and unsayable.*
> *Sometimes the most important thresholds of mystery*
> *are places of silence.*
Of course the science cynic would say
What's the prove of that
As if wisdom needed proof.

Naomi

91 years old
Never had a thing wrong until this.

This small lady looks up at me
Wearing delicate red lipstick
Such thin legs
The football stomach looks incongruous
The ascites being drained
Had her lungs done a while ago.
Ovarian cancer.
I sit
I am in no hurry
And now she can see my face more clearly
rather than my belly.
I take her hand
Touch to communicate she is not alone and find ease
Blackwolf and Jones [9, p. 184] write
  *'Touch is the harmonic healing the grieving spirit craves. A gentle touch on the back, the
  shoulder, the head, the hand tells the receiver more than what can be expressed'*
She tries to be rational
"I've had a good life, the last 20 without my husband surrounded by a good family"
She tries the brave face
But underneath her suffering ripples.
A nurse pops in to check the drainage tap
No sense she disturbs the flow
Naomi declines my offer of a therapy,
She has found a comfortable position
As if that position is precarious,
She thanks me for my attention.
You never know what to expect
When you move into a patient's room
Simply be open to the possibility
in no rush to move on.
No pressure.

Dora Franke

Standing by her bedside
She murmers *I don't think I want a treatment thank you*
Her eyes search mine
'How are you' I inquire
holding her eyes from my six-foot height
the ubiquitous invitation to talk
I could have simply said *OK then* and moved on
But I don't.
I pull up a chair
She talks at length about her husband's dying in the hospice 2 years ago.
How do you feel being here because of that?
Ok, the care Don received was so good.
As if she can now take comfort in her own care.
She is 68
Breast, bowel, bone, and renal cancer spread through her
No pain.
The notes in the green file said she was depressed

Such labels stigmatise and stick influencing the care giver's gaze
Unless mindful enough
I would say she is more preoccupied, wistful, a little fearful.
She knows what is happening to her
And seems ok about that
Perhaps working out old grief
As if preparing to join him.

Mrs Wells

'Good morning Mrs Wells' *I say*
She's been here four weeks now
Now more grey, more subdued
Her breathing increasingly laboured
End stage lung disease
She says in her lugubrious way *just waiting now*
Her husband sits by the window
He endures.
I stand as if standing is my normal pose in passing by
I ask him *how are you*?
He says *ok*
I sense his unease but do not push it.
What else can he say in this waiting room?
I don't ask you if you want a therapy
No need to burden you with the 'No' game we've learnt to play.
Asking myself – what are her needs?
What are her husband's needs?
Not assuming that I know
Knowing what I do know
Murray Cox [10, p. 83] notes
>   He [the therapist] must not confuse the needs of the patient
>   with what the therapist projects from his own experience.
Especially any idea that a therapy is good for them.
I say *it's cold out there, just 2 degrees*
Feel my hand
She takes it and exclaims how cold it is
Her warmth transforming my cold
Caring is a mutual thing
She smiles
I sense she has some peace
I am pleased I didn't pass her by.
We know each other from previous weeks.
She has always declined a therapy.

Belinda

Unresponsive
At first I wondered if you had died
And then your chest moved slightly
Your family about you
Solemn faces searching mine
Who is this stranger at this time?

I have stepped into a death parlour
Perhaps I intrude into this room
tucked away as it is at the end of the long corridor
One can hardly be passing by.
I say who I am
'I'm Chris, the therapist, just passing by to see if I could help in anyway'?
My words spoken from the edge
No chair pulled up to join the throng
No, they don't think so.
Caught up as they are in death's dance
Waiting for the music to play out its final notes.
They thank me.
My compassion with you I murmur
Such words feel right in the moment
As if I needed to say some words to rectify my intrusion
Or express my sympathy
Perhaps both
Having the last word is closure.

George Keeler

Few words spoken between tumultuous tears
His grief for Dandy who died last September
She had collapsed in the bathroom
A brain tumour
Dead in three days
Ripped away from him after 62 years of marriage.
Prostate cancer has spread through his bones
Now – he just wants to close his eyes and not wake up again
Nothing has meaning
Not even his great granddaughter expected soon
Grief obliterates any future.
I sit with him
His spirit broken
Breaking the silence he says *Drink*
His cup empty
What do you like to drink?
Apple juice
I fetch him cool apple juice from the fridge
I do not try to understand him
Or fix his despair with platitudes
That might more comfort me.
Alex James [11] quotes a bereaved woman
   'We were together forever.
   I can't quite believe it was 63 years.
   It has flitted by all too soon.
   I can't imagine going on without him.
   No amount of time would have been long enough for us.
   I wasn't ready for it yet
   and I want to slap those who keep saying he had a good innings'.
Words that help imagine George's suffering

It is enough to dwell with him
My presence a confrontation that life goes on
When he might prefer to be alone
Caught as he is between worlds.
Elias [12, p. 84] informs – 'for some of the dying it might be right to be alone. Perhaps they are able to dream and not want to be disturbed. One must sense what they need'.
George says 'never mind' repeatedly.
Her picture on the table watches over him
Black and white
I say *what message might she give you?*
He sobs *I don't know*
He calms as if she now holds his hand
Easing the broken spirit.

Frank Seymour

Frank puts aside the GWR illustrated text
A railway man of old
Railways his love
but spent the last 20 working years for Charles Forte
I do not ask why the job shift.
Me too an ex railway man
Building bridges and stations
With the Southern engineers
Connection
20 minutes in recollection
Then some talk of the cancer that grips you
and will take your life.
Matter of fact stuff
No emotional release
As if he has already departed his physical body
Mattingly [13, p. 71] writes
> 'but sickness and tragedy have their own curious effects, not least of which is a sort of detachment, a leave taking of the body, a disinclination to care about anything, or a disowning of one's troublesome parts'.
Words that resonate and help frame
He doesn't think he needs a therapy
but then therapy has many shades
we simply dwelt in human contact
beyond the professional and patient labels
Later I say to Wendy *I had a talk with Frank.*
She smiles *He would like that, talking to a man.*
Hospice full of women

We met again next Thursday
'Hello Frank' I say framed within the open door
Chris ... come in
I hover as if in transition
Sit down ... chair over there .....
you can move that stuff off there

The significance of sitting rather than stand as if passing by
With its insidious message 'I am busy'
or worse – 'you are an object'
Sitting is a commitment.
I have time Frank
That's good Chris ... I value our talk
I remind you about the job shift.
They wanted to relocate me to Derby
No consultation
A fait accompli, seeing only the job and not the person
As if standing rather than sitting.
So you decided to quit
You had wanted to be a plateman
But your father's, also a railwayman, defiant no ... too dangerous.
So signals and telegraph it was.
You were envious of your friend who became a plateman.
Frank sucks in between his words
The nasal cannula and the green tube
A constant reminder as you wait for the nursing home to be sorted.
The hospice a waiting room
You must sense I am restless or perhaps you are
Thanks for dropping by and talking.
I guess you don't want any therapy? I say
No, no thank you I'm happy as I am.
Therapy is listening.
Stories are remembering, ordering, healing, connection
The piecing together of a life puzzle
So he can die intact.

Bernard Barker

He barks *you've come at the wrong time!*
A retort that reflects his discomfort
Waiting for a doctor to come to him
Problem with his eye
His anxiety spills *I am too unwell*
in response to my offer of a therapy later
I say *I meet many people who are unwell.*
A rue smile – *good point*
He softens and sees I'm on his side
That he needn't resist me.
That we can form an alliance rather than be adversarial necessary for therapeutic work [14]
No emotional or need to control impasses as Ramos [15] identified as impasses to therapeutic relationships
I can flow with him on his journey no matter the disturbances along the way
I say *I'll find the doctor for you*
He thanks me
Offers me his calloused hand

Rita Pike

Your green file lies on the table.
Opening I read you are 56.
The mood word 'flat' grabs my attention.
'Flat' a word that conjures disturbance of the spirit
The sky is dark outside
Time for my departure
But I will make this last visit.
You have a visitor with you
Perhaps I should not intrude
But my curiosity gets the better of me
My invitation for therapy welcomed with a curt dismissive *NO*
My poise rocked
I am not used to such curt refusal.
Paradoxically I move closer when perhaps I should bow my retreat and apologise for the intrusion.
But I persist and draw attention to the fat robin who flits across the lawn
Am I trying to save face?
Rita cannot see the robin flitting
No matter I say, *I'll leave you to your visitor*
Caught on the hop like the robin I flit away uneasily.
Li argues [16] that relationship should be symbiotic niceness
But Rita is not playing the nice game!
Doesn't she know I am a miner to excavate the deep veins of her suffering?
I say that 'tongue in cheek' but I wonder if an element of truth exists as therapists strut their stuff
Yet I know my presence can put people 'on the spot',
disturb their control when life is itself out of control.
That I was a disturbing stranger
Perhaps Rita had become a stranger to herself facing death
Janet Younger [17, p. 53–4] comments

> *Suffering makes one a stranger ... and the reaction of others is to turn away from this stranger who now lives in a world others may be reluctant to enter ... but when by chance it is suddenly revealed in all its nakedness, people shiver and recoil.*

I rationalise to pull myself free from pique
It is, after all, a reflection of her 'flatness'?
But that would be to reduce her to the symptom
That lies flat in her notes
'Flat' – the tyranny of label that turns her into a deviant [18].
'Flat' – as if I might lift her.
'Flat' – a violation of her spirit as if someone had not understood.
I rarely read a person's notes before seeing the person
To avoid seeing the person wrapped up in labels
But I did this time and learnt a lesson.

Two weeks have passed
The green file reveals Rita may now have brain mets
A new 'label' to explain her 'unfriendly' behaviour
To rationalise her 'disturbance';
She lies on her bed alone idly watching TV

Her red framed glasses a touch of colour to lift the 'flatness'
A slight smile of recognition
Hello Rita? I'm Chris the complementary therapist..
I pause as if to let the words sink in
Do you remember me?
No reply
How are you? I persist
Bored, waiting
Tentatively I inquire *Waiting for what?*
She does not answer.
Turns her head away as if I hit a nerve
You have had some complementary therapy since being here?
Yes
Was it helpful?
Yes
But not today?
No ... but she is not unfriendly.
I'll let you rest
As if again I need to have the last word.
I move away
I wanted to say more but did not know how
I mention this to a nurse
Everyone finds her difficult she says
You shouldn't take it personally
She wasn't like this before.
She suggests its Rita's problem rather than mine.
Comment that reflects the 'dark side of nursing', that points out the stigmatizing effect on patients [19] when we intend, or pretend to be person-centred.
I sense her detachment
Perhaps that is how she copes with dying
Perhaps 'we' don't know her.
As Mattingly writes [13, p. 71] citing Sacks [20, 21]

'But sickness and tragedy have their own curious effects, not least of which is a sort of detachment, a leave taking of the body, a disinclination to acre about anything, or a disowning of one's troublesome parts'.

These words dispel the labels and opens possibility for understanding how Rita might fee,

Another week has passed
Rita is alone, lies on her bed
Viewing TV through her familiar red framed glasses
I like your glasses .....
A slight smile of welcome.
I hover perhaps waiting to be invited to sit
Sitting cannot be assumed
just passing by to say hello,
to let you know I am here today if you would like a therapy?
Her response *No*
I smile *That's fine as well*

She takes my offered hand and I am free.
I wonder if my presence adds to her suffering.
Without doubt suffering is complex
It manifests in many hues that I cannot pretend to know
My ability to ease is limited.

Reflection

The poems capture something of the beauty, mystery and tragedy of caring, its light and its shadow. As I wrote them new images emerged influencing the words I use. In particular I pay attention to how I was feeling alongside the feelings of the patients, reflecting how writing poems stirs the senses as if the words come from beyond the rational mind.

In writing these poems, I had no conscious sense of reflexivity from one experience to the next despite their linear sequence. It is as if I possessed a subconscious inquiry into the nature of holistic therapy where traces of insight from every experience informed me.

Reflecting on the poems as a whole narrative, the words of Murray Cox [10, p. 51] ring in my ear, reminding me that

> 'The therapist must at all times, be himself. He will fail his patients and become either hyper-defensive, or chaotically unbounded, if he does not remain himself as he engages with the patient in the hard work of therapy. It has something to do with a genuine ontological engagement, rather than the adoption of a professional role'.

It is this sense of knowing and remaining myself in relation to the various patients holds the thread between the poems. It is not so much a question of not adopting a professional role but of appreciating the nature of an appropriate professional role. This is true for the person-centred practitioner.

If someone had asked me at the time 'Did you give Naomi a therapy?' I would have answered 'No, she didn't want one'. If someone was to now ask me 'Did you give Naomi a therapy?' I would respond 'yes', a realisation that therapy is more than just giving a physical therapy. It is about being with someone. It is an important insight in terms of what a holistic therapy is. Thus, I do not consider I have 'failed' to give a therapy or feel disappointed if a patient refuses a physical therapy.

It is about appreciating what the person needs and appreciating that we cannot always meet their need [12] despite our best effort. That is the reflective quest to acknowledge and understand the limitation of our skill 'my ability to ease is limited', and strive towards new ways of meeting need [22].

De Hennezel [23, p. 61] made the observation that 'Many of the people I've met at the bedside of the dying feel themselves to be useless and ill at ease in this situation of just being there and not doing anything'.

There is an urge to do something. Her words challenge me to reflect on my attitude as a therapist and the nature of therapy in my quest to ease suffering. Indeed, I wonder if many patients accept therapy because the therapist imposes a demand merely by their presence in their need to justify themselves. Imagine walking around all day grasping a box of aromatherapy oils and unable to use them. How useless might the therapist feel? I can spin the question around and pose 'Is merely giving a "hands-on" treatment therapy?'

I am sometimes challenged – 'Isn't it soft or not academic to write poetry, missing the hard edge of evidence based practice?' My answer is that narrative captures the essence of caring more than any analytical study swamped in statistics. It is immediately available for others to relate to with their own experiences. Thus, narrative in any form challenges the notion of a 'professional text'.

Reflection Through Visual Art

Georgia O'Keefe wrote 'I could say things with colors and shapes that I had no words for' photographed from a building in Boulder, Colorado.

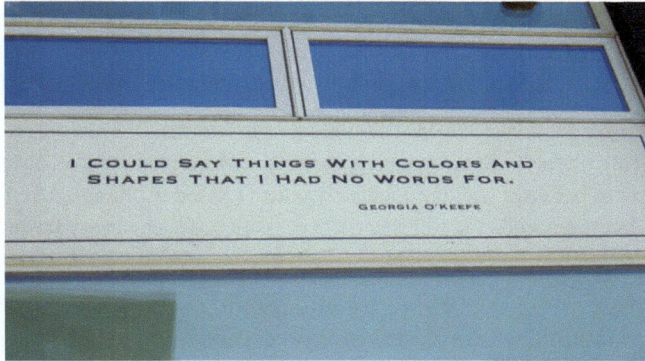

O'Keefe's words reflect that words can limit our ability to express our experience. The reflective practitioner may discover using art enables reflection and constructing narrative through visual forms. Using art such as drawing, painting and photography as modes of reflection shapes and illuminates the narrative. They deepen meaning.

For example, in my narrative 'Smoking kills' [24], I used a series of 12 images of groynes to represent lungs ravaged by lung cancer. I used images of lung cancer and their doom messages from cigarette packets, images of anti-smoking media downloaded from the internet such as 'you can't scrub your lungs clean'. Images that say more than words![ii]

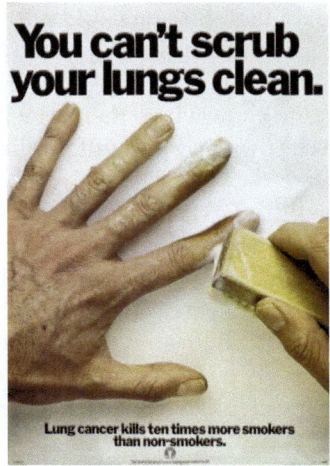

For the men dying of lung cancer portrayed in 'smoking kills', dying was not easy. They might want to scrub their lungs clean but of course they could not. Such images help the author communicate their message and disturb the audience more than mere words.

Studies illuminate how art and poetry enable practitioners to find meaning in their experiences of being with patients [25–29]. Cameron, Phillips, Sawh and Wadey [30, p. 115] illuminate using art to enable students to express their experiences and its potential for group reflection. They note –

'The purpose of the aesthetic assignment is to invite students to participate in a journey that stretches and challenges self in the paradoxes of life experiences. The student begins to engage in a form of "academic play" which gives them permission to "think outside the box" and leads them to ponder, analyze and develop their own perspectives. They apply the theoretical underpinnings of a critical social theory, which includes the values of justice and equity, inclusion, empowerment and respect as related to "lived experience" of their clients. Expression through art brings to life suppressed and repressed feelings, attitudes and beliefs and increases insights and self-awareness'.

Gaydos [31] used collage and group reflection with midwives on a maternity unit in the USA to help them reconnect with their values after a severe period of disruption. She categorised the results as firstly, a clarification of staff values, secondly, she noted (p. 174)

'The collages uncovered previously unarticulated, or unknown, or unaddressed management and care issues. Thirdly unresolved personal issues impacting on practice such as compassion fatigue, interpersonal issues between staff, and fourthly issues related to changes needed and its difficulty and resistance. In other words the full spectrum of issues affecting everyday practice emerged and openly dealt with'.

Moorman [32] used art appreciation as a *visual thinking strategy* with nursing students. Results indicated that students developed ability to see the 'whole clinical picture', to pay more attention to detail, and to explore surface signs for deeper meanings. Sharing their perceptions with peers and guides enabled them to appreciate ambiguity and to speak out especially in a clinical climate where they had felt silenced through fear of judgment by senior nurses. As such, it is not just the art that is important but the sharing of it safely.

Lei reflected with his guided reflection community on how his painting had revealed so much of himself that normally he wouldn't reveal. He felt both vulnerable and elated at his revelation, surprised that his painting could be so revealing and cathartic. It seems as if our bodies hold dark secrets that can only find expression and release through the intuitive and imaginative process, bypassing the censoring ego. Perhaps artists know this well. Spurling [33, p. xix] writes in her biography of Henri Matisse

'He said his portraits uncovered much that he could not have suspected at the start'. 'To sum up, I work without a theory, I am aware primarily of the forces involved, and find myself driven forward by an idea which I can only grasp little by little as it grows within the picture'.

The narrative painter doesn't quite know where their art will take them. They hold onto the plot but the flow of meaning finds its own way as it unfolds like the slow lift of thick morning to reveal the sun and the hills ahead.

Visualisation is more embodied than writing and can better prepare the practitioner for taking envisaged action. Practitioners may be anxious about their artistic skill, sensing that they will be publicly exposed and judged as not very good. Perhaps this is to be expected when they are no longer used to learning through creative play and having to recover their imagination that has been trimmed in the demand to 'grow up' and be rationale.

People within experiences can easily be represented as stick people or thumb prints (see Figure 13.1)[iii]. Both are easy to draw and fun to use [34]. People quickly learn to play again and recover their imagination.

Storyboard

Storyboard is a particular art form of constructing narrative. It was developed in 1930 from the Walt Disney studio as the basis for filmmaking [35]. It typically comprises a number of frames that adequately represent significant moments and insights in the person's experience. Storyboard is a form of narrative visualisation [36], whereby a story is unfolded through a sequence of images. One scene prompts the next. Captions can be written to accompany each frame. Note how the third-year students were inspired by the storyboard of Nurse Bully and the sheep (Chapter 17).

References

1. Loori, J. D. (2005) *The Zen of Creativity: Cultivating Your Artistic Life*. Ballantine Books, New York.

2. Wagner, L. (1999) Within the circle of death: transpersonal reflections on nurses' stories about the quality of the dying process. *International Journal for Human Caring* 3(2), 21–30.

3. Coleman, D., Willis, D. S. (2015) Reflective writing; the student nurse's perspective on reflective writing and poetry writing. *Nurse Education Today* 35(7), 906–911.

4. Polanyi, M. (1958) *Personal Knowledge: Towards A Post-critical Philosophy*. Routledge and Kegan Paul, London.

5. Paramananda. (1991) *A Deeper Beauty: Buddhist Reflections on Everyday Life*. Windhorse Publications, Birmingham.

6. Tuffnell, M., Crickmay, C. (2004) *A Widening Field*. Dance Books, Alton.

7. Winterson, J. (2001) *The Powerbook*. Vintage, London.

8. O'Donohue, J. (1997) *Anam Cara*. Bantam Books, New York.

9. Blackwolf., Jones, G. (1996) *Earth Dance Drum*. Commune-E-Key, Salt Lake City, UT.

10. Cox, M. (1988) *Structuring the Therapeutic Process: Compromise with Chaos*. Jessica Kingsley Publishing, London.

11. James, A. (undated). (nd) *Living with Bereavement*. Right Way Books, Tadworth.

12. Elias, N. (1985) *The Loneliness of the Dying*. Basil Blackwell, Oxford.

13. Mattingly, C. (1998) *Healing Dramas and Clinical Plots*. Cambridge University Press. Cambridge.

14. Mclaughlin, A. M., Carey, J. L. (1993) The adversarial alliance: developing therapeutic relationships between families and the team in brain injury rehabilitation. *Brian Injury* 7(1), 45–51.

15. Ramos, M. C. (1992) The nurse-patient relationship: theme and variations. *Journal of Advanced Nursing* 17, 498–506.

16. Li, S. (2004) 'Symbiotic niceness': constructing a therapeutic relationship in psychosocial palliative care. *Social Science & Medicine* 58(12), 2571–2583.

17. Younger, J. (1985) The alienation of the sufferer. *Advances in Nursing Science* 17(4), 53–72.

18. Trexler, J. C. (1995) Reformulation of deviance and labeling theory for nursing. *IMAGE: Journal of Nursing Scholarship* 28(2), 131–135.

19. Corley, M. C., Goren, S. (1998) The dark side of nursing: impact of stigmatizing responses on patients. *Scholarly Inquiry for Nursing Practice: An International Journal* 12(2), 119–122.

20. Sacks, O. (1984) *A Leg to Stand on*. Summit Books, New York.

21. Sacks, O. (1995) *An Anthropologist on Mars*. Alfred Knopf, New York.

22. Randall, F., Downie, R. (1999) *Palliative Care Ethics* (second edition). Oxford University Press, Oxford.

23. De Hennezel, M. (1998) *Intimate Death: How the Dying Teach Us to Live*. Warner Books, London.

24. Johns, C., Rose-Johns, O. (2017) Smoking kills. In C. Johns [Ed.] *Becoming A Reflective Practitioner* (fifth edition). Wiley Blackwell, Oxford, 301–316.

25. Begley, A. -M. (1996) Literature and poetry: pleasure and practice. *International Journal of Nursing Practice* 2, 182–188.

26. Eifried, S., Riley-Giomariso, O., Voight, G. (2000) Learning to care amid suffering: how art and narrative give voice to the student experience. *International Journal for Human Caring* 5(2), 42–51.

27. Brodersen, L (2001) Creatively capturing care: poetry and knowledge in nursing. *International Journal for Human Caring* 5, 33–41.

28. Vaught-Alexander, K. (1994) The personal journal for nurses: writing for delivery and healing. In D. Gaut, A. Boykin [Eds.] *Caring as Healing: Renewal Through Hope*. National League for Nursing Press, New York.

29. Parker, M. (2002) Aesthetic ways in day to day nursing. In D. Freshwater [Ed.] *Therapeutic Nursing*. Sage, Thousand Oaks.

30. Cameron, D., Phillips, S., Sawh, K., Wadey, P. (2008) Expressing voice and developing practical wisdom on social justice through art. In C. Delmar, C. Johns [Eds.] *The Good, the Wise, and the Right Clinical Nursing Practice*. Aalborg Hospital, Arhus University Hospital, Denmark, 59–72.

31. Gaydos, H. (2008) Collage: an aesthetic process for creating phronesis in nursing. In C. Delmar, C. Johns [Eds.] *The Good, the Wise, and the Right Clinical Nursing Practice*. Aalborg Hospital, Arhus University Hospital, Denmark, 163–178.

32. Moorman, M. (2015) The meaning of visual thinking strategies for nursing students. *Humanities* 4, 748–759.

33. Spurling, H. (1998) *The Unknown Matisse; A Life of Henri Matisse*, Volume 1. 1869–1908. Hamish Hamilton, London.

34. Klutz. (2008) *Thumb Doodles Book*. Klutz, Pal Alto.

35. Canemaker, J. (2010) *Paper Dreams, the Art and Artists of Disney Storyboards*. Hyperion Press, London.

36. Segel, E., Heer, J. (2010) Narrative Visualization: Telling Stories with Data. *IEEE Transactions on Visualization and Computer Graphics* 16(6), 1139–1148.

Notes

i. Reprinted with permission from the Random House Group.

ii. https://ericajayne88.wordpress.com/2009/10/31/are-the-adverts-working/smoking-kills-slowly-v/.

iii. Thumb doodle books (Klutz 2008) offers a useful introduction to using thumbprints. Google 'draw with stick people' reveals several sites offering guidance. For example, http://www.thedrawingwebsite.com/2012/10/10/stick-figures-with-style-basic-design/Also see Edward Segel and Jeffrey Heer – 'Narrative visualisation: telling stories with data (posted online 2010: http://vis.stanfors.edu/files/2010-Narrative-InfoVis.pdf' [accessed 17th December 2016].

CHAPTER 20

Grading Reflexive Narratives

As a teacher and guide, I have read and marked hundreds of reflexive narratives presented as course assignments or dissertations. It became quickly apparent that the existing university grading criteria were not fit for purpose. Assignments are designed to test the student's achievement of curriculum objectives, whether as an essay, portfolio, case study or suchlike, with a deepening interpretation through academic levels.

The student approaches an assignment mindful of the grading criteria set to judge it. Therefore, it must make sense and be easily interpreted. The teacher must talk through the grading criteria with the students so it is understood and any doubt answered.

In designing a grading profile to judge a reflexive narrative, I was mindful that grading a reflexive narrative is marking a piece of unique self-inquiry research. It is the student's personal subjective and contextual journey of being and becoming. As such, they need license to express themselves in creative ways that are respected by markers.

From that perspective, I was further mindful of imposing any criteria beyond demonstrating reflexivity towards realising a vision of practice evidenced with experience. This includes the revelation and exploration of insights. I considered there was no need to grade the application of a model of reflection. Such models are merely heuristic devices towards an end.

The risk with any criteria is that they encourage the student to fit into the criteria scheme that fragments the 'whole', and stifles creativity.

Sparkes (1, p. 223) perspective is informative

'As researchers begin to develop ways to judge auto-ethnography (reflexive narrative), I hope they can resist the temptation to seek universal, foundational criteria least one form of dogma simply replaces another. Garratt and Hodkinson (2) (1998) argue against choosing any list of universal criteria in advance of reading a piece of research. They suggest that the selection of a preordained sets of different paradigmatic rules is not a solution – 'A more constructive way forward begins with the acknowledgment that the selection of criteria should be related to the nature of the particular piece of research being evaluated (2, p. 527). As John Smith (3) echoes, we need to construct our criteria for judging various forms of inquiry as we go along'.

However, constructing criteria as we go along does not help students writing reflexive narratives. They need pointers towards what is expected yet with license to express creatively. My revised criteria (from criteria set out in sixth edition) is set out in Table 13.1. It comprises five criteria with equal grading weight. There is no intended sequencing of the criteria.

However, the first criteria – 'Insights (shown or told) are evidenced through reflection on significant experiences' – informs the student that their insights (learning) must be evidenced by the experience it was drawn from. The second criteria – 'Reflexive weaving of the narrative with a clear focus on its impact towards realising one's vision for practice' – opens the door to creativity interpretation yet with a focus on outcome, the realisation of one's vision. In other words, weaving the narrative has a purpose. The third criteria – 'Critical dialogue with extant theoretical sources to develop, frame and deepen insights and knowing in practice' – focuses the student to critically inform her insights with extant knowledge. By 'critically', the student enters into a dialogue with the theoretical source for its relevance to inform. The fourth criteria – 'Analysis of factors that emerged to either enhance or constrain realising anticipatory action' – demonstrating that the student has anticipated how they could respond differently and factors that might constrain them from doing so. The fifth criteria – 'The narrative is creative, engaging and coherent' – gives rein to creativity. By coherent, I mean the narrative holds together as a whole.

The impact of guidance on enabling the practitioner and co-constructing insights is acknowledged in the criteria of 'Analysis of factors that emerged to either enhance or constrain realising anticipatory action', whereby guidance might be construed as either enhancing or constraining alongside other factors embodied within self and embedded within the practice environment. Considering constraining forces reflects how reflexive narratives are, by their very nature, transgressive and transformative in striving to realise a vision of practice. The grid can be adjusted as a sliding scale depending on the academic level of the student.

Richardson (4) identified five criteria for auto-ethnographic writing: substantive contribution, aesthetic merit, reflexivity, impact and lived experience. These resonate with my own criteria except for specific recognition of dialogue between experience and sources of information.

The grading profile is just my interpretation. As I am sure readers will acknowledge that designing criteria to grade reflexive narratives is complex and yet vital.

Journal Entry 20.1

Recently I read my narrative 'Passing people by' [Chapter 10] to fourth-year nursing students. I asked them to grade the work based simply on their perception. I was given A1, the highest grade. I asked the students if they wrote assignments like mine. They unequivocally replied 'No'.

'Why not?' I ask

Their general response was that they were not taught to write like that. They were caught up in trying to respond to set grading criteria that emphasised applying a model of reflection and the demand for references. Hence, the potential creativity of writing reflexive narrative became lost under a technical rational cloud. The good news was that the students' teachers were present in the workshop and responded positively to the students' feedback. The teachers admitted they could see the creative way theory was linked to the experience and the value of insights. Perhaps change was in the air? Yet, within universities, it is normal to view all assignments from a technical rational bias and consequently heavily weight 'theoretical framing'. Such is the dominance of this approach it seems hard to shift.

Self-assessment

Self-assessment through grading is integral to the reflective process. Indeed, self-assessing grading offers a further level of reflection. As such it is good practice for students to grade themselves. hooks writes [5, p. 16] –

> 'I worked through my tensions around grading by teaching students to apply the criteria that would be used to grade them and then grade themselves so that they could remain aware of their ability to do needed work at the level of achievement they desired ... the difficult part of the process was teaching students to be rigorous and critical in their self-evaluation'.

In my experience, students' self-grading most often has matched my own grading.

Jill's Assignment

Jill's assignment was written as her final assignment studying the BSc End of Life Care programme. The assignment required her to reflect on and draw insight around three aspects of her practice. She works as a night staff nurse in a hospice and chose to write three exemplars around one patient, Sally, concerning touch, the environment and spirituality – all concerned with realising her broader plot of 'How can we create places of healing?[i]' Touch and environment are the focus of the narrative. As you read the narrative reflect on the criteria set out in Table 20.1.

Creating Places of Healing: Reflection on Touch and the Environment

Touch

'This narrative concerns my experience with Sally who struggled to accept her horrific circumstances as life slipped away. Sally was diagnosed with acute lymphoblastic leukaemia two years ago. She underwent a bone marrow transplant, which completely cured her illness. Eighteen months later she developed cutaneous T-cell lymphoma caused by graft versus host disease. There has only been one other case like this reported in the world! Filled with astounded disbelief Sally was left to suffer the consequences of this devastating condition with the knowledge that no curative treatment is available.

On admission to the hospice Sally is in the terminal phase of her illness. Using selective literature, I enhance and substantiate my intuitive awareness that many skills used in palliative care are not formally taught in nursing school but acquired during life experience and personal study. I aim to explore the depths and meaning of touch to gain insight into its therapeutic value. By reflecting on my thoughts, feelings, and reactions of the care I administer, I aim to gain insight to improve my nursing.

The evening reports continues – 'Her skin is burnt all over, each movement causes pain creating many difficulties with her care. She is having trouble coming to terms with her condition'

The words reverberate – perhaps it is us who is having the trouble. But I say nothing.

TABLE 20.1

Assignment Criteria for Reflective Narratives[ii]

	‰	Fail	Pass
		Increasing criticality and creativity ➔	
Insights (shown or told) are evidenced through reflection on significant experiences	20	Insights are not clear with inadequate evidence and analysis from reflected–on experiences to support claimed insights.	Insights are clearly evident with convincing analysed evidence from significant experiences.
Reflexive weaving of the narrative with a clear focus on its impact towards realising one's vision for practice.	20	The narrative has minimal reflexive flow with little sense of realising the practitioner's vision	The narrative has a convincing reflexive flow with clear focus on realising the practitioner's vision of practice
Critical dialogue with extant theoretical sources to develop, frame and deepen insights and knowing in practice.	20	Limited range of sources explored with weak dialogue to inform insights And develop knowing in practice.	A broad range of sources is evident with critical dialogue leading to compelling and creative insight development and knowing in practice.
Analysis of factors that emerged to either enhance or constrain realising anticipatory action	20	Little evidence of appre-ciating the impact of enhancing or constraining factors in shaping responses.	The significance of con-straining and enhancing factors in influencing clinical judgment and action is critically analysed.
The narrative is creative, engaging and coherent.	20	The narrative lacks coher-ence and creativity. Written expression makes arguments difficult to access. Lack of appropriate signpost-ing and planning. Careless referencing.	The narrative is engaging with clear structure and expression. Presentation is concise and creative. Arguments put forward succinctly. Accurate referencing
	100		

Module: Reflective Practice   [Code:] Name of student   first marker   second marker

My mind troubled, I leave the office and wander along the corridor, greeting patients and informing them that I am here tonight. A penetrating nauseous vapour fills the air leading towards an open door. Standing at the doorway my eyes transfix onto the small whispy figure covered only by a thin linen sheet. Her face, peaceful in sleep, disfigured by ferocious, sore red patches which connect and weave their way into every crease and feature of beauty. The main attack centres on her eyes producing a monstrous appearance of two cracked shivering starfish oozing from tenticles. Small mounds of decaying skin cling desperately all around her head reluctant to completely give up and let go. Goose pimples emerge on my arms; my body shudders coldly, ending the momentary glance.

On auto-pilot, I continue to the next room. Disgust and horror overwhelm my mind as I smile at the clean-shaven unblemished tanned face of the gentleman sitting comfortably reading. Conversation readily flows, we discuss the beautiful view from the window but my brain struggles to dismiss the suffering in the previous room.

Sally calls for assistance. She requests I cream a very sensitive sore area on her back. As my hand approaches an invisible layer of heat three inches from her body penetrates my skin. Like entering a hot oven, I carefully make contact with her slippery flesh. The cream dissolves into oil and trickles onto the sheets. With gentle circular movements, my fingers attempt to coat the raw burning tissues of Sally's back, lubricating the rippled surfaces. Feelings of sadness and hesitance are replaced by pleasurable sensations. The moist warmth infuses through the dryness of my hands creating suppleness and ease. In silence, I continue covering any area of need, enjoying the experience of Sally's relaxation radiating through my fingertips.

'That's wonderful: she whispers', 'Your not wearing gloves'.

Startled I question, 'Should I be?'

'Well I'm not contagious but everyone wears them because it's so revolting'.

Sally's reply is nonchalant.

Checking for approval, I ask, 'Would you prefer that I wear gloves?'

With eyes closed Sally relaxes, smiles and mouths, 'No, no it's lovely'.

Continuing our intimate interaction until the peacefulness of sleep encompasses Sally, I leave feeling enriched by this encounter.

Returning to the office, thoughts of gratitude swell my mind. How privileged I am to work in an environment that values and prioritises time with patients. Gone are the days when I was considered a time-waster! De Hennezel [6, p. 61] speaks to me

> 'How often are nurses rebuked for wasting time when they follow their heart's natural instinct and give a little of their simple presence to the sick'.

Even in a hospice I sense the underlying culture that we do things to people rather than essentially be with people.

As morning slowly emerges, I draw back the curtains enabling Sally to witness the beauty of the sunrise over the lake. She smiles whilst beckoning me to her, taking my arm she thanks me for last night. Our eyes meet as I reassure her that I also benefited by creaming my neglected hands.

Sally rushes into conversation about her history and prognosis. As if frightened that I might leave her, she holds my hand tight. With resentfulness she recounts her story, bewildered how or why she has to suffer such torment. Restrained by her grasp, I can only listen; no words are available to explain or bring comfort. Normal responses of stroking the hair or hugging are inappropriate due to causing excruciating pain. Motionless, I stand as the painful darts of information enter my heart and compassion is portrayed through facial expression and contact. Consumed into the depths of reality and truth, I feel Sally's pain opening, disturbing craters in my soul. My mind wanders to things I should put right and others that I want to do before I die [7]. Slowly an awareness of death is expressed [6] observed many times. Like panning for gold, I sieve through each word. Trickling down the mountains of despair is a tiny but clear meandering stream of hope and desire. The simplicity of Sally's needs brings tears to my eyes. Lowering my head, a spontaneous kiss reaches her erupting cheek; fragments of her scabby skin cohere to my lips but I only feel love. Sally mouths a return gesture, smiling we squeeze hands and disengage. 'See you later, I whisper leaving her space'. Sally nods closing her eyes.

Sally's history in report left me dumb struck. What could I say to her that would make a difference, alleviate anguish and help her find peace? As Autton [7, p. 121] agrees – 'In some circumstances words can be more of a hindrance than a help'. By using touch, I relayed my feelings to Sally [8]. I had the intention of achieving connection with Sally through physical contact. Sympathy and empathy can be exchanged by touch as Edwards [9, p. 801] citing Wyshncogrod) explains 'fellow feelings that you and I are one'. I wanted Sally to know I cared, to break down the barriers of being strangers and facilitate her journey of acceptance. Estabrooks and Morse [10] use the beautiful phrase 'bumping souls', which sums up what I wanted to achieve.

Sally and I 'tuned in' to each other through the caring touch [11]. I find amazing peace inside me that so much can be gained without the use of words!

Touch has been categorised as task-oriented, caring and protective [8, 11]. Task touch is the most commonly used by nurses and does not always have the intent to communicate in a positive manner. It can be defined by 'hurried, rough, jarred movements' relaying 'frustration, anger, or impatience' [11, p. 2]. I find this comment disturbing and not true in the hospice. Because of the horrific condition of Sally's skin, I was very wary of how I apply the cream. Taking time to register Sally's reaction to my contact and constantly reassessing our intention, I was able to ensure that we understood each other. To make the mistake of hurting Sally would create fear of me administering treatment and in turn cause anxiety instead of ease [12].

The disgust I felt on first seeing Sally produced intense guilt. The T-cell lymphoma had totally consumed her skin into a revolting, stinking mess. I suppose it would have been normal to reach for gloves. However, I felt they would create a barrier within the touching process, preventing skin to skin contact. I wanted to communicate my acceptance of Sally despite her disfigured body. Autton [7] describes how reassuring physical contact can be transferred by healing massage. Transmissions of pain and touch have joint nerve pathways [8]. The gentle movements of my fingers on Sally's back initiated relaxation and eventually sleep. What better way, during the night, can there be of dealing with personal mental trauma? So often, as hospice nurses, we turn to sedatives to induce sleep but I am learning that giving time to patients is more effective and rewarding. This can be demonstrated clearly in the way that Sally acted in the morning.

If I had created a barrier by wearing gloves, would Sally have received my message? No, I think it would have intensified her feelings of self-repulsion and ugliness. I didn't even consider using gloves. Sadly, when I tried to discuss this with my colleagues, they dismissed the idea and requested that we should all wear aprons as well to protect our clothes! My words fell on stony ground, as if I have touched something deeply threatening, they inherently recoiled from. When they look at Sally, do they only see disgust rather than this suffering woman? The disgust expressed by my colleagues disturbs me. It resonates with the idea of body work as dirty work – the body work behind the screens [13], with the need to protect self from both its physical and emotional impact. The apron protects not just the body but forms an emotional barrier, as if it is death itself touching them. If we choose to work in hospice then such attitude must be confronted, yet with compassion, understanding that this is not easy work. De Hennezel [6, p. 61] writes

> 'Many of the people I've met at the bedside of the dying feel themselves to be useless and ill at ease in this situation of just being there and not doing anything'.

'You might wonder where such attitudes stem from. We need to reorient our values to being with rather than doing to'.

Writing this reflective narrative has heightened my awareness of the physical and therapeutic areas of touch. Chang [14, p. 2] observes, 'touching is an integral part of human life'. Within the nursing environment using touch is a normal, frequent method of administering care both physically and psychologically. Nurses are also allowed to enter the private zones of the individual through intimate touch due to societal agreement [15]. However, consideration must always be given to ethnic background, personal history and social connotations to ensure that touch is appropriate and authentic [8]. Turton [16] reminds practitioners to be mindful of their use of touch and its therapeutic impact. Ochs [17] suggests that we should always ask permission before touching patients or family. I find it more agreeable to continually assess the person's reactions [8]. The meaning of touch is personal and can only be translated by the recipient [15].

Surprisingly, Estabrooks and Morse [10] note, 'One of the most neglected areas of touch in nursing research is the investigation of the touching behaviours of nurses'. These authors suggest that nurses develop their own touching style through individual life experience and training. It is a comfort to know that touching can be a learned behaviour, especially when observing those who appear to have a comfortable natural ability of its proper use.

Environment

Slowly washing my hands in the cream enamel basin, my eyes wander around Sally's room through the mirror above the sink. Wilting, shrivelled stems interspersed by youthful blooms hang from vases. Stagnating in discoloured water, they silently scream for attention. Twisted chocolate wrappers hide between magazines haphazardly balanced on the bedside table. Walkman cables, compact discs and tubes of cream create a 'modern' work of art. 'Get well' cards lie abandoned, children's drawings huddle in a corner and photos of loved ones faces face the window.

An unintentional arena of chaos faces me as I turn around, feelings of claustrophobia creep inside my body. I need some space. Each item of furniture is overburdened with unnecessary clutter. The floor extends storage pads and dressings, red 'infected' linen bags openly display their contents.

Reaching for a paper towel, I dry my hands carefully ensuring that nothing is knocked from the nearby shelf. Gadgets of hygiene engulf the small wash area whilst the sad magnolia walls absorb the atmosphere of dull isolation and neglect. Sally is asleep so I tiptoe away.

Standing outside the hospice a refreshing night breeze hits my skin. A stabbing tightness tightens my chest, Sally finds even ripples of air painful on her burning flesh. She is cocooned in the moist foul smelling warmth of her room. Aromas of freshly mown grass fill my nostrils but Sally's sense of smell has become numbed by continuous stench. Confined to her bed through weakness but craving independence, she is rendered helpless in personally changing her surroundings. I wonder how she would arrange things if able?

Entering the main entrance, a beautiful arrangement of fresh flowers adorn the foyer. 'Welcome' signs invite my arrival and homely décor instils comfort. Windows proudly display wonderful views of nature, a lake, gardens, wildlife and an abundance of glorious, towering protective trees. The corridor turns revealing a quiet area of cosiness to relax, chat with family or befriend other patients. Visually nothing to fear is apparent except the word 'hospice' all around the building!

An intoxicating fetid odour invisibly digests the air, as I get closer to Sally's room. 'Can't sleep' she whispers as I move blankets and clothes by her bedside. 'Can I tidy your room?' slips from my mouth. Sally giggles 'Where will you start?'

Mesmerised by activity Sally remains quiet. Within half an hour her environment evokes order, cleanliness and thoughtful comfort. Nursing supplies are secretly hidden in cupboards. Smeared surfaces now shine with approval. Photos smile at Sally from wardrobe doors and cards hang appreciably overhead displaying their messages of comfort. Wiping tears of joy from Sally's eyes I ask if the room is to her liking, nodding contentedly Sally pours into conversation centred on memorabilia. Time rushes by, twilight creeps across the sky bringing a new day. Exhausted Sally drifts leisurely into the land of dreams.

How many times do I ignore the irritating untidiness of patient's rooms? Actually, the answer is never. Mess constantly annoys me but I don't always clean it up! Neither do I consistently take time to consider how patient feels about their surroundings.

Sally craved her independence but it had been snatched from her. She would have loved to keep her room tidy, bright and cheerful. Her pleasure when seeing her room tidy and family photos smiling at her confirmed it. Yet why had we allowed her room to get in such a mess? It suggests we do not pay much attention to the impact of the environment on her wellbeing. Florence Nightingale turns in her grave.

Sally is vulnerable and silent. The intra-subjective world of the patient is discussed by Sumner [18] who claims the patient becomes vulnerable, in need of help due to illness.

Summer states – 'the patient comes to the illness-induced interaction hopeful that this exquisite vulnerability will be acknowledged' [p. 4]. Hope that this will happen comes from 'a yearning for a recognition or consideration by others of unmet needs' [p. 4]. Morse and Dobernect [19] mention the determination of the patient to endure the unpleasant 'side effects' of illness, in this case the mess in her room. I felt she had lost something of her identity in the mess and that she had become part of the mess.

Loss is described by Robinson and McKenna [20, p. 7] as having three attributes:

- Loss signifies that someone or something one has had or ought to have had in the future, has been taken away.
- That which is taken away must have been valued by then person experiencing the loss.
- The meaning of loss is determined individually, subjectively and contextually by the person experiencing it.

Each point is salient regards Sally. A sense of guilt burdens me that we had let her room get into such a mess. Chris challenges me in the group 'How do I ensure that all staff respect the patient's environment?' 'Can I be influential in changing attitudes?' I like to think so, but I already have a reputation for complaining about care issues. People tend to agree with me but nothing gets changed as if the place is infected with inertia. A focus for future experiences, that is if I persist with reflection after the course is completed. The value of reflection is to lift these things into consciousness, things we take for granted or get complacent about, but then we also get complacent about reflection. We need to establish a regular reflection group at the hospice where such issues can be aired openly and acted upon.

The daily nursing rituals of ward rounds, checking that everything is 'ship-shape' has long gone [21]. In an investigation by Rogers et al. [22] on the sources of dissatisfaction with hospital care, the environment comes right at the bottom of the list! This research included 229 people but only 6 complained about untidiness, or dirty bathrooms. Am I to believe that hospitals and hospices are very tidy, clean places? Unfortunately, we nearly all have personal stories to tell, or have heard disturbing reports to the contrary. Is it good that people are so grateful of our care that they feel unable to express their concerns? Sometimes I feel that in nursing we have gone from one extreme to another. For example, identifying the task of cleaning to a particular person usually, in my opinion, gets the job done, whereas relying on individual commitment unfortunately often doesn't! This is a good example of why the stench from Sally's room had not been dealt with. Everyone had to be aware of its existence, with the exception of Sally, but nobody took responsibility to act.

The sense of smell is the most immediate of our senses due to the olfactory nerve being directly connected to the brain [23]. Smell is also the most fleeting of the senses, fading occurs when one is exposed to a smell for a long time [23, p. 279]. Sally sadly had become a victim of this. I know that Bergamot is one of the most effective deodorising oils [23] so why didn't I take the time to discover this oil and use it? Davis [23, p. 57] also informs that Bergamot is an 'uplifting' oil producing a relaxing atmosphere for the anxious, depressed person. Although Sally had lost her sense of smell, she still could have absorbed the oil into her bloodstream through inhalation via the lungs [23, p. 281]. Music can be used to improve the nursing environment and has been demonstrated to decrease pain, reduce anxiety and promote relaxation [24]. Sally obviously appreciated music, a walkman and compact discs were in her room. Given the potential effectiveness of this non-invasive pleasure, 'it should be offered to all hospital patients in all situations that are known to be stressful. Music improves the mood of patients and may reduce the need for sedatives' [25, p. 9].

My mind fills with a picture of Sally's room. The light is dimmed, Bergamot penetrates the air and soft sounds ripple in the background. Serenity. How easy it is to produce a peaceful haven. So why didn't I achieve this for Sally?

The environment has an enormous impact on both patients and their families. Wuest [26] argues that a broader conceptualisation of environment needs to become a focus for nursing action. I second that!

Commentary

Weaving her reflexive narrative enabled Jill to express herself in a meaningful and creative way. It was a way of finding herself, of bringing the threads of her experiences and insights. Undoubtedly, such writing will have a profound impact on readers and prompts reflection on the readers' own practice especially concerning controversial issues such as wearing gloves, intimacy and attitude of her colleagues. As Jill noted 'Using selective literature, I enhance and substantiate my intuitive awareness that many skills used in palliative care are not formally taught in nursing school but acquired during life experience and personal study'.

In my feedback, I pointed Jill towards Frank's [27] work on remoralisation, as I sensed that Jill's practice with Sally was an act of re-moralisation for both Sally and herself. In guided reflection Jill was challenged whether she could take action with her colleagues as a consequence of these experiences. She was uncertain saying 'I like to think so, but I already have a reputation for complaining about care issues. People tend to agree with me but nothing gets changed as if the place is infected with inertia'.

Such is the power of this narrative that it became a focus for teaching on subsequent programmes, lifting the ineffable into something tangible.

Activity

- Use the grading grid to grade Jill's work at level 3 degree standard.
- What feedback would you give Jill to justify the grade and your own ideas about how her insights could have been developed?
- Consider what insights you gain from engaging with Jill's work?
- Contrast the grading grid with any grading grid you currently use within your practice and reflect on the differences.
- Reconstruct the grading criteria to reflect what you consider would be most appropriate for grading reflective assignments?
- Reflect again on the dichotomy between a technical rational and professional artistry approach and how each perspective might frame reflective grading differently.
- Ask yourself and your colleagues – Do we need grading criteria? What would be the academic fallout of scrapping them?

References

1. Sparkes, A. (2002) Autoethnography: self-indulgence of something more? In A. Bochner, C. Ellis [Eds.] *Ethnographically Speaking*. AltaMira, Walnut Creek, 209–232.

2. Garrett, D., Hodkinson, P. (1998) Can there be criteria for selecting research criteria? A hermeneutical analysis of an inescapable dilemma. *Qualitative Inquiry* 4, 515–539.

3. Smith, J. (1993) *After the Demise of Empiricism: The Problem of Judging Social and Educational Inquiry*. Ablex Publishing, Noewoord, NJ.

4. Richardson, L (2000) Evaluating ethnography. *Qualitative Inquiry* 6(2), 253–255.

5. Hooks, B. (2003) *Teaching Community: A Pedagogy of Hope*. Routledge, New York.

6. De Hennezel, M. (1998) *Intimate Death* [Trans C. Janeway]. Warner Books, London.

7. Autton, N. (1996) The use of touch in palliative care. *European Journal of Palliative Care* 3(3), 121–124.

8. Talton, C. (1995) Complementary therapies: touch-of-all-kinds is therapeutic. *RN* 58(2), 61–64.

9. Edwards, S. (1998) An anthropological interpretation of nurses' and patients' perceptions of the use of space and touch. *Journal of Advanced Nursing* 28, 809–817.

10. Estabrooks, C., Morse, J. (1992) Toward a theory of touch: the touching process and acquiring a touching style. *Journal of Advanced Nursing* 17, 448–456.

11. Fredriksson, L. (1999) Modes of relating in a caring conversation: a research synthesis on presence, touch and listening. *Journal of Advanced Nursing* 30(5), 1167–1176.

12. Davidhizar, R., Giger, J. (1997) When touch is not the best approach. *Journal of Clinical Nursing* 6(3), 203–206.

13. Lawler, J. (1991) *Behind the Scenes: Nursing, Somology and the Problems of the Body*. Churchill Livingstone, Melbourne.

14. Chang, O. S. (2001) The conceptual structure of physical touch in caring. *Journal of Advanced Nursing* 33(6), 820–827.

15. Hickman, P., Holmes, C. (1994) Nursing the postmodern body: a touching case. *Nursing Inquiry* 1, 3–14.

16. Turton, P. (1989) Touch me, feel me, heal me. *Nursing Times* 85(19), 42–44.

17. Ochs, L. (2001) The nurse suggests asking before you touch. *RN* 64(4), 10.

18. Sumner, J. (2001) Caring in nursing: a different interpretation. *Journal of Advanced Nursing* 35, 926–932.

19. Morse, J., Doberneck, B. (1995) Delineating the concept of hope. *Image: Journal of Nursing Scholarship* 27, 277–285.

20. Robinson, D., Mckenna, H. (1998) Loss: an analysis of a concept of particular interest to nursing. *Journal of Advanced Nursing* 27(4), 779–784.

21. Biley, F., Wright, S. (1997) Towards a defence of nursing routine and ritual. *Journal of Clinical Nursing* 6(2), 115–119.

22. Rogers, A., Karlsne, S., Addington-Hall, J. (2000) All the services were excellent. It is when the human element comes in that things go wrong': dissatisfaction with hospital care in the last year of life. *Journal of Advanced Nursing* 31, 768–774.

23. Davis, P. (2000) *Aromatherapy A-Z*. C.W. Daniel & Co., Saffron Walden.

24. McCaffrey, R. (2002) Music listening as a nursing intervention: a symphony of practice. *Holistic Nursing Practice* 16(3), 70–77.

25. Evans, D. (2002) The effectiveness of music as an intervention for hospital patients: a systematic review. *Journal of Advanced Nursing* 37(1), 8–18.

26. Wuest, J. (1997) Illuminating environmental influences on women's caring. *Journal of Advanced Nursing* 26(1), 49–58.

27. Frank, A. (2002) Relations of caring: demoralization and remoralization in the clinic. *International Journal of Human Caring* 6(2), 13–19.

28. Kearney, M. (2008) *A Place of Healing: Working with Suffering and Dying*. Oxford University Press, Oxford.

Notes

i. The idea of 'places of healing' reflects the influence of Michael Kearney's 'A place of healing' [28] used as a seminal idea within the holistic module.

ii. The grading grid has been adapted from the bespoke grading grade I constructed for the Osteopathy Professional Doctorate. The original is shown as Table 11.2. The adaption reflects how all such reflective tools are continuously scrutinised for their efficacy to reflect the essential nature of reflection through representation as a reflexive narrative.

PART 3

Student Narratives

Students wrote these narratives on various academic courses. They offer:

1. Exemplars of constructed and creative reflexive narratives.
2. Evidence of the efficacy of guided reflection towards guiding students to realise their visions of practice, notably person-centred practice. In doing so, the narratives reveal the nature of person-centred practice and barriers to its realisation.

CHAPTER 21

Awakenings: Guided Reflection as 'Reality Shock'

Introduction

Without doubt, many practitioners suffer various degrees of burnout resulting in fatigue, low morale, stress, anxiety, disillusionment or whatever adjective fits the bill. Burnout is a state of physical, mental and emotional exhaustion. It can occur when you experience long-term stress and feel under constant pressure[i]. One cause is 'reality shock', especially those new to the profession where expectations do not match with reality creating dissonance [1]. In the following narrative 'Awakenings', Aileen reveals how guided reflection enabled her to reveal her reality shock and burnout and begin to understand and resolve it.

'Awakenings' is constructed from an amalgam of her three assignments whilst undertaking the becoming a reflective and effective practitioner course.[ii]

Awakenings

The First Assignment

People live in crises that ripples across their beings below the surface of conscious thought. These ripples can be observed by paying attention to the signs, yet most people live in a state of partial visibility, as if wrapped up in themselves to keep the tension from exploding. Reflection is my trigger to release this tension. Johns and Freshwater [2, p. x] state that reflection 'gives us wings to soar as we emerge from our cocoons'. I certainly feel that I am at that stage. I sense reflection is my opportunity, that window which Johns [3, p. 9] describes as 'a window to look inside, to know who I am as I strive towards understanding and realising the meaning of desirable work in my everyday practice'. I am beginning to associate reflection as permission to break from 'performing' to consider the 'performance' and the need to plan future 'performances'.

After our first guided reflection session, I wrote in my journal

> I sat in a room full of strangers stating I had left nursing in the '70s because I didn't like it. With that came the realization that after all the studying, all the work, I still felt the same way! It washed over me, a strange experience, a flooding sensation from foot to finger tips. Physical and deeply emotional. I tried to explain in a later session of clinical supervision with my ward manager ... 'but you're a good nurse Aileen, very professional, everyone says so, etc'.

... Yes, but it is the professionalism in the armour I use to keep myself together through a multitude of experiences I find exhausting, stressful, distasteful and frustrating. Nursing is far from my expectation, my personal practice is not what I want, it is confined by so many limitations. All my idealism forced to the recesses of my mind, never perhaps to be realised. I have always had the capacity to marginalise myself, never good at conforming to satisfy others. What am I now doing? More studying. Why? Will this provide some key to unlock disappointment, or will it be a balm to bring about acceptance of what is, and where I'm at?

Reflection so far seems to raise more questions, but can I answer some? I am unable to separate myself from my practice. So much of nursing is personal, the professional may separate the personal side, but the personal fragility provides much of the human touch. There is not much opportunity to personalise the rigid routines of the ward routine. Much verbal encouragement is given, but little happens. The routine continues, the relentless routine. Probably there is safety in the routine, and a workforce of long serving nursing assistants who pride themselves on maintaining the routine, continue the past and reduce the future; although I work with people who would reshape what we do. I need to reshape what I do, because it swallows me like a whale. This all seems negative, but I feel more positive in expressing my doubts. I am aware of my feelings within myself daily. I am not complacent about the issues that affect my feelings about my job, but maybe I am worn down.

This reflection was much needed cathartic therapy. Heron [4] felt catharsis enabled the dissolving of scars from emotional vulnerability. Valentine [5] said that nurses and women were nurturing, caring, loving kinds of people – the antithesis of confrontation. This does not allow for the integration of assertiveness as a personal trait. I believe that many women like myself are skilled at being assertive but consciously choose to use alternative traits to deal with certain issues to reduce exposure to vulnerability. By this I mean I can reflect on several ways of dealing with my dislike of my current situation, but know that I will not act alone, or completely independently, choosing just for myself, since the consequences affect far more people than myself. Bendelow [6] found that by avoiding conflict, it is turned inwards and experienced as stress, a feeling I relate to, knowing that stress and frustration are constantly with me at work.

My reflective account shows a lack of energy throughout. Peers (from the group) described feelings of sadness, hopelessness and profoundness. I also revealed some of myself and the conflict I felt within, to weigh what I would like to change personally against the reality of what I work with daily. I felt that this group of people saw me then as helpless and hopeless. Yet this is wrong! People who know me well would laugh at that suggestion. Yet honesty causes me to acknowledge my restrictive upbringing, strong on conforming (though I do not always do this), doing what is right, not challenging, with little meaningful communication. All this leads me to feel I have long fought to be different and yet fundamentally remain the same.

Graham [7] talks about a sense of humanness and personal identity belonging to the patient. I would argue that the nurse too, has the right of personal identity, especially during reflection and essentially during practice. Social groups (such as our reflective group) are very important in maintaining a sense of humanness. I think this ties in well with the fragility I talked about. I know I am fragile; that makes me sensitive to myself and others. Humanness allows us to remember that fragility is part of being human.

The Second Assignment

It occurs to me that at the point of narrating my journal, I had viewed my professional manner as armour to hold myself together, but with reflection I review my original feelings and now wonder if this was a valuable tool to prove to others my sense of capability, sense of responsibility, etc. With the unfolding of my reflection, I begin to see how my notes illuminate and transmit meaning to theory. My personal learning curve is increasing as I start to see beyond myself and understand liberating the tight rein on my emotions. Clearly I am incongruent with my beliefs and have been guilty of holding back, to my own cost. Although I hold strong beliefs related to equality of opportunity, personal rights, etc. I was submissive in order to conform and be accepted. This perception, I now feel is distorted and I struggle to make sense of my feelings. Miller [8] cited in Oakley [9] identified characteristics that develop from belonging to a dominant or subordinate group, which helps me underpin my difficulty in changing my situation while nurses continue in the subordinate group of submissiveness, and the culture in my own environment is managed, based on submissiveness and ever coping!

My recent experience would have been less stressful had I been myself from the onset and unafraid, but I was brought up to practise self-sacrifice – 'You can't always have what you want', and I have transferred my upbringing to my career, fearing I could not make wrong right and I should sacrifice my own values to be employed. There is now within my recognition to change. I have highlighted fundamental problems and surfaced my tension. I can see how important my need to bring to the surface the underlying value systems from my past which are valued as crucially important to change. Johns [3] was so right about being unable to cleanse ourselves from our histories.

In my reflective group, I am the junior grade. I remind myself that I am merely an E grade, especially when I listen to reflections from others that highlight attempts for managerial grades to rule over others with patriarchal supremacy. I believe Newman [10] when she says that who people are can be read as a pattern rippling across the surface of their being, and just as I read my own ripple (guided by my supervisor), I can read those patterns in my group, and I vary in response. I am ambivalent, frightened and bloody-minded all at once in sharing my thoughts with theirs. I feel I began as a qualified nurse after a difficult training period, where there were definite attempts by the college to make life more difficult when I 'fought' them on several issues that I felt strongly affected my values. In this way, I felt first hand their power over me and the effect it wielded over my future. I currently reflect on whether that experience so affected me that I lost my autonomy to express my opinion without fear of punishment. This view has been further supported by experience within the team I work. The reality of the situation means I must work with 'what is', yet I carry some bitterness, a useless emotion, which always adds to life's path and saps my energy to grow. Yet I can sense some fluttering within me to grow, and this may encourage me to seek a new job in due course. I can relate to Moira's experience (in the group) and feel in her story my own.

When I shared my reflection within the group, I was offered the visual image of a jungle: to cut space in the undergrowth using a machete or to sit in the trees dropping anger into the space below. I am amazed at how effective this visualisation has been. I have developed my own pattern of dropping coconuts on people I feel anger towards. It is surprising how many coconuts I have dropped! This has made me aware that I do hold on to anger, not only towards myself but also towards others, especially those I cherish and value. I think I am very self-critical and know I can be caustic and hostile and so have avoided confrontation. I need to 'prick the bubble' in order to let go the anger I hold onto.

I can see that the questions will continue in my reflection because, although one can consider the contradictions and debate ways forward, there is then the need to make choices. I stand in front of a bridge I must cross. That is, making the choice. For me, I think it is essential that I make the correct one, as my personal well-being will depend on it. It seems I must repair some confidence along the way.

Johns [11] asserts that reflective practitioners interpret extant knowledge for its relevance to their practice. Watson [12] states that it is necessary to use theory as a lens for reflective seeing to help bring the mountain and the marsh together; the mountain being Schön's [13] hard high ground of technical rationality, whereas the marsh is Schön's enduring metaphor for the messy indeterminate nature of professional practice. I feel I have inhabited the depths of the marsh but can now see and find meaning in the mountains and their relationship with the marsh in the wider landscape. In realising this, I understand more of how my feelings impact so strongly on my practice. However, this is not an automatic process. Rather, it is an extremely complicated one, a long therapeutic journey where I will look back on this analysis as crude and unskilled as I become more proficient. I have acknowledged my own discomfort but also surfaced some strengths in my abilities. I have shown a pattern in my life. There is much truth that learning through experience is arduous work [11].

The Third Assignment

I pick up my journey some four months later. My group guide commented on his awareness of my tentative steps in becoming more positive and affirmative of myself both as a person and as a practitioner. This feels true. I am aware of subtle and real changes taking place. One major change has been the acquisition of a new role with promotion. This was a result of realising the tension and frustration in my previous role where I was unable to meet my practice potential or any personal satisfaction. Guided reflection has given me the opportunity to allow myself time and space to 'spring clean' emotions long held onto, deep within emotional depths. The theme of these emotions has been ever present in my reflections. Now my reflective practice feels like a new dawn, a new horizon of opportunity towards realising my therapeutic potential.

I return to Johns' comment [2] that reflection gives us wings to soar, as we emerge from our cocoons but that this was balanced alongside many arduous years of being many things to many people where I arrived exhausted from the emotional labour of dealing with other peoples' feelings and regulating my own emotions James [14]. Over time I have been able to create the time and space to recover from emotional entanglement, having come to recognise that nursing is almost parasitic in the way it takes psychological reservoirs of one's personality and that one needs a strong sense of self to recharge our batteries. When evaluating emotional work, what we say depends on who we are talking to, what shared knowledge may be assumed and what kinds of reaction are anticipated [15]. My own emotional work has been influenced by many complicated personal and practice events. Initially, as a newly qualified nurse, I found the stress of coping with adults attempting such behaviours as self-mutilation and suicide draining and isolating since there was little opportunity to explore feeling, especially in a unit where such behaviours were an almost daily occurrence. One positive aspect of listening to others' reflecting is to realise my stresses are shared by others. At the same time, I was nursing my mother who died of cancer, my son left home to go to the university, and I changed jobs and my batteries went flat. Emotions are fruitfully seen as embodied existential modes of being. Work commitments and a busy lifestyle contributed to me carrying them as baggage – picking them up and dumping them at as time allowed, but not exploring them, letting them go or renewing them. Work spent considering this now is charging my batteries. I have come to recognise how dangerous my lack of self-interest in sorting them may have been, and if I am honest, I can see how I reduced myself as a practitioner by capping my true feelings as this extract from my journal illustrates:

> 'Don't hold my hand, please don't hold my hand, I cannot hold yours. You are dying and you know it. I know it too – I see it in your eyes. I know you are frightened. Your fear is not within the layers where most people hold onto theirs, when they are not well. No, it is on the surface, covering you. It is beyond your skin all around you in the room. I feel it. I know it and I must cope with it. I do everything to make Margaret comfortable. The position, the pillows, the light, the warmth. All are considered. A sip of water, a fumble with the charts, take the blood pressure, keep the oxygen

nearby. Soothe the relatives, say the right things. Are you watching me? I'm good, you can tell I've done this before. They think I'm an expert and unaffected. There are no experts in this and the effects mix with my own bereavement.

Her hand is so fragile, small and like a bird's shaking as life flows away. How large my hand seems. Ugly next to Margaret's. Every time I approach the bed she tries to grab my hand – she is seeking reassurance. I know I must hold her hand and show reassurance in my eyes. I say something soothing but I am not there. I think now as I write all the hands I've held and wonder if anyone will be there to hold mine. When you think about how many people we love in our lives that hold onto our hands, parent, partners, children, no wonder Margaret wants hers held now as she dies'.

As a nurse, I have held many people's hands during times of pain and stress. It is never easy to do. To me it connects you so physically with them. I think I am exposing more of my shadow self but I am cautious since there isn't enough guided reflection space to deal with it all, and like others, this year I worry about the impact of coping with newly surfaced emotions. Zerwekh [16] wrote that it is always a turning point when nurses can find and celebrate humanity and competence that at first may be hidden by suffering and degradation. She says nurses search for ways to validate people who have lost faith in themselves or who no longer believe in their own power. I'm searching in my practice for their humanity and mine. If I must find it to be considered an effective practitioner, I may fail, but if I work amongst people who can see how elusive this achievement is, I can relax in being human and frail ... my recurring theme. Possibly I am becoming a more effective practitioner because I accept fragility. I have learnt that while I can create a therapeutic environment for others to release their emotions, I am not a machine and must therefore find appropriate expressions of my own in order to be available to others. I use the being available template as a mirror to see myself[iii]. Do I like the reflection? I like it more. I recognise now that I am very strong and have coped with much, and those aspects of me that show fragility are warm, human and okay. Life experiences force me to be more honest about who I am and what and why I contribute to others as I do. Having previously looked in some depth at the gender issues and prevailing attitudes between doctors and nurses, I concur there is a definite set of constraints as to what nurses are able to do for patients and for themselves.

It seems realistic to say that some of my reflections have been painful, and I have had to think about managing myself during reflection. If I am hard on myself does that follow I am hard on my patients? I have discussed being less hard on myself and know that the kindness I extend to others can be extended within, but the barrier is not altogether down. Chapman [17] concluded from Menzies-Lyth's work [18] on the ritualistic practices utilised by nurses to protect themselves from anxiety, that individual behaviour attempts to defend one from the primitive anxieties evoked by death, dirty tasks and intimacy are simply avoiding the real issue that causes the anxiety. I have found myself attempting the protection, yet overtly steering myself from ritualistic practice in the hope of achieving more holistic care; being much more comfortable with a strong belief that patients are people with minds and soul and feelings, and not object bodies given up by medical domination.

My reflection on my experience with Margaret shows the tension between my performance to respond to her need as I interpreted it, and the deeper levels of myself that constrained me. Cultural patterns of avoidance, the forbidden topic of death, govern interactions around dying patients in hospitals [19]. This surely contributes little support for the nurse who cares for these patients, attempting somehow to support patients, relatives and others, whilst managing their own emotions throughout. Fortunately, I find myself thinking about many issues in a different way, attempting to step free of ingrained cultural and socialisation limitations. Now I am beginning to see how restricted I have been.

Watson [12] said that reflective caring practice helps us to stop and think, to pause in the midst of action. I have certainly done much of that. Watson felt this resulted in us being more aware, more mindful, authentically present, allowing a re-direction. She likened it to being a simple shifting of one's consciousness from being harried, hurried or rushed, to being still, to finding one's quiet centre. When I think of this I am inspired to be calm yet the days are often so hectic. I was known to those who knew me well that I want peace in my life, but the reflection I have laboured at this year makes me think that the peace I seek is here in the quiet centre of myself; and if I had the courage to exorcise my shadow self I would find more peace. In response, my guide said 'the shadow self does not need exorcising, it needs embracing because it tells us important things about ourselves'. Through reflection, I come to acknowledge and value my shadow self and integrating it within. Perhaps on this level, we most need the challenge and support of guidance.

During my first assignment, I realised I was at a bridge that I must cross successfully to maintain my own mental health. Now I view myself crossing that bridge reflecting on Johns' words [2, p. ix] 'assure your bridge is strong with a well defined plan'. Truthful reflection (or in other words that I am deluding myself) has helped me focus on my plan and I begin to see what the future could hold, and more importantly, there is now a time for me to be kinder to myself.

I have changed my job. I was not prepared to continue in a restrictive routine that didn't recognise individual patients' needs. I reflect on how guided reflection has cared for me and how that caring is about enabling the other to grow [20]. I've grown by becoming more self-determining, by choosing my own values and ideals, grounded in my own experience. This shows a personal right (and insight) to become whole (if that is fully achievable). It fills me with confidence that the person I am, while unique and independent, is okay and that I now feel less isolated from other practitioners, which shows progress since I previously commented on feelings of isolation.

In the group, I have explored relationships amongst work colleagues and have come to a better understanding how affected my well-being. I was seen as a confidant and lent on for support, yet needed much support myself, more than I had realised and would admit openly. I was seen as capable, yet often questioned that of myself, feeling that my integrity and logic opposed others. While I am guilty of using others in the workplace, I too have been used and exploited by friends and superiors. Even when such exploitation was overt I tolerated it, but les so now. I/we must find better ways of supporting each other [21].

I wrote in my journal –

> 'That my time on the Unit has been fraught with frustration and I have seen myself wanting to be more involved, often part of a routine I disliked, of events that I wanted to challenge and part of a team whose support varied …. Yet again nothing is certain, I cannot be sure my choice of job will be better. I often ask myself why do I put myself through so much'.

Already I see events repeating themselves, yet I do see them and work towards responding differently even as the less than welcoming reception has left me guarded and confused, wondering at the psychological cost. My sensitivity is re-emerging, depleting my batteries yet again, and yet the opportunity to reshape something is not lost on me, and I am able to utilise new reflective coping strategies, ensuring not to absorb too much. Let them keep their prejudices and problems that are not mine. Reflection has equipped me with so many intrapersonal and interpersonal skills, but it is written here for the reader to see that there is a great turmoil between what I am and what I do.

> It's not that I am black and blue
> Nor any shade that's blurred from view
> Its just that when I want to care
> to show for you that I am there
> The nurse that I am just doesn't dare

But there is a new and changing me
a person grown who now can see
the callous cruelty of what was done
the right to care, but live, have fun
and in doing that change the job for which I trained
so there's more of me and less that's drained.
I'm not where I want to be
I want more, I want to be free
to give to others better choice to start
to practice life and work from the heart
a sense of self in all they do
that's not dependent on hierarchy such as you!

The ghosts I have carried from my experience as a student nurse are not laid to rest. I am trying, but they are still not exorcised. The poem reflects my hope that nurses will drop this need for devotion and sacrifice and come to understand that the best ones have a right to life as well. The final verse reflects my fervent wish to have a role in shaping the experience of beginning nurses so that ultimately more will be able to challenge the hierarchical structures and professional dominance that have restricted me and no doubt countless others from realising our therapeutic potential and destiny. Then the mountain and the marsh may well come together.

Commentary

The narrative is an ontological quest for Aileen to find and renew herself. There is a tremendous sense of pathos in this narrative that I am certain many practitioners can relate to but have never expressed. Guided reflection opened a space for Aileen to release her feelings. What spilled out was a confessional of a self that had become constrained, conditioned, conformed, afraid, exhausted, frustrated, helpless and drained of energy. As she describes it, 'my batteries had gone flat'. She illustrates how reflection was a path back to herself, unravelling herself from the binds that constrained her and what she valued. It gave her power to recharge her batteries. Guided reflection was a cathartic and therapeutic experience. It shows just how battered practitioners can become working in routinised and unsupportive environments that lose sight of the human factor. Aileen noted within her guided reflection group that 'one positive aspect of listening to others reflecting is to realise my stresses are shared by others'. By revealing such deep issues, it gave permission for her peers to reveal theirs, where perhaps before they slid along the surface of experience rather than penetrate its depths. Of course, many practitioners do cope as best they can and become conditioned as survival. But some, like Aileen, rail against it at such cost.

Aileen finds her voice that sheds light on her shadow, a voice accepted and nurtured through guidance and which connected her to her authentic self. She was able to find meaning in her experience of 'reality shock' whereby recovery and resolution became possible where possibilities for the future emerged [16], a turning point where she could find and celebrate her humanity and competence that was hidden under layers of her by suffering and degradation [13]. Guides cannot prescribe what the practitioner chooses to reveal. Neither can the guide set out a therapeutic stall about what is acceptable to share. The guide and practitioner work with 'what is'. In Aileen's experience, the guide holds her hand, despite Aileen's resistance to having her hand held either literally or metaphorically, to help her pull herself out of the swamp. Guided reflection doesn't set out to rescue her but to enable her to rescue herself. The swamp doesn't disappear but it can be viewed differently so practitioners can discover a more positive way to practice in it. Belenky et al. [22] considered that women need to be reconnected to communities of caring such as Aileen's guided reflection group. Aileen did have clinical supervision with her ward manager where she tried to reveal her predicament only to be told – 'but you're a good nurse Aileen, very professional, everyone says so, etc'. The ward manager saw only what was on the surface not the turmoil lying beneath.

Reality shock can be mitigated within the reflective curriculum (Chapter 14) whereby students graduate with understanding of the contradictions between reality and vision.

References

1. Kramer, M. (1974) *Reality Shock; Why Nurses Leave Nursing*. Mosby, St Louis.

2. Johns, C. (1998) Preface. In C. Johns, D. Freshwater [Eds.] *Transforming Nursing Through Reflective Practice*. Blackwell Science, Oxford, 1–20.

3. Johns, C. (1988) Opening the doors of perception. In C. Johns, D. Freshwater [Eds.] *Transforming Nursing Through Reflective Practice*. Blackwell Science, Oxford, 1–20.

4. Heron, J. (1975) *Six-category Intervention Analysis*. Human Potential Research Project. University of Surrey.

5. Valentine, P. (1995) Management of conflict: do nurses/ women handle it differently. *Journal of Advanced Nursing* 22, 142–149.

6. Bendelow, M. (1983) *Managerial Women's Approaches to Organizational Conflict: A Qualitative Study*. Unpublished Doctoral Dissertation. University of Colorado, Denver.

7. Graham, I. (1998) Understanding the nature of nursing through reflection. In C. Johns, D. Freshwater [Eds.] *Transforming Nursing Through Reflective Practice*. Blackwell Science, Oxford, 119–133.

8. Miller, J. (1977) *Towards A New Psychology of Women*. Beacon Press, Boston.

9. Oakley, A. (1984) The importance of being a nurse. *Nursing Times* 83, 24–27.

10. Newman, M. (1994) *Health as Expanded Consciousness*. National League of Nursing, New York.

11. Johns, C. (1995) Time to care? Time for reflection. *International Journal of Nursing Practice* 24, 1135–1143.

12. Watson, J. (1998) A meta-reflection on reflective practice and caring theory. In C. Johns, D. Freshwater [Eds.] *Transforming Nursing Through Reflective Practice*. Blackwell Science, Oxford, 214–220.

13. Schön, D. (1987) *Educating the Reflective Practitioner*. Jossey-Bass, San Francisco.

14. James, N. (1989) Emotional labour; skill and work in the social regulation of feelings. *The Sociological Review* 37, 15–42.

15. Frith, H., Kitzinger, C. (1988) 'Emotional work' as a participant recourse: a feminine analysis of young women's talk in-interaction. *Sociology* 32, 299–320.

16. Zerwekh, J. (1995) A family caregiving model for hospice nursing. *The Hospice Journal* 10, 27–44.

17. Chapman, G. (1983) Ritual and rational action in hospitals. *Journal of Advanced Nursing* 8, 13–20.

18. Menzies-Lyth, I. (1988) A case study in the functioning of social systems as a defence against anxiety. In: *Containing Anxiety in Institutions: Selected Essays*. Free Association Books, London. 43–85.

19. Glasser, B., Strauss, A. (1965) *Awareness of Dying*. Aldine, Chicago.

20. Mayeroff, M. (1971) *On Caring*. Harper, New York.

21. Johns, C. (1992) Ownership and the harmonious team; barriers to developing the therapeutic team in primary nursing. *Journal of Clinical Nursing* 1, 89–94.

22. Belenky, M. F., Clinchy, B. M., Goldberger, N. R., Tarule, J. M. (1986) *Women's Ways of Knowing: The Development of Self, Voice, and Mind*. Basic Books, New York.

Notes

i. https://mentalhealth-uk.org/burnout/.

ii. This course is set out in Chapter 14.

iii. See Figure 5.3.

CHAPTER 22

Voice as a Metaphor for Transformation

Introduction

Helen is a staff nurse working in an adolescent orthopaedic unit. She is a student on the 'Becoming a reflective and effective practitioner' programme (see Chapter 14 for details).

Her narrative is structured through the development of voice as a metaphor for empowerment and transformation based on the work of Belenky et al. [1] (see Chapter 8).

To remind readers, Belenky et al. set out five levels of voice:

- Silent voice
- Received voice
- Subjective voice
- Procedural voice: connected and separate voices
- Constructed voice

Helen's Narrative

Moving Out of Silence

Initially, when I reflected on experiences, I recall feeling downtrodden by doctors and undervalued by other members of the multi-disciplinary team. I identified a need to become more assertive. By reflecting on situations that exposed my lack of self-confidence, I was able to become more in tune with my feelings. Prior to incorporating reflection into my practice, I found the easiest way of dealing with conflict was to accommodate the other professional's opinions. In doing so, I felt I was failing both my patients and myself. After experiencing a number where doctors ignored what I had to say, my relationships with them became a focus for reflection. The difficulty I had in giving them feedback or challenging their perspective when I knew it was not in the patient's best interests was undermining my integrity and compromising my practice. I lacked confidence in entering a discussion with a doctor and yet felt frustrated when he or she did not recognise my experience. Sharing these experiences within the guided reflection group, I came to realise I needed to become skilful in creating and sustaining collaborative relationships with doctors rather than reacting against my self-oppressed state and being marginalised as 'stroppy'. Drawing on work by Cavanagh [2], I began to reframe situations of conflict with doctors as opportunities for collaboration whereby a mutual exchange of ideas and respect would enhance patient care. So, the task I set myself was to illuminate my transformation through three particular experiences.

Jack

I suspected Jack had dislocated his hip. As the incident occurred at the weekend, I informed the doctor on call. I explained my concerns to him, yet he felt the leg looked in a good position. He did not know Jack at this time, and I considered his observation had been insufficient. However, I did not question his judgement or knowledge of Jack. I felt even more frustrated when I subsequently discovered that Jack's hip was indeed dislocated and he would require further surgery to correct this. On reflection, I realised I did not communicate my observation of Jack in a direct way. I hoped that the doctor would interpret my concerns and engage in further discussion about Jack. He failed to do so, and I lacked the confidence to pursue my concerns. I framed this within Stein's [3] doctor–nurse game in which the nurse shows initiative and offers significant recommendations in such a way that the doctor can make the decision (as if it was his own judgement), thus minimising any threat to the doctor's dominance (or God like ego). Failure to play the game is 'hell to pay', and I was strongly motivated to avoid conflict, like the majority of my peers [2].

Roxanne

Some months later I confronted a team of doctors about their inappropriate decision to discharge Roxanne. I was concerned that the doctors were being too hasty and explained that Roxanne had only just got her brace (following a spinal fusion) and that she had not slept in it or been seen by either the physiotherapist or occupational therapist. The senior registrar turned to me with an indignant look and asked why it was taking so long to get the patient prepared for discharge. I immediately felt the conflict. I felt put down and embarrassed and felt these feelings were a consequence of not playing the doctor–nurse game. Yet I refused to be put down. I asserted (perhaps blurted out) that it was wrong to let Roxanne think she could go home when rehabilitation had hardly begun! I realised that although being assertive (and here I might simply say 'confrontational' because I am conscious that the assertive person does not carry the emotions I was feel at the time) is an important part of giving feedback, the strategy one employs to stimulate discussion is equally important. I did not want to be seen in any adversarial way but to be involved in the decision about Roxanne's discharge – in other words, moving from a competitive mode of managing conflict to a collaborative mode. Yet it takes two to tango, and the registrar was not in a dancing mood. I believed they disapproved of my direct manner and sought to reassert their power by undermining me – 'hell to pay'. Chapman [4] has highlighted how doctors use humiliation techniques to keep nurses subordinate within the status quo. Johns [5, p. 37] states that 'despite mutual recognition by both nurses and doctors that the focus of the work should be collaborative towards meeting the patient's need, the reality is that such issues become clouded in professional concerns about power and control'.

By taking the moral high ground of patient interest, I was able to challenge the power-invested interests of the doctors and help them see Roxanne as a vulnerable person rather than as some object in the bed availability quota. This experience was transformative because in the guided reflection group I could begin to acknowledge my voice and power: that I could confront and win even though I might eschew winning as desirable. It was necessary because of the lack of professional collaboration. To be heard, I had to shout; otherwise, my timorous voice would be discounted.

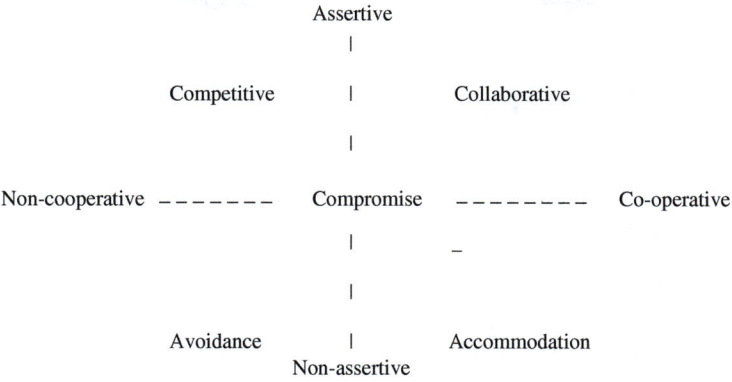

FIGURE 22.1 Styles of managing conflict grid.
Source: Adapted from [11]/scl.cornell.edu.

Many of my peers within the group related to these stories with their own similar stories. The group guide posed the question – 'how is it, you nurses, have been socialised to have no voice in such situations? Do you, (addressing all of us) perceive yourselves as subjected to medical dominance as many commentators have suggest?' [6–10]. The weight of evidence cannot deny this history, as my own lived experience and that of my colleagues testify that this issue is still alive. Why have educational processes failed to pay adequate attention to social forces that stifle nurses' voices? Is it because our teachers' voices have also been stifled? Or is it simply seen as a normative state of affairs and therefore not an issue to consider? These are vital questions to pose and ponder, for, as my experiences illuminate, a self-perceived sense of subordination and a silent voice are major barriers in my realisation of desirable practice.

As my self-esteem grew, so did my desire to assert my own beliefs about practice. I began to voice my feelings and opinions. Through the process of reflection, I was constantly challenged to open my eyes and view my practice more critically. I had always to justify the way I felt, thought and responded within situations. My received voice lay in tatters – even though I had been unaware of it in the way I perceived and responded to situations of conflict. The different styles of managing conflict were a reflective revelation: to position myself within the Thomas and Kilmann conflict management grid [11] (Figure 22.1) and critically analyse each of these positions and how I fitted within them. Which position did I desire and why? These are such simple yet such profound questions.

What knowledge I had been filled up with was scrutinised for its validity within each experience I shared. My assumptions were laid bare. Literally I was taught to think for myself. It gave me the confidence to express my own feelings and views about things. It was both scary and exciting.

Avoidance is non-assertive and non-co-operative characterised by a negation of the issues and rationalisation that attempts to challenge the situation is futile.

Accommodation is non-assertive and cooperative where the individual gives up their own needs to others for whatever reason.

Compromise is realising that every involved party cannot be satisfied and setting aside one's personal views to resolve the conflict.

Competition is pursuing one's own needs at the exclusion of others leading to win-lose resolution.

Collaboration involves the effort to solve conflict to a mutually satisfying conclusion leading to win-win resolution.

Claire

The issue of conflict was again central to the experience I shared in the group about Claire. She was recovering from a spinal infusion. The incident occurred during a night shift whilst I was taking my break. Claire was incorrectly moved by an inexperienced agency nurse. Claire subsequently became distressed and was crying in pain. I was upset that Claire should suffer unnecessarily and angry that the nurse had moved her when I had previously explained the need for caution during the handling of patients following spinal surgery. I felt responsible because I was Claire's named nurse and knew that she trusted me. I assumed that Claire blamed me for what had happened and tried to reassure her by promising that the nurse would not move her again. In my journal, I summed up my anger with the words 'professional incompetence'.

Reflecting on this situation, I became aware that my angry response was influenced by my protective feelings towards Claire. I blamed myself foe her distress. When I shared this experience within the guided reflection group, I felt challenged when I was asked how Claire felt about the incident. I didn't have an answer to that challenge, as I had not encouraged Claire to discuss her feelings. I was too wrapped up in my own anxiety. My belief that she thought I had let her down was purely speculative. Since the incident I have been 'stewing in my juices' locked into my anger and being unable to resolve my conflict. This experience has increased my self-awareness that my emotions profoundly affect my responses to a situation. I really need to know myself better so I am better equipped to deal with such situations more appropriately. I thought I could handle conflict more easily following Roxanne's experience but this experience showed me I still had much to learn. In the group, I was encouraged to reflect on my relationship with Claire and in particular my protective stance towards her and other adolescents. What type of relationship did I desire to have with them?

Ramos's [12] research into the nature of the nurse–patient relationship highlighted two impasses to developing a truly therapeutic relationship. The first impasse is concerned with power – the need to control the relationship. The second impasse is concerned with emotions: the need to protect the patient. It seems, on reflection, that I was stuck in both impasses. And yet I felt that Claire and I had many characteristics that typify what Morse [13] describes as a 'mutual connected relationship'. For example, I involved her in decisions about her care. However, I must reluctantly admit I did see her primarily in terms of her medical condition – what Morse describes as a 'therapeutic relationship' rather than as a suffering young woman. I was Claire's nurse and she was my patient, and in this incident, I was primarily concerned for her safety and the repair of her spinal fusion.

Through the group dialogue, I realised I should have empathised with Claire's experience and addressed her needs and not merely tried to reassure her that the agency nurse would not move her again. I felt ashamed in the group that I could be so blind when the contradiction was so obvious. It was like a flash of recognition! Suddenly, and perhaps for the first time, I really felt I knew myself and the impact of myself on relationships. Utilising the 'Being Available template' (Figure 5.3) I sensed the significance of knowing and managing myself and knowing the person behind the patient to be person-centred.

Speaking with Both Separate and Connected Voices

From the perspective of connected knowing, I must confess I am as guilty as the next nurse in seeing Claire in terms of my nursing interests, and yet I would have always described myself as empathic. Reading and discussing Belenky et al.'s [1] concept of connected knowing was very revealing and disconcerting in light of my experience with Claire. No one said that learning through reflection was easy!

I have also illuminated the way I am now framing my experiences within the context of theory, and holding that theory up for critique for its value to inform my practice. For example, I reject Morse's [13] idea of types of relationships. From a holistic perspective, there can only be connected-type relationships; the other types are merely descriptive failures of the connected relationship.

Ann

This experience took place some months after my experience with Claire. Anne had been admitted for an arthrogram of her left hip. She was a tomboy. She hated the pop group 'Take That', whom the girls in the bed space either side of her loved, and whose latest video they were playing when Ann arrived. Immediately I sensed that Ann was uncomfortable in her new environment. In response I offered her the opportunity to move into another bed space. Ann ignored me, and her mother said 'it takes a while for her to settle in'. Paradoxically, the mother's glib reassurance heightened my concerns. In response I decided to pursue forming a 'connected relationship' with Ann. However, when I asked her about her hip and knee pain and how her injury had occurred, she was reluctant to talk to me. Her hobbies were football and riding her bicycle. I asked her if her pain restricted her hobbies and she replied 'A bit'. I felt frustrated and wondered what was bothering this young person. I decided to give her some space and observe during the afternoon. When I spoke to her later this evening, she still seemed totally uninterested in me.

The following morning when she was scheduled to go for her hip arthrogram, she became very distressed an abusive. Clearly under that undemonstrative exterior was a frightened young woman I knew nothing about. I had rarely experienced such a negative response when trying to form a relationship with a patient. My head was buzzing with ideas about gaining her confidence. I wanted to know what she was feeling, what was bothering her and why she appeared not to like me. I felt despondent. Sharing the experience in the group I was again challenged if I was still responding to Ann as a patient and not as a young woman with a life outside the hospital. Even asking about her hobbies was related to her hip and knee injury and pain. I had also assumed that Ann would be interested in me and want to develop a relationship. Why should she? Perhaps I was just another authority figure intent on telling her what to do? As it was, she was not willing to play my game. The more I tried to connect with her the more she tried to evade me! Again I felt despondent: had I not learnt anything from Claire's experience? Had I embodied a way of being that defied change? The idea that just because we come to see something differently doesn't mean we can change the way we respond hit home.

Much of the literature about knowing the patient refers to the notion of 'clicking' [13–15] as an 'immediate rapport between patient and nurse' [15]. Morse [13] suggests that 'clicking' with a patient n evokes the development of a deeper relationship. However, I could find little literature that discusses the relationship that does not click. Johns [16] suggests that all relationships can be viewed along a reciprocal-resistance continuum yet, for one reason or another, either the practitioner or the patient resists this development. I felt Ann was resisting me and as a consequence I failed to get on to her wavelength, which left me feeling I had failed.

The group challenged me to consider how else I might respond. I know from previous experiences that disclosing aspects of my own life has enhanced a relationship. In other words, I become a human being and not just a nurse. It is interesting to speculate how Ann would have responded had I done that with her. I feel it would have changed the focus of conversation away from her treatment. I felt the group gave me permission to break out of the nurse mode to experiment, to be creative, to take risks, to liberate myself to be me rather than some nurse caricature. Yet there is no recipe for success. With some people, such as Ann, it may not be possible to develop the desired relationship. I must guard against imposing a type of relationship or thinking I have failed.

Finding My Constructed Voice

The last experience I shared in the group concerned Angela. When I went to admit Angela, it struck me that I was clutching her medical notes and nursing documentation. As I sat down next to her. I consciously left those files at the end of the bed and focused on her as a person. The first 15 minutes of our conversation centred on Angela's journey to the hospital and her first year at university. Our discussion progressed naturally to the reason for her admission and how she felt about her treatment and the future. Finally, I turned to the nursing documentation and decided I had obtained more information about Angela than I would have done pursuing the assessment formula.

My letting go of the need to control meant that I was able to flow with the moment. I really believed that Angela and I 'clicked' and connected. When I admitted Angela, the ward was not so busy as usual, giving me more time to be with her. Yet, in saying that, do I fall into a trap of justifying that time alone made this possible rather than my mind-set? Perhaps having time did create the space to be with Angela, but I can now appreciate the value of giving this 'task' more time. I can see the way we never value this 'talking time' in the pressures to get work done and yet knowing the person is fundamental to nursing them from a holistic perspective. All my colleagues value seeing the person as an individual and yet the contradiction between this value and ward practice is stark.

Through this experience, my vision of nursing has been scrutinised and strengthened, building on the insights gained from nursing Claire and Ann. By using the metaphor of voice, I feel I have become empowered to practice more in tune with my values than previously. Before, I felt I needed to be in control and hence reduce the person to a patient to be controlled. Paradoxically, by letting go the need to control, I am less anxious and more creative, more able to realise desirable practice. When I speak with colleagues, I speak with a more knowledgeable, empathic and passionate voice! I hope my experiences have illustrated this journey of empowerment and transformation.

Reflection has enriched my practice and enabled me to develop new skills. It has enabled me to unlock some of the dilemmas and confront the barriers that impeded my practice. This takes an inquiring mind because a practitioner must be ready to challenge their actions and develop new ideas. I no longer feel defeated by the constraints of management and resources, nor do I view myself as a 'mere' staff nurse. I have gained an inner sense of purpose and a desire to provide effective care. The no man's land between reality and desirability has decreased as I continue to face new challenges that arise in my work.

Reflection

Helen noted – 'as my self-esteem increased so did my desire to assert my beliefs'.

As she comes to know and realise her beliefs as a lived reality, so her commitment to realise person-centred practice is nourished and grows. She became more available to her young patients as evidenced through the sequence of experiences. She became increasingly assertive in her knowing informed by relevant theory that helped her frame her insights and expand her empathic lens to see the patient's experience.

Helen's utilisation of Belenky et al.'s development of voice [1] reveals the significance of using appropriate frameworks to structure narrative development. The stages of voice became signposts of development, something tangible to work towards realising her vision person-centred practice. The narrative points to the awareness that the person-centred practitioner speaks with a constructed voice.

References

1. Belenky, M. F., Clinchy, B. M., Goldberger, N. R., Tarule, J. M. (1986) *Women's Ways of Knowing: The Development of Self, Voice, and Mind*. Basic Books, New York.

2. Cavanagh, S. (1991) The conflict management style of staff nurses and managers. *Journal of Advanced Nursing* 16, 1254–1260.

3. Stein, L. (1988) The doctor nurse game. In R. Dingwall, J. McIntosh [Eds.] *Readings in the Sociology of Nursing*. Churchill Livingstone, Edinburgh.

4. Chapman, G. (1983) Ritual and rational action. *Journal of Advanced Nursing* 8, 13–20.

5. Johns, C. (1994) Constructing the BNDU model. In C. Johns [Ed.] *The Burford NDU Model: Caring in Practice*. Blackwell Science, Oxford, 2–60.

6. Friedson, E. (1971) *Professional Domination*. Aldine Atherton, Chicago.

7. Hughes, E. (1971) *The Sociological Eye: Selected Papers*. Aldine Atherton, Chicago.

8. Capra, F. (1982) *The Turning Pint: Society and the Rising Culture*. Fontana, Lincoln.

9. Buckingham, J., McGrath, G. (1983) *The Social Reality of Nursing*. Adis, Sydney.

10. Brunning, H., Huffington, C. (1985) Altered images. *Nursing Times* 81(31), 24–27.

11. Thomas, K., Kilmann, R. (1974) *Thomas Kilmann Conflict Mode Instrument*. Xicom, Toledo.

12. Ramos, M. (1992) The nurse-patient relationship: themes and variations. *Journal of Advanced Nursing* 17, 496–506.

13. Morse, J. (1991) Negotiating commitment and involvement in the nurse-patient relationship. *Journal of Advanced Nursing* 16, 496–506.

14. May, C. (1991) Affective neutrality and involvement in the nurse-patient relationships: perceptions of appropriate behaviour amongst nurses in acute medical and surgical wards. *Journal of Advanced Nursing* 16, 552–558.

15. Fosbinder, D. (1994) Patients perceptions of nursing care: an emerging theory of interpersonal competence. *Journal of Advanced Nursing* 20, 1085–1093.

16. Johns, C. (1999) Caring connections: knowing self within caring relationships through reflection. *International Journal for Human Caring* 3, 31–38.

CHAPTER 23

The Beast and the Star: Resolving Contradictions Within Everyday Practice[i]

Introduction

This narrative was written by Ruth Morgan, a community nurse team leader, based on her final assignment on the 'Being and Becoming a Reflective Practitioner' programme (see Chapter 14).

The Beast and the Star

There was something remarkably brazen about the manner in which Heather moved to our area; something outrageous in her assumption that all services would instantly be at her beck and call without a warning or even a few days notice. Inevitably she chose a Friday afternoon.

The surgery was alerted to Heather's imminent arrival by a last-minute phone call from a 'friend'. We were told that Heather lived alone and was paralysed. She was on her way from Luton and needed the services of the district nurses. The address given was that of the local travellers' site. Somewhat alarmed, I decided as team leader of the district nurses to contact our equivalent service in Luton for further information. Her existing nurse, Claire, turned out to be in complete ignorance of the forthcoming move, despite having visited Heather that morning. The picture she painted was very negative. Heather and her family had the reputation of being uncooperative and difficult, so much so that the nurses always visited in pairs. Her complex needs involved the services of the district nurses, social services and caring agencies once or twice daily, along with medical loans of essential equipment.

By the time we met as district nurses for our Monday morning meeting, we had received further negative reports of Heather. Trexler [1] warns that critical communication between staff can validate, justify and reinforce difficult or deviant labels put on patients. Sadly, our discussion deteriorated into unconstructive criticism of Heather's reported behaviour. I recall that no attempt was made to understand her difficulties or her tragic situation, and she was quickly denounced as demanding and ungrateful. We had rapidly succumbed to the trap of pre-labelling a patient whom we had never met. Corley and Goren [2] describe such stigmatisation as 'the dark side or nursing', resulting in patients being marginalised and their quality of care being compromised. This was reflected in the grudging visit to Heather that was carried out by two of the team, Wendy and Elaine, following the meeting. Geographically, Heather had moved into Wendy's patch and would therefore be her responsibility. Unfortunately, the unhelpful mindsets of the nurses that morning, together with Heather's rude, aggressive responses, proved disastrous and resulted in reinforcing her negative labelling.

By Tuesday morning, the team were practically in revolt. Wendy, next in seniority to me, was particularly appalled and tense. She positioned herself firmly in the 'power' chair to take charge that morning. I have noticed how she appears to need to be in a physically powerful position when stressed and needing to take control. The ensuing discussion was full of vitriol against Heather 'must get her off our list', 'can't have this' and 'must get her sorted'.

Stories were compared about the horrors of 'gypsy' behaviour, tales that displayed judgemental attitudes and drew sweeping conclusions about physical dangers for us on their site. The travellers, as a body, were effectively 'etherised upon the table' by the critical analysis, and the souls of their people were left to 'evaporate into thin air' [3, p. 29]. Having no previously bad experiences of gypsies, I listened in disbelief, but I felt unable to argue with conviction. Looking back, I wish I had had the courage to challenge views being expressed. It may have at least steadied the tide of opposition sweeping Heather's way. Trexler [1] comments that an individual from a socially oppressed or stereotyped group is more likely to be stigmatised as deviant than a similar personality from a more 'acceptable' group.

The team appeared to be whipping itself into a frenzy with a momentum that was alarming and unnecessary. We e-mailed the doctors to alert them to the difficulties Heather was presenting us in terms of our ongoing time and resources. As she was not yet registered as their patient, Heather, Wendy held out a fleeting hope that they would refuse to accept her on their list. After all, 'Why should we have to do her?' asked Wendy resentfully.

Putting this down in black and white exposes its immaturity and selfishness, an attitude we so often loftily condemn in others, especially the doctors. The action of putting pen to paper has enabled me to 'freeze the action' and recognise the hypocrisy behind the question [4, p. 151]. The doctors, however, showed no interest in our difficulties and, to this day, have not asked how we are managing. Unfortunately, this lack of concern heightened our escalating resentment and demonstrated the lack of mutual support and cohesion with the surgery team. Caring behaviour and awareness of individual and collective emotion are necessary group 'norms' for strong effective teams [5].

Wendy was so disturbed by her difficult visit to Heather the previous day that on Tuesday she insisted I accompany her. This created difficulties for me because I needed to attend Peter, a dying patient, at the same time. Inwardly I believed that any one of the junior nurses in the team could have supported Wendy and that her insistence on my attending undermined them. However, I was unable to assert my view, and so I avoided open conflict in favour of an outwardly 'harmonious team' [6]. It left me with intrapersonal conflict, however, as I struggled with the contradiction between my commitment to Peter and the louder demands of Wendy. Feeling pressurised, I complied with the more powerful voice and went with Wendy to meet Heather for the first time, leaving Peter to wait. Co-operating with Wendy and negating my own wishes was an accommodating way of managing the conflict. It prevented disagreement and nurtured my own need for acceptance and approval [7]. However, it left me feeling voiceless and resentful, stuck in the sterile trap of having to put another's needs before my own [8].

My first impression of Heather was of a very angry, truculent lady. She was obviously antagonised by Wendy who could not open her mouth without a rude, aggressive response. I had not realised Monday's visit had gone so badly wrong. I introduced myself and, in the face of silent hostility, tried a pleasant but form approach to her care. Heather remained unremittingly disagreeable, issuing constant demands and instructions and refusing to respond to initiations of conversation. Questions about her care were met with defiance aimed directly at Wendy – 'I told you yesterday', 'your supposed to be the nurse' and 'you never believe what I say'.

I challenged the last sentence and was told that Wendy had an attitude problem to her 'sort of people' and would not listen to her. This in fact reflected the truth and is a warning about how much of ourselves we give away. Despite now being impeccably pleasant, Wendy was clearly today in a no-win situation.

I felt I had to challenge Heather's constant stabs of hostility: 'you know we can't work together like this, don't you?'

In hindsight, I can see how this rather patronising question simply escalated her sulky, intransigent mood, and now recognise the 'parent/child game' in process. Heather was clearly in 'child mode', having a tantrum, in response to our 'critical parent' position [9–11]. Wendy at this point left the room to fetch some water. I unconsciously switched to 'nurturing parent mode'.

'What happened to you Heather?'

'A road accident' came the brief reply.

There was silence followed by tears welling up in Heather's eyes. I felt able to put my arm briefly round her shoulders to comfort her before Wendy returned. The 'child' having found the nurturing parent felt more comfortable and the atmosphere changed dramatically. Heather became noticeably contrite and more co-operative.

'I'm sorry nurse at the way I behaved. I'm not normally like that' aimed Wendy.

'That's alright, I'm sorry too. Let's both make a fresh start' a conciliatory reply from Wendy, accepting her part in the hostilities.

At the time I was staggered by Heather's complete capitulation, while Wendy, amazed, assumed I had delivered an extremely effective lecture whilst she was out of the room. On reflection, 'reading the riot act' would have entrenched us further in the 'critical parent/sulky child' game we had been unwittingly playing. The question about the past actually focused on Heather's situation rather than on her behaviour and helped her feel less defensive. Her response to my 'nurturing mothering' role was that of a repentant child looking for approval. Harris [10] explains that these games are played as a defence against to protect the individual from the painful 'I'm not OK' position that we learn in early childhood. Underpinning the game is a child needing a parent for approval in order to feel 'I'm OK'.

An uncertain calm ensued which was instantly rocked by the arrival of two efficient social workers. They needed to carry out an assessment of Heather's needs to enable her to receive her personal care from carers. Once established, this care would relieve us of the non-nursing duties we were carrying out. Heather was resistant to matter-of-fact attempts to discuss her needs, refusing to consider any areas of difficulty for the carers. Those who are chronically sick often feel their mounting losses are misunderstood or minimalised by professionals and, as a result, experience acute emotional isolation from them [12]. Perhaps Heather's defensiveness was actually the sign of a healthy spirit refusing to be crushed by the negative signals she perceived around her, signals which left her feeling discounted and devalued [12].

I left the stalemate to continue my nursing calls. This log visit had put huge pressures on a day which became additionally fraught due to Pater's death and Wendy's ongoing angst. Heather's aggressive behaviour to Wendy, and even the apology, had simply escalated the stresses and anxieties Wendy felt about visiting her. My one experience of Heather had been more positive and I instinctively wanted to care for her. I felt unbalanced by the demands placed on me seemingly by everyone, and by the absence of any personal support.

The following day, Wednesday, Wendy was back in the 'power chair' for our team meeting, firing bullets of instructions. I can see now how her inability to manage Heather was driving her into bullying tactics. In terms of transactional analysis, she was replaying the childhood behaviour of demanding her own way now, in order to feel 'OK'. She had notified our nursing manager, Jean, that we had a 'dangerous' visit on a gypsy site that put our personal safety at risk. She directed us to back up her statements by maintaining a principle of two trained staff at Heather's house each day over the next four days while she was off-duty. She refused to consider my suggestions of other combinations of staff despite the fact that it would reduce the burden on us. I suspect now that yielding to any alternative views would have risked weakening her fragile position. In the unconscious nature of game playing, I played the 'indulgent parent' placating the 'child' by allowing the bullying. It saddens me now to recognise the inherent weakness and low self-esteem her aggression belied. 'In the swamp of powerlessness breeds the virus of aggression' [13, p. 20]. Understanding this at the time would have reduced the power of Wendy's behaviour and enabled me to challenge her demands more appropriate and compassionately.

Following Wednesday's meeting, Wendy and I visited Heather and the atmosphere was more relaxed than on previous visits. I was concerned that for five days now the care of Heather had monopolised two nurses for nearly two hours each time, to the detriment of other patients. Unfortunately, our time problem was not going to be resolved once the carers began their care because Heather had made it clear that she still needed us twice daily to deal with her bowels. I noted that, despite this claim, she had refused bowel care on two of the five days so far. I tried to explore other ways of managing her care, complying with her needs (demands) and reducing our time commitment. This was an attempt at a win/win style of interaction seeking mutual benefit for both parties. However, it deteriorated into a win/loose conflict in the face of Heather's inflexibility and my lack of options [14]. Heather appeared totally unsympathetic over our time issues and the needs of other patients. They would simply have to wait. I tried to move her from that position but recognise on reflection that the unfortunate tome of my question alienated her further.

'How would you feel if you were left to wait while we nurse others first?'

She inevitably rejected the implication that her demands affected the care of other patients. Again on reflection, I loaded the canon even more by mentioning that I had to leave a dying man to visit her the previous day. She remained unmoved.

My attempt to appeal to Heather's better nature failed because it promoted our power and her need. Price [15] explains that humans can reach a state of disequilibrium in response to the stress of chronic illness making them appear non-compliant and irrational. Price suggests addressing this by abandoning external goal setting and exploring instead the individual constructs and personal objectives of the patient. In this way, a level playing field is drawn and the relationship is reinforced as one of equals. It would also have helped pull us out of the 'parent/child game', clearly again in full swing between Heather and myself by giving us the opportunity to reframe the relationship as 'adult/adult'.

Our stalemate was interrupted by the arrival of Debbie, the social worker, presenting Heather with yet another critical parent figure. Heather behaved like an uncooperative child in response to Debbie's clear assertive comments about her care. At the time I recall admiring Debbie's no-nonsense directness, but further reading has enabled me to appreciate the likely impact of her approach on Heather, who was probably made to feel like an object, a job to be performed. Thorne and Robinson [16] highlighted the clash of perspectives between professionals and those receiving their care. They found that patients were often fraught with frozen anger, suspicion and intense vulnerability as their wishes were disregarded. They found that patients felt affirmed and validated by being trusted by their health professionals to direct their own illness management. In the absence of such affirmation, patients lost any naïve trust that health care providers worked in their best interest, and learnt to make their needs known in an assertive and unequivocal manner. This, of course, clarifies much of Heather's demanding behaviour and shines a more negative light on Debbie's approach.

Matters with Debbie were further complicated by the electricity supply being cut off, disabling the electric bed and preventing Debbie from carrying out necessary moving and handling assessment. Without this assessment, the carers, starting their care the following day would have to leave Heather in bed. Heather, now in totally intransigent mood, flatly refused to allow Debbie to return that afternoon to carry out the task and so doomed herself to paying the price. It could be argued that, as professionals, our controlling attempts to manage Heather's care drove her into a belligerent position from which she would lose face if she backed down. The result was an unproductive lose/lose interaction in which both Debbie and Heather failed to achieve their goals due to the determination on both sides to 'stick to their guns'.

I felt noticeable less anxious going to work the next day knowing that Wendy was off-duty. Tensions in the team over Heather had been monopolising every morning meeting and then bleeding forward into the remainder of the day's work and relationships. My unspoken conflict with Wendy was draining me more emotionally than the issues that created it. I also now detect a secondary desire within myself to 'sort out' the team in her absence! Over the following days the team willingly tried various combinations of workers (nurses, students, carers) for Heather's visits, making better use of resources but going against Wendy's express wishes. The success of this should have enabled me to approach Monday's meeting more positively. Instead I felt stressed and anxious anticipating Wendy's furious response. It seems senseless now to have gone about things in this way rather than thrashing out our differences before hand. Analysing it, I realise my inability to confront Wendy left me powerless against her bullying tactics and voiceless in negotiating heather's care. I therefore took the short-term easy option of acting in Wendy's absence, exacerbating the problem by reducing Wendy's control of the situation and thereby increasing her need to bully. Struggles of 'interpersonal conflict and power relationships' [17, p. 196] were now in play and Heather had become a pawn in the battle between us.

Wendy again seated in the 'power chair', reacted to our change in tactics as predicted. The meeting prickled with antagonism in which other team members became involved, Elaine openly disagreeing with her. Wendy sought sanctuary in the role of victim, which pushed her into demanding 'child mode'.

'I can only work in this unreasonable situation if things are done my way' (subtext – I am the one who is suffering).

This common game is one in which the 'victim' searches either for a 'persecutor' to inflict wounds and justify her rejected view of herself, or for a 'rescuer' to offer help and support her belief that I can't cope on my own [11]. Useless now to try and explore her agenda and negotiate agreement [18]. Wendy was too busy with self-pitying stories in an attempt to galvanise supporters. The 'game' marched on and I was forced to turn to our manager, Jean, to help us through the issues. A meeting was organised for the next day and, feeling threatened, Wendy asked me to stop Elaine from attending. I refused, stating firmly that it was a team issue and we should all be there. I note how quickly Wendy capitulates when I actually make an assertive response.

The whole team were present. We moved into a different room from our usual office and sat at a circular table with Jean taking control. The usual tirade of negative, judgemental views about travellers were expressed, mainly by Wendy but supported by Chris and Dianne. How much valuable time had we expended on such unproductive angst over recent days? Given the success of our visits in Heather's absence, I was taken aback by the support Heather got from Chris and Dianne. It perhaps demonstrates the power of bullying behaviour, causing others to swing over to her side. On reflection, I realised I must adopt a different attitude to Wendy in future. Over the years I have learnt to manage her tirades by 'carrying' her until she inevitably calms down. However, as I now consider the cost to my own peace of mind and the inhibiting effect on team dynamics, I realise that the price of this strategy has become too high.

Jean, the manager, swinging between 'adult' and 'critical parent' role, batted off many of the unreasonable demands and attitudes being expressed until eventually we were able to discuss the actual management of Heather. In the light of the evidence of the last few positive visits, Wendy was forced to back down from her insistence on two qualified nurses for each visit and agree to double up with carers when possible. In view of the drain on our time, we decided to offer Heather visits on alternative days with check phone calls on the intervening ones.

This seemed reasonable in view of the wasted visits, we had already made when Heather had not wanted bowel care and had not attempted to let us know. Wendy, for no sensible reason but hanging on to a remnant of control, insisted that the weekend day should be a Saturday, even if the alternate day fell on a Sunday. Sheep-like, we succumbed to her bullying and verbally agreed, knowing it could not work in practice. Furthermore, after discussion, the decision was made not to offer Heather any out-of-hours nursing support because of the position and 'dangers' of the site where she lived. I had not sensed any danger or threatening behaviour on my visits and felt this decision was unjust and motivated by stigmatising behaviour. Trexler [1] finds that exclusionary reactions are common amongst nurses against those labelled 'deviant'. I am reminded of a poignant sentence from Ron Kovic [19, p. 99] in his autobiography 'Born on the fourth of July' as he lay imprisoned in his paralysed body, labelled by his nurses as demanding

'I am alone again. I have been lying in room 17 for almost a month. I am isolated here because I am a troublemaker'.

It fell to me to take the decisions of our meeting to Heather to gain her consent. As a result of the ongoing process of this reflection, and feedback from sharing this extended experience in my university-guided reflection group, I felt better equipped to communicate with both Heather and Wendy. I have become increasingly aware of the need to develop a relationship of reciprocal trust with Heather, involving the abandonment of professional decision-making in favour of soliciting Heather's views and perspectives. Nowadays we talk very eloquently about 'gaining patient compliance' as a means of achieving good healthcare, but this viewpoint has been challenged by Taylor [20], who views it as a means of maintaining professional power. She recommends working towards 'concordance' in nursing where nurse and patient jointly agree gaols and plans of action in an open relationship or partnership. This promotes trust between both parties, which fosters self-confidence, self-esteem and the 'achievement of wellness in chronic illness' [16, p. 787].

The responsibility of Heather was gradually sliding from Wendy to me, a shift I welcomed as Wendy and Heather were unlikely to achieve any comfortable rapport. Now I had the job of approaching Heather with decisions already made about her care, hardly the spirit of an open relationship discussed above! However, I endeavoured to negotiate in a collaborative manner, seeking mutually satisfying solutions to our differing views [7]. It was an attempt to achieve a win/win conclusion to the conflict between Heather's demands and our resources.

We succeeded in making compromises, both yielding in some issues and standing firm in others. I made a specific effort to spend more time building a relationship with Heather to reduce the status differential between us. Finding things in common has strengthened this: our age, the age of our children, even the highlighting of our hair on the same day! According to Walker et al. [21], 'humanising' myself in this way helps to foster friendship and provide a sense of support. I felt immensely honoured and encouraged by a sudden invitation from Heather – 'Would you like to see my wedding photos?'

As a result of this reflection, I have also given more considerable thought to how I can work more effectively with Wendy. She has many strengths and assets she brings to the team, in particular her organisational skills and her genuine interest in individual team members. I have felt in the past there have been benefits in avoiding outright confrontation with her and in 'carrying' her through stressful situations. However, the sudden insight I had to the insecure emotions behind her bullying caused a fundamental shift in thinking for me, as if a light had been turned on inside. My own powerlessness diminished and I recognised an opening for constructive dialogue. I wonder now if she almost wants reasoning out of her 'panics'. In recent issues regarding Heather, I have made sure that I have expressed my views. The resulting discussions have not been totally harmonious but at least they have been more open and honest. I feel the whole team has benefitted from exposing the conflicts than from hiding behind a façade of togetherness [17]. My change in thinking has also caused me to be more assertive in other areas of difference between us, enabling us to negotiate mutually acceptable solutions. Johns [22] points out that collaboration does not happen automatically: it has to be actively created.

I have now recognised an amazing paradox: we have both been reinforcing each other's weaknesses. Our different behaviours actually stem from similar roots of self-doubt. Wendy's bullying tactics and my anxiety to please have both been attempts to promote ourselves in the face of underlying poor self-esteem [8]. My avoidance of confrontation has stemmed from a fear of losing popularity but it has also perpetuated Heather's bullying and established a vicious circle in which I stay approved and Wendy has stayed powerful.

Moore [3] discusses how to 'care of the soul' by discovering and understanding the paradoxes within human nature. He reminds us that transformative change can only come about through understanding the hidden depths of our personality. We cannot just make ourselves want ourselves to be. He points us to the loathsome beast in Greek mythology known as 'Asterion', a name which paradoxically means 'star'. The same contradiction of ugliness and beauty is found in the profound hidden roots of individuality. The 'beast' and the 'star' jostle within each of us.

> 'It is the beast, this thing that stirs in the core of our being, but it is also the star of our innermost nature. We have to care for this suffering with extreme reverence so that, in our fear and anger the beast, we do not overlook the star' [3, p. 21].

As I continue to develop my practice as a team leader, I now recognise that ignoring or denying the 'beast' within us is counterproductive. The beast of self-doubt and low self-esteem needs recognition and acknowledgement before any transforming change can occur. The solution lies in establishing 'norms' as a team that recognise and understand individual weaknesses, to uncover the shining stars which lay in the shadow of the beast. The effect of rediscovering compassion for ourselves is to renew and facilitate our love and care for others [13]. We all benefit, each other, the patient and ourselves!

Last Sunday I visited Heather as usual. She lay very still, crumpled in bed. For a heart-stopping moment I wondered if she was breathing. I was reminded of the fragility of her life and wondered what on earth all the conflict had been about.

Reflection

This is a narrative concerning conflict due to issues of authority and values. Without doubt, much of reflection is triggered by conflict between colleagues. It reveals the significance of developing the therapeutic team with shared values and collaborative ways of working whereby 'who is in control' is deflated. As Ruth noted 'Johns [22] points out that collaboration does not happen automatically: it has to be actively created'.

Not easy when practitioners have learnt a particular way of being.

References

1. Trexler, J. (1996) Reformulation of deviance and labelling theory in nursing. *IMAGE: Journal of Nursing Scholarship* 28(2), 131–135.

2. Corley, M., Green, S. (1998) The dark side of nursing: impact of stigmatizing responses on patients. *Scholarly Inquiry for Nursing Practice: An International Journal* 12(2), 99–121.

3. Moore, T. (1992) *Care of the Soul.* Piatkus, London.

4. Street, A. (1995) *Nursing Replay: Researching Nursing Culture Together.* Churchill Livingstone, Melbourne.

5. Druskatt, V., Wolff, S. (2001) The relationship of theory and practice in the acquisition of skill. In P. Benner, C. Tanner, C. Chesla [Eds.] *Expertise in*

Nursing Practice. Springer Publishing, New York, 29–47.

6. Johns, C. (1992) Ownership and the harmonious team: barriers to developing the therapeutic nursing team in primary nursing. *Journal of Clinical Nursing* 1, 89–94.

7. Cavanagh, S. (1991) The conflict style of staff nurses and nurse managers. *Journal of Advanced Nursing* 16, 1254–1260.

8. Dickson, A. (1982) *A Woman in Your Own Right.* Quartet Books, London.

9. Berne, E. (1964) *Games People Play.* Penguin Books, London.

10. Harris, T. (1967) *I'm OK- You're OK.* Arrow books, London.

11. Stewart, I., Joines, V. (1987) *TA Today: A New Introduction to Transactional Analysis.* Russell Press, Nottingham.

12. Charmaz, K. (1983) Loss of self: a fundamental form of suffering in the chronically ill. *Sociology of Health and Illness* 5(2), 168–195.

13. Dickson, A. (2000) *Trusting the Tides.* Rider, London.

14. Covey, S. (1989) *The Seven Habits of Highly Effective People.* Fireside, New York.

15. Price, B. (1996) Illness careers: the chronic illness experience. *Journal of Advanced Nursing* 24, 275–279.

16. Thorne, S., Robinson, C. (1988) Reciprocal trust in health care relationships. *Journal of Advanced Nursing* 13, 782–789.

17. Johns, C. (1996) Understanding and managing interpersonal conflict as a therapeutic nursing activity. *International Journal of Nursing Practice* 2, 194–2000.

18. Sebenius, J. (2001) Six habits of merely effective negotiators. *Harvard Business Review*, April, 87–95.

19. Kovic, R. (1976) *Born of the Fourth of July.* Corgi, London.

20. Taylor, B. (2002) Nurse-patient partnership: rhetoric or reality? *Journal of Community Nursing* 16(3), 16–18.

21. Walker, A., Wilkes, L. M., White, K. (2000) How do patients perceive support from nurses? *Professional Nurse* 16(2), 902–904.

22. Johns, C. (1999) Caring connections: knowing self within caring relationships through reflection. *International Journal of Human Caring* 3(2), 31–38.

Note

i. The narrative was previously published: Morgan R., Johns, C. (2005) The Beast and the Star: resolving contradictions within everyday practice. In C. Johns, D. Freshwater [Eds.] *Transforming Nursing Through Reflective Practice* (second edition). Blackwell Publishing, 114–128.

CHAPTER 24

Shifting a Nurse's Attitude to Deliberate Self-harm Patients in an Accident and Emergency Department

Introduction

Jane approached myself to guide her BSc Nursing studies dissertation. She had previously studied the 'Becoming a reflective and effective practitioner' course[i]. She wrote in her dissertation – 'I chose to work with Chris in a guided reflection relationship because reflection had become such a meaningful learning milieu for me. Reflection had enabled me to access and analyse my practice leading to insights that had influenced my subsequent practice'.

Session 1: Beginnings

In our first session, issues surrounding deliberate self-harm patients (DSH) were not initially on my mind, or so I thought. Chris simply began by simply asking 'how I was' and inquiring if there were any issues emerging from my practice in Accident and Emergency that might be a potential focus for my study. I had not anticipated what might arise and to my surprise anxieties about DSH patients tumbled out.

Something happened a few weeks ago. I haven't really thought long and hard about it yet. I have some nagging doubts about what happened. I think it's been easier to ignore it and put it to the back of my mind. On a recent shift, I dealt with a man who had deliberately cut his arm. I still feel uncomfortable about the whole way I responded to him. It was a night shift, around 3 in the morning. I went into the cubicle to carry out his treatment. Until this point, I had not met this man. All I knew about him was that he had deliberately cut his arm. He required sutures. On reflection, I am aware that I prejudged him, stereotyped him. His deliberate act of self-harm irritated me before I met him. I went into the cubicle and communicated the necessary information with him; I was 'professional', and I tried to hide my feelings but felt 'empty'. He was excluded from any feelings of compassion that I am able to feel for other patients. Prior to commencing treatment, he asked if it would hurt. I felt his was a ridiculous question, why should I care if it hurt? I found my irritation bubbling to the surface and in answer to his question I replied 'the local should numb the pain of the stitches but it must have hurt when you did it!' I wasn't asking a question that required an answer. I now realise it was a way of communicating my feelings, a reprimand for his behaviour. Although my response makes me feel uncomfortable, I wonder if compassion would encourage him to continue with such futile acts time again and again. Mutilating you're your own body is such an alien concept. It seems such a waste of time stitching someone up likely to repeat the injury.

Chris asked me if I had any idea why I felt this way? I hadn't really thought about it. It's frustrating when you see the same patients returning over and over again; they never seem to recover. Chris suggested that perhaps I didn't see the ones who do recover because they don't come back for treatment, that perhaps my frustration lies with my inability to 'put things right'? Are such patients manipulative? He challenged me to examine whether my role boundaries required me to 'patch up the damage', or whether DSH patients require a more therapeutic approach? I had to admit that I didn't feel I had enough knowledge to distinguish between manipulative and non-manipulative patients. I said 'They obviously have reasons for their behaviour but I find it difficult to respond'.

Chris responded 'What sort of reasons?'

I said 'I didn't know. There could be a million of reasons. The environment doesn't help. The A&E environment is very challenging, for example, a nurse may find herself comforting grieving relatives one moment and the next trying to come to terms with the fact that the person in front of them has tried to take their own life, or inflicted harm on themselves.'

Chris then challenged me 'Are some patients more worthy of care than others?'

That put me on the spot. I know I should treat everyone with the same care and compassion, but in reality, I do treat these people differently. The very fact that I do is upsetting: it doesn't meet my own philosophy of care, and they are not feelings I expected to have when I embarked on my nursing career. I care, that's why I entered the profession; it distresses me that I can't be more therapeutic with this patient group.

Chris pursued the topic 'Does anything else influence your reaction to these patients?'

I had spoken about my mother in the past. She suffers from a progressive debilitating condition and I constantly witness her failing health. She doesn't deserve it. Why do fit and healthy people injure themselves? Chris could see I was upset. Gently he prodded

'Do you think this subject will be too emotive to tackle?'

I agreed it would be very emotive but that I should attempt to understand why I feel this way and work to change the way I deliver care to this patient group and hopefully deliver care in a therapeutic way.

Looking Back

Looking back on this session, it seems amazing how talking for an hour can turn my world upside down. It was powerful! I realised I had concerns working with DSH patients that had laid dormant, perhaps waiting for the right time to be expressed. I suspect that if I had not been in guided reflection at this moment in time, these issues would never have been expressed. They are difficult and disturbing to face up to. Through our previous work together somehow, I had implicit trust in Chris and knew I could reveal this side of my practice. I knew he would not judge me in any way.

Sharing my experience resulted in me asking various questions of myself such as – 'Why do I have difficulty with offering the same level of care to this patient group?' I realised that my negative prejudice and detachment in care giving with this group of patients affected their wellbeing.

Watson [1, p. 225] highlights this – 'We see glimpses indicating that the nurse's presence and consciousness, attitude and behaviour can affect the patient, for better or for worse'.

Wrapped up in my self-concern I simply was not available to them. From this first session, I take with me the need to know more about DSH. I will use my experience in a positive way and try to be more mindful of what I have learnt when faced with another DSH patient.

Chris utilised the 'being available template' (see Figure 5.3), whereby the practitioner seeks to be available to the other to help them find meaning in their health-illness experience, to guide them to make best decisions about their life and assist them as necessary with skilled action to meet their life goals. The extent the practitioner can be available is determined along six dimensions:

The extent I hold the intent to realise my vision of practice moment by moment

- The extent I know the person
- The extent I am concerned for the person
- The extent I can respond with appropriate and skilled action to meet their health-illness needs
- The extent I am able to manage my involvement within relationship with poise
- The extent I can create and sustain a supportive environment

Of these dimensions, I really sensed the fundamental contradiction between my practice as it was and the holistic way I wanted to be. To acknowledge myself as uncaring was deeply shocking and yet confessing this was a relief. I knew that my clinical gaze had been on the symptoms of 'harm', averting my gaze from the person. I realised during the guided reflection session that I do care about DSH patients, and I did want to develop this area of my practice. Realising that I didn't care for these patients in the way I should was distressing, and even though I may find this research difficult and lay myself open to vulnerability, I care enough about my practice as a whole to resolve this contradiction.

Concern is the motivational expression of caring. Concern creates possibility within the caring relationship [2]. The greater my concern, then the greater the possibility with my relationship with the patient and their family. When a practitioner's concern becomes numbed, then reasons for this can be explored and understood, and concern nurtured to become again a strong passion and motivational force.

The other side of concern is poise. Chris expressed poise as the empathic ability to be fully present yet without taking on board the other's suffering as their own. I could sense the possibility of emotional turmoil if I had opened myself to the DSH patients. No wonder I kept my distance and yet, I do care deeply, it is an aspect of my practice I feel I am good at with other patients. Perhaps that is why I felt bad. I know I have the potential to transform this side of me. My eyes and heart are open.

Reflecting on the environment I recognise the negative attitude to DSH patients is endemic. They are not popular patients. Chris points me towards unpopular patients literature, notably papers by Hughes [3] and Eastwick and Grant [4] entitled 'normal rubbish' – about time wasters in A&E. Do I see DSH as time wasters? Chris challenged me about what I know about DSH. Not much to be honest. So, following the session, suitably motivated I commenced a preliminary exploration of the literature.

DSH is a term used interchangeably with parasuicide. Arguments surround the various terminology used. Fairburn [5] criticises terms such as parasuicide believing they are used to suggest a person's intent to die, when arguably the range of injury a person can carry out upon themselves is wide ranging and not always life threatening. For the purpose of this research, the preferred term is DSH.

Anderson [6, p. 92] also utilised this terminology in a review of self-harm and suicide, stating: 'The term deliberate self-harm encompasses behaviours where the patient can be considered suicidal, such as taking an overdose, self suffocation, self strangulation, wrist cutting, drowning, etc. However the term also used to refer to acts a young person may engage in, but where suicide may not be the intention'.

DSH is one of the top five causes of acute medical admissions for both males and females [7]. With the majority presenting at general hospitals, 150,000 attendances occur per annum [8].

McLaughlin [9, p. 7] notes that 'The casualty department is usually the first port of call for these patients. Such high incidence rates can cause stress on both nursing and medical staff and could influence the attitudes they hold in relation to attempted suicide'.

It is estimated that in the UK, one person every day contemplates suicide [10]. The Government Green paper 'Our healthier nation' outlines targets for the reduction of suicide rates [11]. Research and literature surrounding the attitudes of nurses and other health professionals in both A&E, and surprisingly, psychiatric units, suggest that an improvement in attitudes is needed to improve patient care and reduce suicides. How then is this to be achieved if the literature suggests that attitudes are incongruent with desirable practice? Alston and Robinson [12, p. 206] state that when responding to suicidal patient – 'the nurse may hold attitudes which lead to fear, anxiety, absence of empathy and anger'. I can identify with that.

An article by Fiona Lynn, a woman with a history of self-harm writes – 'Needing stitches was a nightmare. I felt embarrassed and shamed about being stitched up by a nurse whose comments, or lack of comment, made me want the ground to open up to swallow me' [13, p. 56].

Reading these words had a big impact on me. Lynn heard the nurses' attitude without a word being spoken. Her words confronted me to view DSH from a different perspective.

Session 2: Avoidance

I met Chris again four weeks later. I have reconstructed our dialogue from notes Chris made during the session he gave me for verification.

Chris: 'What's happened since we last met?'
Jane: 'Nothing, I have had no contact with any DSH patients'.
Chris: 'Why is that?'
Jane: 'I don't know really, interactions just haven't happened'.
Chris: 'No DSH patients have been through the department when you were on duty?'
Jane: 'Well, yes plenty of patients, there always are, but I was busy with other patients. No, that's not really true. I suppose if I'm honest I've been avoiding them'.
Chris: 'Avoiding them?'
Jane: 'I haven't really thought about it. On reflection I suppose it's easier, isn't it?'
Chris: 'Perhaps you deliberately use avoidance to give you more time to unravel your belief system before you wade in again?'
Jane: 'I admit I have been avoiding them but I haven't analysed why. I do feel that I need to grasp more understanding of the subject. I don't want to hurt anyone by saying the wrong thing'.
Chris: 'I think this period of avoidance is a positive step towards understanding yourself. How do you feel about the two sessions we've had? Any insights emerging for you?'
Jane: 'I can acknowledge my negative prejudice towards DSH patients. It was a relief to admit that I feared the next interaction'.

Reflection

The session began with negative feelings about avoiding contact with DSH patients. During the session, I realised I had been avoiding contact with DSH patients for a specific reason. Chris suggested that I had used avoidance as a mechanism because I needed more time, that it was a step to unravelling my belief system. He realised this period of avoidance was a necessity and that it was significant on my journey of reflection. Carveth [14] believes avoidance is used by nurses when the prospect of a difficult patient arises. Whilst avoidance provides a protective mechanism for the nurse from life and death issues, avoidance can be painful for a patient who may already feel isolated [15].

Having explored the literature, I realise I am not alone. Many nurses have difficulty with this patient group although I mustn't fall back on that as a rationalisation for my negative attitude. The work of Corley and Green [16] identified the way in which nurses stigmatise certain patients, including those who are suicidal. This results in nurses distancing themselves from these patients and minimising the contact they have with them.

Jameton [17] describes this as 'the dark side of nursing' their contact with them. I conclude from Corley and Green's writing that, amongst other reasons, the overriding factor for my thoughts/feelings/actions is my upbringing, my nurse training, and my life as a whole, that have moulded my beliefs and moral opinion. I now understand that I need to view patients and respond beyond the 'label', to see these DSH patients as people, as individuals, needing help.

Chris has challenged me to see examine my boundaries as an A&E nurse, whether my role only required that the damage was 'patched up'? I realised now that I knew my feelings, however, well hidden, are picked up by patients and this ultimately affects their care. Corley and Green [17] cite Younger [18], who suggests that nurses protect themselves from being overwhelmed by suffering by distancing themselves from the sufferer. I feel I distance myself for more than one emotional reason: fear, anger, resentment and lack of empathy come quickly to mind. Distancing myself from patients has certainly been a tactic I have used in the past. I am beginning to understand that I used this as a way of protecting myself.

I felt that one significant issue was a growing sense of empowerment to act according to new beliefs and changed attitudes. As Johns [19] understands it, reflection is first concerned with coming to an understanding of the way things are. Secondly, it is concerned with becoming empowered to change self and practice whereby I can act in tune with my beliefs and values. Thirdly, it is concerned with transformation; the realisation that self has changed and contradiction has been resolved, even as new contradictions emerge. Whilst the 'Being available template' offers me a model to frame my transformed self, Chris suggested an 'empowerment' model might help frame my emergence. He talked through several potential approaches to review. I chose Kieffer's [20] 'Attainment of participatory competence through four phases of involvement framework' (Figure 24.1).

Phase	Development
Era of entry (birth of struggle against conflict)	Birth of emergence of participatory competence. Integrity violated, provoking and mobilising sense of frustration and powerlessness towards an empowering response.
Era of advancement (continuing struggle)	Maturation of empowerment through extension of involvement and deepening understanding through intensive self-reflection with the help of an external enabler.
Era of incorporation (continuing struggle)	Reconstructs sense of self as author and actor in environment. Learning to confront and contend barriers to self-determination leads to a sense of mastery and competence in the individual's sense of being.
Era of commitment (continuing struggle)	Adulthood of participatory competence – integrates new possibilities and insight into reality in meaningful ways.

FIGURE 24.1 Kieffer's framework for participatory competence.
Source: Adapted from [20].

I am currently at what Kieffer terms 'the era of "entry"'. Kieffer explains that an individual who moves through this stage is motivated because they have experienced an emotionally significant or symbolic episode. Particularly significant was the comment that 'the wound must hurt when he cut himself, so why was he worried about the pain of stitches?' Kieffer states that this symbolic event triggers a period of reactive engagement. Chris is the catalyst at this stage, helping me through understanding and my new commitment to convert my negative attitude into a positive attitude, liberating my trapped energy for the task ahead.

Session 3: Moving from Avoidance to Connection

Chris picked up on the issue of avoidance from the last session: 'When we last met you realised that you had been using "avoidance" as a coping mechanism. Has anything new developed?'

I replied that I realised I was using avoidance was a step forward in itself. I acknowledged how I have been using 'avoidance time' to get my thoughts together. Now I want to work out how I would overcome this first hurdle and try and care for DSH patients more in tune with my holistic values. Chris pressed me to be clear about my holistic values – I say 'it is to be available to all my patients irrespective of the cause of their compromised health'.

Chris asked if I have cared for any DSH patients since we last met? Yes I have! In fact I went out of my way to nurse a DSH patient. I spoke to my colleagues on shift and asked if I could 'take' DSH patients. It wasn't what I expected at all. I took the handover of a DSH patient and went into the cubicle explaining what clinical procedures were needed. I acted in a way that I wouldn't have previously. I gave what I hoped was a warm smile. I pushed negative feelings to the side.

Chris interjected 'Just remind me of those feelings you usually experience when dealing with a DSH patient?' I responded that self-harm is a cry for attention, not as 'deserving' as my attention and care as other patients. They are often time wasters when I could be helping someone who really needs it.

Chris noted that we have already discussed why I felt that way. I understand my past experiences had made me feel that way. I do want to do something about it, as hard as it is. I had asked Andrew, the patient, very directly why he had taken the overdose. He said his life was a mess, that his mother didn't care. He was thin, emaciated, and I felt sorry for him.

Chris asked how I felt asking him why he had taken an overdose? I admit I felt very, very clumsy. I stumbled over my words. I felt hot and uncomfortable. In fact I began to relive these feelings with Chris. He recognised and acknowledged this, simply asking

'Why do you think you felt like that?' I said I knew that if Andrew had answered my question, I wouldn't have known how to respond. I didn't do any psychiatric training. I wouldn't be able to fulfil his needs. He might ask for something I cannot give. I would have exposed as a fraud.

Chris pushed me 'What do you usually do when you don't have an answer?'

I said 'Well, I suppose I ask someone for help.'

Chris said 'So, if a DSH patient asks for something you struggle to respond to, you could refer to a colleague to help? Your statement that he might ask for "something I can't give; is significant."'

I paused before answering, pondering the depth of this question. I responded 'I suppose what I really means is that he or she may ask me to understand them, have knowledge of whatever disorder or mental illness they may have. I don't think I have it inside me to understand. I want to change. I want to give more than clinical care, but I find these patients mentally draining. It's scary to think that someone can be so desperate!'

Chris affirmatively reflected back my words: 'Okay, so you feel clumsy but that must have been important to Andrew. He has a past history of this sort of thing?'

I responded, 'Yes, he has done it several times before.'

Chris pushed home the point: 'So what does that tell you? Do you view him less seriously? Or more seriously? You said you felt sorry for him, why?'

'Previously, before looking at the facts and figures in the literature, I would have viewed him as an attention seeker, taken him less seriously than another patient. I have discovered since we last spoke that individuals may inflect harm many times, sometimes over long periods of time. Eventually, a significant number will actually commit suicide, so maybe this helps me understand a little. I felt sorry for him because, apart from his appearance, he was very apologetic, he was compliant with his "clinical care".'

Chris drew links with our previous discussion around the concept of the 'unpopular patient' asking: 'He was a good patient?' I had to admit reluctantly that he was.

Pursuing the point Chris said: 'It's rather interesting that you liked him and stated that he was compliant. Perhaps if he had been non-compliant in some way or "abusive" you may have not liked him, felt so warm towards him'.

Chris reiterated the literature that explored the concept of 'good and bad' patient, notably a paper by Kelly and May [21]. Patients who comply 'do as they are told' by the nurse or doctor. He suggested I might explore this paper. As time was drawing to a close, he asks if there is anything else I want to discuss? I was happy with what we've covered. I think anymore would be too much for me to take in.

Chris recapped: 'Although you felt clumsy, you feel positive about your interaction and feel that you can learn from this experience and move forward? Perhaps you can think of a way to ask patients like Andrew why they have self-harmed in a different way, for example using a "cathartic" approach- asking them what has upset them so much that they felt the need to hurt themselves. Or perhaps a very direct approach is appropriate for a particular patient? John heron's work is a useful reference'.

Jane: 'I think I would be happier to frame the question in a different way but my nerves got the better of me.' I replied: 'I would be happier to frame the question in a different way, but my nerves got the better of me'.

Chris sensed that Andrew didn't mind from what I had told him. He felt the most important thing is that I wanted to ask, and I had asked, breaking through my avoidance and becoming more available to Andrew.

Reflection

This was my first contact with a DSH patient since the interaction I shared in session one. The dialogue reveals that this interaction, although not perfect, was a positive experience. The main clinical issue is my lack of knowledge surrounding psychiatric nursing, although I now feel empowered to change.

Picking up the issues from the session, I have read the work of Kelly and May [21]. They suggest that it is typically assumed that negative attitudes held by nurses, for whatever reason can be corrected through training. However, if negative attitudes had been 'corrected' surely there would not be an abundance of literature highlighting negative attitudes amongst nurses? Sociologists such as Conrad [22] claim patients are treated according to class, attitude or illness. Kelly and May [21, p. 154] state – 'it is unlikely that problems in nurse-patient relationships will prove amenable to simplistic prescriptions because the cause of those problems is endemic of social interaction itself.'

The literature led me to the same answers: 'the answer is not simple', a wider view must be taken, 'medical models' are too rigid. I am constantly led to 'reflexivity'; it would seem that to reflect, to know self, to be open to all possibilities will ultimately resolve my original question and unravel my belief system. Chris suggested that I consider why I liked Andrew and asked if it was because he was apologetic and compliant with his treatment. Trexlar [23, p. 132] described 'difficult' patients as those who are perceived to act in a deviant manner, and that such patients respond by adopting expected role behaviour that results in 'stigma and social isolation that reinforces the original behaviour and may leads to secondary deviance and validation of the nurses judgment of the patient'.

If Trexlar is correct in her assumption, perhaps nurses and society play some part in patients who repeatedly self-harm. Perhaps, as nurses, we perceive such behaviour as unacceptable, and this is picked up by patients who continue with deviant behaviour, or at least they do not know how to respond differently.

Perhaps Andrew tuned into me. He was a young man with a past history of harming himself and who was familiar with the attitudes and responses of medical staff. Perhaps he manipulated the situation by turning himself from 'deviant' to a 'compliant' patient to provoke a caring response. Nievaard [24] cites Kiesler's [25] classification of interpersonal behaviour, describing how attitudes of hospital patients are divided into four main groups:

- Dependent
- Self-reducing
- Cooperative
- Rebellious

Perhaps compliance is a mix of self-reducing and cooperative, whereas deviant is a mix of dependent and rebellious. Recognising my use of negative labels, all labels are perverse because they are linked to a behavioural response.

Whilst understanding that Andrew's compliance did effect my response to him, my response was empathic and this comes from the dawning of understanding. I have learnt that not all individuals who self-harm do so with the intent of dying. The reasons for self-harm vary and it is carried out under differing circumstances across a broad spectrum of individuals [26]. However, as Hawton and will reveal that truth. Hawton and Fagg noted [7, p. 1409] – 'someone who has attempted suicide is a hundred times more likely to commit suicide than the general population within the following year'.

I may never fully understand DSH but I can change how I interact with this patient group. Never before have I asked a patient 'Why?' Perhaps I would have dealt with another less compliant DSH differently? Maybe. New experiences

I feel empowered to bridge the theory-practice gap, as well as being confident to examine myself. I would have said my beliefs did not affect patient care. I now know that my beliefs do affect not only my ability to care. Furthermore, I now believe that previous patients have been aware of my negative feelings, something I would have previously denied.

Session 4: Confronting My Resistance

I shared my experience with a patient who made me feel really angry. Karl had taken an overdose. His notes revealed that he had taken a near fatal overdose 12 months previously. This really brought home the seriousness of Karl's feelings to me. I am attempting to view all DSH patients as 'serious', but it was easier to view Karl seriously because of his history. I went into his cubicle, feeling open, wanting to help, wanting to be cathartic. I asked 'what upset you so much today?' 'Something must have really upset you to do this to yourself.' Karl didn't want to talk to me. He ignored me, he didn't even look at me with his face averted to the wall. I looked at the situation and asked myself 'how is Karl feeling? What is his main concern?' His brother and mother were also in the cubicle so perhaps he didn't want to talk in front of them. I asked if they would mind leaving. I then asked Karl again, and again he ignored me. I asked if he could at least look at me. I felt my anger rising but felt that I managed it well.

Chris asked 'Why did you feel so angry?' I didn't answer so he further asked: 'Was it because he ignored you?'

I replied: 'Yes, that's it and he wouldn't even look at me. There I was making all the effort, a big effort. I felt like I was falling flat on my face. Why was I even bothering? The fact that I wanted to help had no effect on Karl, he wasn't interested.'

Chris affirmed the way I understood and managed my anger. 'What happened next?'

I said I told Karl that I could see he was upset, but if he wanted to talk later I was here. I told him I would come back and see him later and would be available to talk if he wanted to.

Chris again affirmed my response 'So you sent him a very positive message to Karl. You let him know that you cared and were available to him. Are you placing too much emphasis on the fact that he wouldn't talk?'

I sensed that Chris was suggesting I had reacted to being rejected when I had made such an effort. I replied: 'A couple of days later I reflected further on this experience in my journal. I had calmed down by then and realised that one of the reasons I wanted to talk with him because I had a need to understand. I know that Karl's reasons for DSH is not the same as everyone's but I thought he could give me some insight. The other reason for feeling angry was simply that it had taken me courage to offer myself, to make myself available to him, and yes, you're spot on, I did feel rejected. Ego stuff!'

Again Chris was affirmative: 'But you managed yourself within the unfolding moment. You negotiated both your own resistance and Karl's resistance. That's a big change in you'.

Reflection

I now feel happier, more comfortable and appreciate my interaction through new eyes. I understand that I rushed in with a cathartic approach with high expectations. I now realise that's alright that Karl didn't want to talk. It wasn't the right time for him and I can reassure myself that he will have the opportunity to talk when he is ready because, in his case, admission to hospital was required. Again, the empathy I am beginning to feel is in itself motivating me towards achieving more. The most important thing is that Karl knew I cared. I felt I managed my rising anger so it did not affect Karl's care.

My anger came from the fact he didn't need in the way I anticipated. I understand he just needed a caring response and nothing more. My residual negative feelings have evaporated. I can now explore myself at a deeper level and go beyond my anxiety, as if facing a great white shark in a steel cage.

I utilised the 'Being available template' as a way to view myself moving along each of the six factors that determine how available I was with Karl:

Knowing What Is Desirable

I have a much clearer vision in my mind, and aware of my vision within-the-moment – what Chris describes as intentionality, in particular to treat Karl in the caring way I would treat any other patient. Holding a vision is a very powerful idea. It is liberating and makes everything more meaningful. I wonder why I have not thought about before. I sense it is because my practice is driven by tasks to do around symptoms and treatments rather than by values and knowing the person.

Knowing the Person

I made a huge effort to connect with Karl. Perhaps on reflection, it was an unpolished effort but the intent to know him as a person was there. Chris had informed me of the Buford reflective cues (see Chapter 6). The first two cues are:

- Who is this person?
- What meaning does this health event have for the person?

These cues are helpful guides. However, in A&E, when someone is admitted in a life-threatening condition, the emphasis is on saving lives. In my experience with Karl, we had moved beyond that phase. Knowing the person is informed by ideas from DSH literature, and that helps me understand why Karl may have withdrawn and turn his head away from me as he did. I shouldn't have expected him to be compliant like Andrew. All people are unique sand respond differently, yet my tendency has been to categorise people – 'DSH patients'.

Concern for the Person

It is interesting the way my vision fuels my concern. I was genuinely concerned for Karl. He really did matter to me and yet I could see how my own concerns were getting in the way – that I became concerned for myself as reflected through my sense of being rejected.

Knowing and Managing Self's Involvement with the Person (poise)

My experience informs me that poise is a precarious thing – why else did I feel anger and yet I could contain it within the moment. This awareness is a new thing for me. As Ramos [27] noted, the blocks to therapeutic relationships with patients are due to issues of emotion and control. Before I had kept my distance through labelling and aversion and now I felt entangled, as if I do not know to respond on a cathartic level. I am experiencing a great sense of motivation.

In understanding and managing my own concerns, I was more able to negotiate my own resistance as well as his resistance to me. I could see that both Karl and myself resisted each other because I had not tuned into his wavelength adequately. As Chris suggested, I need to imagine a space between Karl and Myself so I can see these things unfolding, yet remain available to Karl even as he resists me.

The Aesthetic Response

I feel I walk a tightrope of learning new skills of being available to a DSH patient. I imagine such skills are transferable between patients but I know otherwise because of the emotional context. I recognise that to be available to Karl, I first had to be available to myself – poised, confident, and skilful, especially in catharsis.

Creating and Sustaining an Environment Where Being Available is Possible

I tried to provide the best environment in the given circumstances.

He was in a private cubicle. I asked his relatives to leave allowing him and I let him know that I wanted to care for him. I am aware I have not yet explored attitudes to DSH patients with my colleagues and yet that is vital to change our collective practice. I accept that responsibility bat a later stage. But first I must get my own house in order.

Session 5: Nurturing My Concern

I was looking forward to sharing and examining my thoughts and feelings with Chris in session 5, because I felt I had made real progress. Chris started the session by asking what I had share since our last meeting. First, I shared my insights about the DSH literature I had explored. Then a new experience – a man in his forties who has taken a large overdose. He had visited his estranged wife and when she refused to let him into the house he sat down in her garden and took a massive overdose. She wasn't aware that he was still in the garden and some hours later a passer-by called an ambulance. To say that 'I interacted with him is debateable. I carried out his clinical care but he was unconscious, quite ill in fact, so I didn't actually speak to him'.

Chris asked how I felt about the man. I felt really sad. Sad that he felt so desperate. Sad that he could die. Sad that maybe he didn't mean to kill himself. Perhaps he just wanted his partner to come outside and talk. I felt sad that his estranged wife would probably feel guilty and blame herself. Just incredibly sad. Then I saw the seriousness of DSH, the desperation, and the waste.

Chris said 'This is new for you, this sympathy?'

I had felt sad when DSH patients have died in the past, but perhaps not as sad as, for example, a victim of a road traffic accident or a child. I feel different now. Reflection has made me feel different about all sorts of things, not just in the workplace; its bigger than that! A combination of these sessions, keeping a journal and learning about DSH are beginning to affect my thought processes and the way I interact with this patient group.

Reflection

This experience was very significant. I found myself caring for this man at a time when everything I've been thinking about is falling into place. Through understanding, my whole attitude is changing. My belief system and moral opinion is being replaced by new values, brought about these profound insights.

I now consider I have entered Kieffer's second stage 'Era of advancement'. Kieffer [20] identified three quite distinct and necessary elements needed to successfully move into this stage:

1. The focus and stability of a mentoring relationship as reflected in my relationship with my supervisor – Chris has been extremely stable and has focused on relevant and significant issues.
2. The supportive peer relationships within a collective organisational structure. Most of my peers have been curious and supportive of my research. I hope that my research on an individual level will induce a collective action towards change.
3. Critical understanding of social and political relations that I have gained through critically exploring the DSH Literature, giving me a deeper understanding of DSH.

I would add that this stage is marked by a non-return to previous ways of being. I am mindful of myself with SH patients to revert to previous ways of being. Such is the power of insight to change me.

Session 6: Realising Right Attitude

Chris started by reviewing our last session and asking about new interactions. I felt very comfortable, relaxed and exhilarated. I had been waiting to tell Chris about another interaction with a DSH patient that had gone really well.

A young man in his twenties. He arrived in the early hours of the morning, he had taken some paracetamol tablets, not many, but he was very distressed. He kept saying sorry and apologising for wasting the nurses' time. I found that instead of offering no reply to this statement or giving a half-hearted 'you're not wasting anyone's time' I actually wanted to talk to him. I sensed he wanted to talk; he had financial worries and girlfriend problems. It all tumbled out very quickly. I was only supposed to be carrying out triage, – a two- to three-minute assessment to categorise his problem that dictates how quickly someone should be seen by a doctor. But I found myself talking to him for at least 15 minutes. The department was not busy, so instead of handing his care over to someone else, I took him into a cubicle and continued to talk. At all times during my interaction, I was aware of my concern for him. I felt tender towards him. I had a strong desire to help by simply listening. I know he appreciated my concern for him and I know he felt my concern was genuine. He had to stay in the department for several hours waiting for results of blood tests before he was assessed by a doctor who discharged him. His friend was going to stay with him overnight and ensure he attended an out-patients appointment in the morning.

Chris felt this was a very positive experience. He asked: 'Why do you think you wanted to talk with him, what surfaced your concern, why did you feel tender?'

I expect my reply sounded rather glib: I was conscious of reflecting within the moment, of reading his pattern. The more concern I felt the better I felt. I wasn't hiding anything from myself. I viewed him as a person not as a condition. Using the Buford model cues, I ask myself 'Who is this person?' 'What does he need for me at this moment?', 'How can I help him?' These cues help me to focus on him as a suffering human being and able to transcend any lingering prejudice I have for people who deliberately self-harm.

The word suffering is Chris's word – he feels suffering encompasses the whole person and doesn't discriminate in that we all suffer to varying extent. The word is evocative of compassion, that the carer's human response to suffering is compassion.

Reflection

I am happier now I am more available to patients. My belief system is very different from when I commenced this self-inquiry. Focusing on the third element of the Being Available Template – 'concern for the person', I am more motivated to care, to express my empathy and am discovering that such expression opens up new possibilities for the relationships I develop with DSH patients. While I believe my care remains balanced. I am discovering that the more I 'give' the more I 'get' from shared relationships. My beliefs and values have been exposed and examined for their meaning and relevance. My response to DSH patients has changed: there is a positive shift towards more congruent practice.

Session 7: Knock Back

Commencing session 7 I was feeling quite 'down' about my recent experiences but felt comfortable enough about my relationship with Chris to discuss what I considered to be fairly negative interactions.

I said: 'I feel as if I've taken two steps forward and three back! I don't know where to start. I've had what I consider a very negative experience and a positive one, and I don't understand why. I know that I shouldn't blame myself, but I do feel guilty about the negative interaction I had'.

Chris suggested I start with the negative experience first.

'Well, the shift was really busy; it was over the New Year period that a young girl presented in the department after taking an overdose. Her friend had recently committed suicide. She was hysterical, I could not calm her down. At the start of our interaction, I reminded myself that here was a young girl who had lost a friend in traumatic circumstances. As I already said the shift was busy, and there were other patients close by who were very ill. To be fair to this patient and other patients, I needed to calm her down. I had conflicting priorities; my other patients needed a quiet calm atmosphere, but I needed to take control with this young girl but I was failing. The more hysterical she became the more irritation I felt, my anger was rising up inside me. I thought she was silly, a "drama queen". Obviously I understood she was grieving for her friend, but I was under pressure, it was two o'clock in the morning, and I think alcohol a part to play in her behaviour'.

Chris said 'So she wasn't a "good" patient then?'

'No! Her father wasn't any help either! He had also been drinking and their relationship did not come across as particularly close. I hoped the father would calm her down, but he seemed to cause yet more hysteria. I felt she needed to be told her behaviour was unacceptable. I told her I wanted to help but couldn't if she wouldn't let me. Nothing I tried worked. As I felt I had made no connection with her and that I could not manage my feelings or was responding in the patient's best interests, I felt it best to hand over her care to someone else, to remove myself from the situation. It was best for the patient and myself to be removed from the situation. She was moved away from the poorly patients. The second nurse was firmer than I was, the girl eventually calmed down, I don't know what happened after that.'

Chris wondered if I had adopted a parental role with her because her mother was absent and her father useless? Whether I had taken on the role of a critical mother to tell her off?

I felt Chris's challenge. I am learning his tongue in cheek style of guidance of gentle but astute confrontation. Being positive to his challenge I responded 'No, I wasn't conscious of taking on a parental role but, being a mother myself, it is an easy role to fall into. Anyway, if I did unconsciously take on a parental role it didn't work, did it? I didn't even get to the point of thinking about deliberate harm!'

Chris asked about the other patient I had mentioned.

'This is where my confusion lies. A few days later another young girl, about the same age came into the department. She was at school, bought in by the class teacher; she had taken a small overdose. I was completely different with her, I was able to talk with her, let her know my concern was genuine.

Chris asked what factors made this interaction so different?

"It was a day shift 9 or 10 in the morning and quiet in the department. I had time"'.

He asked if I thought the busyness of the department made a difference in the way DSH patients are treated?

'I'd like to say no but every ward, every department works under pressure. When it's busy it's impossible to give that little bit more. As awful as that sounds, time is an influencing factor. We all try to make time, to make the most of our time, but sometimes it isn't often enough'.

Chris asked if any research supported that idea and I was able to cite a significant literature that pointed to the influence of time on practitioners' attitudes towards DSH patients. Chris picked up this point, noting that having time affected me with the second girl. He wondered if it being a day shift, I was more receptive to her needs because I wasn't tired as I can be on night duty? Certainly having time, I did not feel the pressure of competing demand. I was able to ask her why she had self-harmed and we discussed other things that she could have done instead of taking the tablets. She had taken them because her mum wouldn't let her visit her boyfriend the night before. I don't think she did it to manipulate her mum, I think she did it because she so desperate about not seeing him. She agreed that a preferable course of action would have been to talk to someone; a nurse, a teacher, her mum, or a friend. I think she actually learnt from the experience, she took something positive away with her.

Chris asked if I had adopted a parental role? In this case I had yet this was ok because she was frightened; she needed comforting. Chris agreed, noting that the parent–child pattern of communication [within Transactional Analysis] can be therapeutic when the practitioner is mindful of adopting that pattern rather than simply reacting to the situation because it evokes a maternal response and yes, my response was reactive – I see your point that emotional reaction reflects the way I had absorbed the girl's suffering as a mother does for her child and may have obscured appropriate decision making. So – what accounts for the difference in my response to these two young girls? The first girl outside my emotional limits the second girl within them. I feel bad.

Chris twisted this around, suggesting that my first experience was also positive because I learnt from it? I said 'That's perhaps a better way to look at it'.

Reflection

My response to the second patient was more congruent with my newly developed values. With the first patient, within the unfolding moment I felt I could not manage my own concerns and care for the patient. It was in the patient's best interests to receive care from another nurse. She deserved better. I feel good about that now with hindsight. At the time I felt I had failed her and worse, failed myself.

In exploring the variables of the session with Chris, we recognised the impact of time and workload, and time of day as significant. Greenwood and Bailey [28] state that the majority of DSH patients present to A&E departments 'out of hours' confirmed by an audit of DSH time presentation. They suggest this may contribute towards negative attitudes due to difficulty in accessing psychiatric services 'out of hours'. My own experience also confirms this fact. This means that on a night shift it is typical to care for at least one DSH patient. During the night shift 'enthusiasm' may not be at the same level as during the day thus leading to a more negative approach and being less available to these patients.

The human response it to critique each other on meeting for the first time. McLaughlin [9, p. 1111] states –

> 'Nursing can readily lend itself to the rapid formation of attitudes towards those who come into contact with it'.

McLaughlin further suggests that initial contact, in addition to confidential information about the patient, can lead to negative attitudes that influence the quality of care and jeopardising the development of a therapeutic relationship. This I know for myself as reflected vividly through my self-inquiry. The focus of my self-inquiry has largely been on my relationships with DSH patients and yet the environment of care – issues, such as time, attitudes of staff, workload, time of day, the quality of the physical environment are all significant in my being available. Without doubt, the young girl benefitted from being moved from the 'resus' room to another. The resus is a large room equipped with several beds used for patients requiring life saving interventions. The resus room may have been very frightening for her, not ideal for intimate conversation about life and death. Moving her into a single room provided privacy for both her and her family but also for the other patients. She also benefitted from a nurse who was able to manage her own concerns and was tuned into the girl.

A few days later I met another girl, also around 15 years old who had overdosed. This time I was happy with the way I responded and cared for her. I was able to do this because of the insights gained through guided reflection.

Mezirow [29, p. 223] (extracted from a pile of papers on reflective practice that Chris suggested I read) noted:

> 'Our meaning structures are transformed through reflection, defined here as attending to the grounds (justification) of one's beliefs. We reflect on the unexamined assumptions of our beliefs when the beliefs are not working well with us, or where old ways of thinking are no longer functional. We are confronted with a disorientating dilemma, which serves as a trigger for reflection. Reflection involves a critique of assumptions to determine whether the belief, often acquired through assimilation in childhood, remains functional for us adults. We do this by critically examining its origins, nature and consequences'.

My belief system had not been working for me. This triggered reflection has changed the meaning in the way I deal with patients. This meaning is revised and is still changing with each experience and new knowledge. This is made valid by the very fact that the next interaction provoked a caring response. Obviously, variables are different. It was during the day. Quite early in the shift, the workload was light and I could concentrate on her care. Throughout my interaction, I remembered the other teenager. Again, I was dealing with a girl verging on hysteria, quite difficult to deal with; our interaction could easily spiralled into a negative experience for both of us. However, whilst managing my own concerns I successfully met her needs. I no longer fear involvement with such patients. As Benner and Wrubel [2] believe, connecting with my caring is one of the most effective coping resources.

Deeper Reflection

From the outset of this self-inquiry, I was concerned that any changes I made to my practice in relation to DSH patients would leave me vulnerable. Benner and Wrubel [2] believe that emotions can no longer be viewed as interruptions. By this, they mean emotions have significance and content in their own right and that respect for knowledge and wisdom is gained if the individual allows their emotions to direct their thoughts and attention. They state –

> 'Attending to emotion offers the possibility of bringing past interpretation of the situation into the present, where past history can be reinterpreted and reconstituted' (p. 96).

How true. As a result of my understanding about my beliefs, a host of factors including cultural and religious beliefs emerged that influenced the way I was responding to DSH patients. Being brought up in a predominantly Christian society with strong cultural beliefs about self-harm and suicide has impacted on me. As recently as 1961, suicide and attempted suicide fell into the same category as murder and there were a number of prosecutions.

Decriminalisation in 1966 did not lead to any great change in the prevailing Christian ethic even as the world became more secular. As McLaughlin [9, p. 1112] states –

> 'In the Judeo-Christian cultures there has always been a belief that suicide is reprehensible and ethically wrong'.

Other factors contributing to my previous belief system included my experiences with DSH patients. Now I can see that these relationships were always tinged with anger. Accepting my mother's failing health and the seriousness of her condition dissolved some of my anger. I recognised that because I worked in an acute area, I had fallen into a trap of measuring, quantifying, prioritising patients and their conditions. Fear that lacks of knowledge would make a bad situation worse played a part in my incongruent practice.

Creating a Positive Attitude Environment

Later I convened a debate with my A&E colleagues in response to their interest in my study. They were divided in their own feelings about DSH patients. Whilst some felt they firmly understood and treated the patient group in exactly the same way they would any other. I wonder if they distort their reality? It is not easy to face up to uncaring. Some found themselves, perhaps like myself somewhere in the middle, lacking real knowledge of self-harm and experiencing difficulty in caring for such patients. Some felt that DSH were time wasters and manipulated both nurses and the medical system. One colleague stated that she was 'resigned' to nursing DSH patients. I asked her to explain and she said that the only DSH patients we met were those in crisis. She further explained that we never saw patients who got better or recovered. The comments made were similar to those documented by Anderson et al. [30] on the attitude of medical staff towards the suicidal. These authors state –

'Nurses and doctors do not support the notion that suicidal behaviour reflects mental illness' (p. 8).

One staff nurse who took part in the research commented –

'Sometimes I think they are timewasters – occasionally, and quite selfish. If you have good reason to self-harm that's that ... but if not then I think it's quite selfish'

These were some of my own thoughts prior to my self-inquiry. The debate with my colleagues enabled thoughts and feelings to rise to the surface and whilst I was not able to change my colleague's opinions, perhaps a seed was sown, a seed that may surface later at a time that is right for the individual to address their own contradictions. When others choose to address their own contradictions, perhaps a paradigm shift from the normal approach to a different approach will occur. If and when this happens, a paradigm shift from the normal medical approach to a holistic approach will occur. The debate helped prepare the ground for growth.

Anderson et al. [30, p. 2] suggested that attitudes towards DSH patients are complex, multidimensional, and the interaction between nurse and patient will depend on the belief system of each other. Repper [31, p. 11] discussed the important role of A&E staff with DSH patients – 'Poor information and communication systems, lack of knowledge about suicide; negative attitudes towards people who self-harm does not help the rising number of patients presenting with DSH ... A&E staff must become more involved with education/training where negative attitudes are challenged'.

My insights into my practice with DSH patients have significantly shifted my practice. I am mindful.

As I interact with these patients, and more genuinely available to them. I hope that my research will challenge others towards enabling others to find a more therapeutic way of responding to DSH patients in A&E.

Without reflection I could go no further than to superficially question this contradiction I had ignored and yet bubbled uncomfortably beneath my calm, confident surface. Chris had challenged me earlier to identify the nurses' role in A&E. Is it holistic or merely patch work? I take the view it is holistic. I know better that my response to the DSH patient does makes a difference; that compassion and non-judgmental acceptance works better than indifference or worse, rejection and thinly veiled contempt.

Moss [32, p. 616] states –

'If nursing is to attain the status of an independent profession it must identify and rectify the factors that influence nursing attitudes'.

Only when practitioners like myself resolve contradiction can they realise their visions of practice as a lived reality and lead more satisfactory lives. In acknowledging and confronting my prejudice, I have discovered myself as a person and that this, in itself, naturally leads to 'tuning' into others and their needs. It is astonishing to realise such self-neglect and yet I sense that nurse education gives little emphasis to developing and sustaining effective therapeutic relationships, especially with what be construed as the 'difficult' patient.

All experience is positive if we can learn from it. My learning has travelled a full circle, described by Gadamer [33] as an oscillating cycle that continuously evolves.

My empowerment to act came from within because I could no longer live with the contradiction, once that protective veneer had been torn off within guided reflection with Chris. I had a choice to retreat or push forward. But in reality, I had no choice because where would I have retreated to? My cover was blown!

So, I chose to push forward, to face up to my vulnerability with the challenge and support from Chris.

As Kieffer [20] clearly acknowledges in his framework of participatory competence, the role of the external enabler is vital (see Chapter 8). As Johns (2004) notes 'it is not easy to see beyond the normal self'.

Emancipation, or the realisation of my changed self was affirmed quite recently. Through understanding myself I became empowered to transform my practice.

My arms around a woman in great distress, crying a steady stream if tears, suddenly I realised I genuinely cared. I had not needed to prompt myself about the best verbal response. We were talking as I carried out clinical observations but I was so 'in tune' with this woman I instinctively knew what she wanted from me. I sat next to her and her tears began. She physically moved towards me; I believe she sensed my empathy and genuineness. As I circled her in my arms, I felt emotional, I felt sadness for her but realised the truth in Ramos's words [27, p. 504] – 'nurses described an emotional identification which was real, not devastating to the nurse, but a motivator'.

I felt very positive as if a burden had been lifted from my shoulders. Ramos describes such a relationship as a reciprocal relationship and the very cornerstone of nursing care. I wanted to hold this woman because she needed me to hold her and I felt very comfortable doing so. With this interaction came the realisation that I had moved through the 'Era of incorporation' and attained entered Kieffer's [20] final stage – 'Era of commitment'. Kieffer believes that individuals may struggle at the stage as they try to integrate personal knowledge and skills into everyday situations. The reader will already be aware of my struggle to integrate newly acquired knowledge through shared dialogue and patient interaction. Maybe I am being optimistic about reaching this level of participatory competence. It has, after all, been a relatively short journey. My 'new self' is still to be tested for its robustness in face of more difficult interactions.

Commentary

Jane's narrative reveals her living contradiction between her values 'what she came into nursing to do' and the reality of her negative attitude towards DSH patients. Through guided reflection she strives to unpick her attitude, to understand it and transform it. It was not easy learning. Her narrative also reveals the impact of guided reflection in enabling her through reconstructing dialogue with her guide. It is courageous and committed work.

References

1. Watson, J. (1999) *Post-Modern Nursing and Beyond.* Churchill Livingstone, Edinburgh.

2. Benner, P., Wrubel, J. (1989) *The Primacy of Caring.* Addison-Wesley, Menlo Park.

3. Hughes, D. (1979) Normal rubbish: deviant patients in casualty departments. *Sociology of Health and Illness* 1, 90–107.

4. Eastwick, Z., Grant, A. (2004) Emotional rescue: deliberate self-harmers and A&E departments. *Mental Health Practice* 7(9), 12–15.

5. Fairburn, G. (1995) *Contemplating Suicide: The Language and Ethics of Self-Harm.* Routledge London.

6. Anderson, M. (1999) Waiting for harm: deliberate self-harm and suicide in young people – a review of the literature. *Journal of Psychiatric and Mental Health Nursing* 6, 91–100.

7. Hawton, K., Fagg, J. (1992) Trends in deliberate self-poisoning and self-injury in Oxford 1976–1990. *British Medical Journal* 304, 1409–1411.

8. Hawton, K., Catlin, J. (1997) *Attempted Suicide: A Practical Guide to Its Nature and Management.* Oxford University Press.

9. McLaughlin, C. (1994) Casualty nurses attitudes to attempted suicide. *Journal of Advanced Nursing* 20, 1111–1118.

10. McLaughlin, C. (1991) Parasuicide counselling in casualty departments. *Nursing Standard* 6, 15.

11. Department of Health (1998) Our healthier nation; a contract for health. HMSO (London).

12. Alston, M., Robinson, B. (1992) Nurses' attitudes towards suicide. *Omega* 25(3), 205–215.

13. Lynn, F. (1998) The pain of rejection. *Nursing Times* 94, 27.

14. Carveth, J. (1995) Perceived patient deviance and avoidance by nurses. *Nursing Research* 44, 173–178.

15. Eldrid, J. (1988) *Caring for the Suicidal*. Constable, London.

16. Corley, M., Goren, S. (1998) The dark side of nursing: impact of stigmatizing responses on patients. *Scholarly Inquiry for Nursing Practice* 12, 99–121.

17. Jameton, A. (1992) *Nursing Ethics and the Moral Situation of the Nurse*. American Hospital Publishing, Chicago.

18. Younger, J. (1995) The alienation of the sufferer. *Advances in Nursing Science* 17, 53–72.

19. Johns, C. (2004) *Becoming A Reflective Practitioner* (second edition). Blackwell Publishing, Oxford.

20. Kieffer, C. (1984) Citizen empowerment: a developmental perspective. *Prevention in Human Sciences*, 84, 9–36.

21. Kelly, P., May, D. (1982) Good and bad patients: a review of the literature and a theoretical critique. *Journal of Advanced Nursing* 7, 147–156.

22. Conrad, P. (1979) Types of medical social control. *Sociology of Health and Illness* 1, 1–10.

23. Trexlar, T. (1996) Reformulation of deviance and labeling theory for nursing. *Image: Journal of Nursing Scholarship* 28, 131–136.

24. Nievaard, A. (1987) Communication climate and patient care: causes and effects of nurses' attitudes to patients. *Social Science and Medicine* 24, 777–784.

25. Kiesler, D. J. (1983) The 1982 interpersonal circle: a taxonomy for complementarity in human transactions. *Psychological Review* 90, 185–214.

26. Roberts, D. (1996) Suicide prevention by general nurses. *Nursing Standard* 17, 30–33.

27. Ramos, M. (1992) The nurse-patient relationship: theme and variations. *Journal of Advanced Nursing* 17, 496–506.

28. Greenwood, S., Bradley, P. (1997) Managing deliberate self-harm: the A&E perspective. *Accident & Emergency Nursing* 5, 134–136.

29. Mezirow, J. (1981) A critical theory of adult learning and education. *Adult Education* 32, 3–24.

30. Anderson, M., Standen, P., Nazir, S., Noon, J. (1999) Nurses' and doctors' attitudes towards suicidal behaviour in young people. *International Journal of Nursing Studies* 37, 1–10.

31. Repper, J. (1999) A review of literature on the prevention of suicide through interventions in Accident and emergency departments. *Journal of Clinical Nursing* 8, 3–12.

32. Moss, A. (1988) Determinants of nursing care: nursing process or nursing attitudes. *Journal of Advanced Nursing* 13, 615–620.

33. Gadamer, H.-G. (1979) *Truth and Method* (second edition). Sheed and Ward, London.

Note

i. See Chapter 14.

PART 4

The Performance Turn

First, there was the reflective turn. Then, the narrative turn and then the performance turn.

CHAPTER 25

Jane's Rap: Performing Jane's Journey Towards Shifting Her Attitude to Deliberate Self-harm Patients in an Accident and Emergency Department

Introduction

Clare's reflexive narrative 'Life begins at 40' (Chapter 18) has a rhythm whereby she could easily perform her narrative. Imagine her sitting on a stool reciting the narrative to an audience. Before she commences, she invites the audience to dialogue with her. As she reads, she moves about the stage. Perhaps she engages others to act out different scenes. Perhaps she uses images as background or even music. She pauses at certain moments to heighten the impact of what she is saying, giving the audience a moment to reflect and digest. She draws her audience into the performance. This is significant in terms of the audience dialoguing with and gaining their own insights. As Mattingly [1, p. 8] notes –

> 'It [narrative] casts events in a particular light that allow the audience to infer something about what it is really like to be in that story ... it persuades by seducing the listener or reader into the world it portrays, unfolding events in a suspense-laden time in which one wonders what will happen next'.

Performing narrative is creating drama to engage its audience. Art, poetry, metaphor and music embellish and create drama. Quotes from literature can be screened and read silently by the audience to absorb rather than spoken. Posing questions is another strategy to create pause, breaking the monological flow. Following pauses, the audience are more expectant of what follows. Music might be background music. It can be an aspect of the performance where the performer pauses and plays some music integral to the text. For example, I introduce the performance of 'My mother's death' [2] by playing Jim Reeves song 'Welcome to my world'. Jim Reeves was my mother's favourite music and the words 'welcome to my world' depict moving from her home into a care home and ultimately her death following a fall and broken leg. As such, the music creates an immediate mood. 'Live' music can accompany a performance as if a play between music and words whereby the music extemporises in dialogue with the text.[i] Performance is a more active way of dialoguing with an audience rather than reading the narrative. It opens a dialogical clearing where meaning can be contested through dialogue with its audience, as an active part of the performance. Gray, Ivanoffski and Sinding [3, p. 57] note –

> 'Audience members thus become co-producers of the drama, not through action, but through the meanings they bring to the performance and the meanings they construct from the performance'.

Dialoguing with an audience opens a further level of reflection. The author may have implanted potential insights into their narrative they are not aware of. The audience can read between lines, pick up clues, use their imagination and pursue them, challenging the practitioner's interpretation of their reality.

Someone reading a narrative cannot easily dialogue directly with the practitioner unless an on-line facility to facilitate communication is set up, whereas audience feedback from performance creates the opportunity for practitioners to get a sense of the impact of their work on their audience [4].

Performing narrative is listened through the senses. It enables an audience to sense the author's experience and insights, moving beyond a cognitive to a more embodied and emotional understanding. It is more intense and immediate than reading a narrative that draws more on the rational mind. It enables the practitioner to sense their own insights and express their associated feelings more dramatically than the written word.

To compare the impact of reading and listening to the same narrative, I arranged for four conference attendees[ii] to read my narrative prior to performing it. The four people all agreed that listening was a different experience to reading. It was more intense, more visceral, more engaging plus the benefit of ensuing face to face dialogue.

The audience can be primed to view the performance as the 'spark' to reflect on their own experiences leading to a sharing of stories. Park-Fuller [5] terms this as 'Playback theatre' as participatory viewing. This opens the gateway to social action so that when the audience departs, they have a strong sense of how the performance and dialogical engagement might impact on their own practice.

To help 'spark', I pause and prod the audience, to disturb them with my words and voice and voices of others. I deliberately emphasise what I feel are particular aspects of the narrative to focus and disturb the audience and create dilemmas in their mind. Some of the audience may well take offence if the narrative challenges their own sacred cows!

The audience may ask – 'What was all that about?' And I answer 'What do you think it is about'? In other words, performing narrative does not intend to be a passive experience. If so, I have failed. However, some audiences can be so passive no amount of enticing can stir them.

I know that audience can struggle to dialogue, as if overwhelmed by what they have experienced. Perhaps they are intimidated by the expectation to engage in dialogue. I usually give the audience a short break following the performance to digest it, giving some time to process what they have experienced. It is not necessarily easy for an audience to respond immediately to what they have just experienced especially when they are expected to respond. I often ask the audience prior to the performance to note just one or two things about which they might like to dialogue. This also encourages the audience to pay more attention. Active audience participation opens a way into dialogue by asking those who participate to reflect on their participation and then opening up to the whole audience. A useful technique especially when dialogue is stifled.

The very nature of reflection is to expose the conditions that underlie and influence everyday practice, notably those conditions that constrain realising one's vision. Thus, the practitioner is mindful that their narrative and performance is political. As Madison [6, p. 277] asserts, performance is

> 'An act involving potential struggles and negotiations over meanings, identity and power. A site where the performance of possibilities occur'.

The focus of dialogue is 'How can the contradictions between practice as exposed and the practitioner's vision within the performance be reconciled?' not just for the performer but also for the audience to co-create insights that move the audience to take action.

Viewing the narrative as a call for social action may seem extreme for the student writing a reflective assignment but even so, it is worth the student bearing in mind the wider potential authority of their narrative towards social action.

As Jane noted in the previous chapter –

> 'I hope that my research will challenge others towards enabling others to find a more therapeutic way of responding to DSH patients in A&E'.

Left written on a shelf Jane's assignment would simply gather dust. Being published, it exposed it to a wider audience [7]. As a performance that has been performed widely, both nationally and internationally, it invokes dialogue and subsequently more influential.[iii]

Jane's Rap

Introduction

I constructed Jane's rap as a performance narrative from her undergraduate post-registration dissertation (Chapter 24). Narrative privileges the narrator's voice. Thus, the voices of the self-harm patients referred to in Jane's dissertation were not heard. Logistically, it would be difficult for the self-harm patients to voice their own perspectives but perhaps not impossible if the narrative was initially conceived as a collaborative working with the persons involved from the outset.

In the performance, I give voice to the self-harm patients through empathic poems composed by Colleen Marlin who gives their voices a neutrality. The poems invoke a real sense of the self-harm patients' experiences. They heighten the sense of drama and open up perspective to the performance.

Jane's rap has been performed in conference, educational and workshop situations. My preferred approach is to recruit eight people to represent the eight voices of the self-harm patients. These have been both psychiatric nursing and drama students. The stage is arranged in a spiral with eight chairs. As I read the text, I move from chair to chair as the co-performer reads the poem. The performance is structured through the eight guided reflection sessions between Jane and myself as her guide. Note – quotes in italics are shown on a power-point to be read by the audience. This creates silent moments for the audience to digest. Thirty minutes is allocated for ensuing dialogue.

The text is constructed as a sequence of lines. In the performance, I pause briefly at the end of each line as if to open up the spaces between the lines for the audience to sense.

Jane is performed by one person. A second person (optional) could perform as 'Chris' to emphasise the process of guided reflection.

Pp 1>

Jane's Rap

A journey through guided reflection towards shifting her attitude towards deliberate self-harm patients within an accident and Emergency department.

The students enter and sit in their allocated chairs accompanied by music. When all are seated, I move onto the stage.

Pp 2> Session 1

Reflection has become meaningful for me.
Anxieties about my attitude towards deliberate self-harm patients trigger this self-inquiry.
I tell a story.
'Night shift, around 3 in the morning.
This man, he had deliberately cut his arm.
Needing sutures.
I recoiled.
I tried to hide my feelings but felt empty.
No compassion.
He asked if it would hurt.
My irritation bubbling to the surface
'Must have hurt when you did it' I retorted
What a wanker!
Such a waste of time stitching him up.
Can't waste compassion it would only encourage him to do it again and again.......'
Chris asks 'Could you act differently? Did you prejudge him? Stereotype him? Are some patients more worthy of care than others?'
He's put me on the spot.
Does he want a confession?
But then I know I should have treated him with compassion and that I didn't bothers me.
Chris asks 'Is this too upsetting?'
I answer 'No, well, yes a bit.'
Chris inquires 'What is your role, what are your values? Do you merely patch up or care?'
Shifting uneasily in my seat, I mumble something like 'The environment doesn't help.'
It's a lame excuse. He knows it too. The lid is off. Do I expect absolution?
Do I patch up or care?
I sense the cutter's blade and shiver.

CHAIR 1

I find myself here, bleeding and scared,
Wondering if I've gone too far.

'Will it hurt' I ask,
unable to bear more pain.
Too much already
An interminably long night of it
Until the blade offered respite
Sweet, however briefly

She gives 'the look'
I can't alienate her
Fear I already have
She thinks I must like pain
To do this,
But she sleeps at night
Soft, empty,
In a peace I rarely touch

Voices in my head won't let me
Images I can't shake
Somersault of flailing limbs
Kick my feet out from under
Until I look to the blade
To find where I am
In the heart of the mess

She probably takes an aspirin for her rare headache
Aspirin doesn't begin to touch the roar in my skull
No volume button on the noise
Too loud too much too hard

That determined black dog,
I'm at its mouth, in its bite, vulnerable ...
The blade
The only tool to cut myself loose from
Being chewed to death

She probably thinks I want to die
When all I want is peace
A minute without
The press of what comes at me ...

She thinks I like pain
In truth, I can't stand any more
And to silence it,
I cut, I tear, decidedly, determinedly,
To feel something
As normal and comfortable
As the touch of metal to skin
Cold sharp
Beautiful, for a second to feel that ...

With the blade in skin, the roar softens, bearable ....
And now, I want to disappear myself
Or her, looking at me as she is
As if I am scum
And have no right to drip my blood
On her polished, pristine floor.

Looking back – it's amazing that – talking for an hour can turn my world upside down.
Dormant concerns spring to life, my negative prejudice to DSH patients exposed. Wrapped up in self-concern I was not available to him.
Chris inquires 'How much do you know about self-harm?'
I answer 'Not a lot. I need to know more.'

Pp 3>

'The term deliberate self-harm encompasses behaviours where the patient can be considered suicidal, such as taking an overdose, self suffocation, self strangulation, wrist cutting, drowning, etc. However the term also used to refer to acts a young person may engage in, but where suicide may not be the intention' [8, p. 92].

Pp 4>

'The casualty department is usually the first port of call for these patients. Such high incidence rates can cause stress on both nursing and medical staff and could influence the attitudes they hold in relation to attempted suicide' [9].

Pp 5>

'Fiona Lynn a woman with a history of self-harm' writes – 'Needing stitches was a nightmare. I felt embarrassed and shamed about being stitched up by a nurse whose comments, or lack of comment, made me want the ground to open up to swallow me' [10, p. 56].

Fiona Lynn's words speak to me.
She heard the nurses' attitude without a word being spoken.
It helps me view things from a different perspective, hitting home the point.

Pp 6> Session 2

Chris inquires 'What's happened since we last met?'
I answer 'Nothing, I have had no contact with any DSH patients'.
He responds 'Why is that?'
I answer 'I don't know really, interactions just haven't happened.'
He persists 'No DSH patients have been through the department when you on duty?'
I answer 'Well, yes plenty of patients, there always are, but I was busy with other patients. No, that's not really true. I suppose if I'm honest I've been avoiding them'.
He gives me the word back 'Avoiding them?'
I answer 'I haven't really thought about it. On reflection I suppose it's easier isn't it? I haven't analysed why. I need more understanding of the subject. I don't want to hurt anyone by saying the wrong thing. Cock it up'.
Chris inquires 'Avoidance is a positive step towards understanding yourself. What insights have emerged?'
I answer 'Acknowledging my negative prejudice towards DSH patients. To be honest it's a relief to admit that I feared the next interaction'.
Voices ring in my ear.
The dark side of nursing exposed by Corley and Goren [11]
Chris shines a light
Lends me the torch
Reflection is first understanding
Second empowering
Third transforming
The confession less threatening
His parting shot – Bring me a DSH story
Oh Yes my lord

Pp 7>

'Avoidance is used by nurses when the prospect of dealing with a difficult patient arises' [12]

Pp 8>

'Whilst avoidance provides a protective mechanism for the nurse from life and death issues, avoidance can be painful for the patient who may already feel isolated' [13].

Pp 9> Session 3

I had gone out of my way to nurse this DSH patient. His name was Andrew.
Not what I expected at all.
I went into the cubicle explaining to him what clinical procedures were needed.

I acted in a way that I wouldn't usually.

Gave a warm smile.

Pushed my negative feelings to the side.

Let him tell his story.

It reminded me of those negative feelings that self-harm is a cry for attention, not as 'deserving' of my care as other patients.

They are often time wasters.

I could be helping someone who really needs it!

I asked Andrew very directly why he had taken the overdose.

He said 'My life is a mess. My mother doesn't care.'

He was thin, a little emaciated, I felt sorry for him.

Chris inquires 'How did you feel asking him why he had taken an overdose?'

I answer 'Very, very clumsy. Stumbling over my words, feeling hot and uncomfortable'.

He again gives me back a word 'Why clumsy?'

I answer 'Well, if Andrew had answered my question, I wouldn't have known how to respond. I didn't do any psychiatric training; I wouldn't be able to fulfil his needs. He might ask me for something I can't give. I would have been exposed as a fraud'.

Chris challenges 'Is that "he might ask for something you can't give" significant?'

I answer 'Well, I mean, he may ask me to understand him, have knowledge of whatever disorder or mental illness they have. I don't think I have it in me to understand. These patients drain me. It's scary to think that someone can be so desperate. He's done it several times before'.

Chris inquires 'So what does that tell you? Do you view him less seriously?'

I answer 'Previously, before dwelling in the literature, yes, an attention seeker, that individuals may inflict harm many times, sometimes over long periods of time. A significant number will commit suicide. I felt sorry for him because, apart from his appearance, he was apologetic, he was compliant with his clinical care'.

Chris challenging 'Perhaps if he had been non-compliant you may not have felt so sympathetic towards him?'

How true.

I squirm.

My competence hung out to dry.

Chris inquires 'What do you usually do when you don't have an answer?'

I answer 'I would ask someone for help'.

The politically correct answer to keep him off my back.

Andrew had been compliant, perhaps through experience of his many A&E visits. Perhaps I was manipulated?

I may never understand DSH but my attitude and response to DSH patients is changing.

Never before had I asked a patient 'why?'

Perhaps I would have dealt with another, less compliant DSH differently?

Maybe.

New experiences will reveal that truth.

I now know that my beliefs and attitude do effect my care.

So many patients must have suffered because of my ignorance.

Facing the truth is not easy.

CHAIR 2

The great pass-off – 'I don't want him you can have him,
he's too dark for me'
The new nurse face lunging in at me
A mask of warm smile
She's been practicing in the mirror

And her words, awkward, scripted
'why did you take an overdose?'

Why do you think?
'Cuz I'm so g-d happy,
'cuz I'm living such a brilliant fuckin' life ...

I can't answer, you wouldn't want me to
This dark of mine, risky, infectious

Tighten your mask, nursey,
Keep your distance from the germ of my substantial discontent

She asks as if she wants to know
But she doesn't ...
The truth would crack her mask

She's vaguely afraid of me
I can sniff it
And my life, like my fridge,
Smelly, empty, save for the sodden take-away containers

In the eyes behind the mask
I see her judgment,
She thinks I want attention ...

I must be good now
Give her something of what she wants.
So maybe she can do something
For me
If I'm very good
I'll be good.

Between sessions I read

Pp 10>

> 'It is unlikely that problems in nurse – patient relationships will prove amenable to simplistic
> prescriptions since the cause of those problems is endemic of social interaction itself' [14, p. 154].

Pp 11>

I read

> 'Difficult' patients as those who are perceived to act in a deviant manner. Such patients respond
> by adopting expected role behaviour that results in stigma and social isolation that reinforces the
> original behaviour and may leads to secondary deviance and validation of the nurses judgment of
> the patient [15, p. 132].

Pp 12> Session 4

Karl had taken an overdose.
I'm upset.
He nearly died a year ago.
The seriousness of DSH hitting home.

I moved into his cubicle, being open, wanting to help, using catharthis.

That's a new word for me!

I said 'What upset you so much today? Something must have really upset you to do this to yourself'.

I oozed compassion.

He rejected me.

His face averted to the wall.

His mother and brother watched me.

I asked them to leave.

I asked Karl again.

Still he ignored me.

I felt my anger rising.

I fell flat on my face.

Chris sympathetically inquires 'What then?'

I said to him 'I'm available if you need me'.

Conveying my concern for him.

Finding my poise.

I'm learning that poise is a precarious thing.

I cannot dictate the pace or expect his compliance.

I move through the emotional and power impasses that impede therapeutic relationships that Ramos identified [16].

CHAIR 3

Walls tighten
The press of your diagnostic gaze
My head in a vice

You, in nurse fashion, ask
'What upset you so much today?'
Today ...
Not only today ... everyday.

You want me to talk,
I can't, can't breathe
Can't risk wasting precious air on stupid words
They won't be enough for you anyway

You send my family away
Thinking now I'll talk

To you?
In your peach polyester uniform?
So you can do, what,
Feel better about your own sweet life
Tell my woes at your dinner table and tsk tsk
At the hardship that doesn't touch you
All safe, smug, employed ... loved.

You press again
I turn away, conflicted

Don't want to answer and
Satisfy your curiosity
As you crane your neck
At me, poor victim of an awful accident

And yet
To answer, ... to dislodge this stone blocking my airway
Inch it in your direction,
What it would unleash,
A geyser of bile would land on your hospital frock
And never wash out
With all the chemical laundering
It's just not safe ...

I turn to the wall
So you can't see
I want to cry

'I'm here if ...' you say, before leaving
As if ...

Pp 13> Session 5

A man in his forty's.
He had taken a large overdose.
He had visited his estranged wife and when she refused to let him into the house he sat down in her garden and took a massive overdose.
She wasn't aware that he was still in her garden.
Some hours later a passer-by called an ambulance.
To say that I interacted with him is debatable.
I carried out his clinical care, but he was unconscious, so I didn't actually speak to him.
Chris inquires 'How did you feel about him?'
I felt sad, sad that he had felt so desperate, sad that he could die, sad that maybe he didn't mean to kill himself but just wanted his partner to come outside and talk, sad that his ex wife would probably feel guilty and blame herself.
Just incredibly sad.
Then I saw the seriousness of DSH, the desperation, the waste.
Chris inquires 'This is new for you isn't it, this sympathy?'
I had felt sad when DSH patients had died before, but not as sad as say a victim of a road traffic accident, or a child.
Now I feel different.
Reflection makes me think differently about all sorts of things, not just in the work place, it's 'bigger' than that!
Through understanding my whole attitude is changing.

CHAIR 4

I can breathe underwater
Weight of cool liquid on me under me in me
Can't open my eyes
Yet I see
I was walking through her garden
To her door

There to tell her of my love
My continuing astonishingly intense love
Unprepared for her face, cold at her door,
Her finger
Pointing me away ...

I thought we could work it out try again

And I think I sat down in her garden
On a chair we'd picked together ...
Weary
Smell, sicky sweet
Can something smell purple?
My insides bruised purple
By the bash of heart on ribs
So uncomfortable
That look
Eyes, steeled blue

I waited
For her to remember she loves me
And now, under water, my lungs full
Storm warning ...
I near drown in tears ...
Taste salt or something

Some sounds far off
Roar of motorboat ... no,
Wheels rolling ... away

Why is everything going away?

And off there
As far away as the sounds, a shimmer ...

Someone has come to fetch me
Wish someone here
Could reach out
Hold me, save me
My wait over

Pp 14> Session 6

A young man in his twenties.
Early hours of the morning.
A paracetamol overdose
Not many, he was very distressed.
He kept saying sorry, apologising for wasting the nurses' time.
I sense he wants to talk.
He had financial worries and girlfriend problems.
It all tumbled out very quickly.
I was only supposed to be carrying out triage but talked to him for 15 minutes.

The department was not busy, so instead of handing his care over
to someone else, I took him into a cubicle and continued to talk.
I felt tender towards him.
I had a strong desire to help by simply listening.
I know he felt my concern was genuine.
Being mindful, reading his pattern.
Transcending any lingering prejudice.
Focussing on him as a suffering individual human

CHAIR 5

I took a few pills
More than I intended
But sleep wouldn't come ...

I'm sorry I'm taking your time
Sorry you're looking at me
All solicitous and concerned

I took a few tablets too many
Sorry ... I have financial troubles
Sorry ... my girlfriend would rather be
With him or anybody but me

I have such a sorry life
And you see how sorry it is
And feel sorry for me

I've swallowed bitter poison
Now my blood is sharp with it
And I messed up your day
Sorry I caused you to miss coffee break.

Sorry, most, perhaps,
That I am still alive
And aware of all this ...

Pp 15> Session 7

Just as I was feeling confident ... knock-back.
Two steps forward and three back!
Where to start?
Two experiences – one negative, one positive one
Chris suggests 'Tell me about the negative one?'
It was a busy shift over the New Year period.
A young girl overdosed.
Her friend had recently committed suicide.
She was hysterical.
I couldn't calm her down.
Reminding myself that here was a young girl who had lost a friend in traumatic
circumstances.
Pressure from within to calm her down.
Conflicting priorities, other patients needed a quiet calm atmosphere,

I needed to take control with this patient and I was failing.

The more hysterical she became the more irritation I felt.

Alcohol a part to play in her behaviour.

I thought she was silly, a 'drama queen.'

Losing sight of her 'grieving', under pressure, two in the morning,

I was tired.

Chris notes 'So she wasn't a "good" patient then?'

I answer 'No! Her father wasn't any help either! I hoped he would calm her down, but he seemed to cause yet more hysteria.

Nothing I tried worked, no connection with her, couldn't manage my feelings.

I felt it best to hand over her care to someone else, to remove myself from the situation. She was moved away from the poorly patients.

The second nurse was firmer than I was.

The girl eventually calmed down.

I don't know what happened after that.'

Chris inquires 'Had you adopted a parental role with her because her mother was absent and her father "useless"?'

'No ... at least I wasn't conscious of taking on a parental role but, being a mother myself, it is an easy role to fall into.

Anyway, if I did unconsciously take on a parental role it didn't work, did it?'

CHAIR 6

The nurse tries to quiet me,
With a 'there, there, pat pat' of words and hand

I might have died
It happens
My friend did,
An error in judgment
Consumed enough to take her out
I almost went too
Unwittingly, unwillingly,
Oh God oh God oh God ...
I need to cry, get it?
Like the newborn, shocked, relieved
To be here after all ...
Slapped up side the head.
Oh, the nurse is truly annoyed now.
She feels powerless against
My waves of hundred proof emotion,
Drop a match and see what happens.
Her anger nothing compared to the fire of my fear

I could have died
And she wants me to calm down ...
Then frustrated, hands me over to
A tough cookie, too like my own mother
One whose look demands, insists
There's no more consoling ...
Instead, an unspoken

'shut up, or else ...'
I understand.

I slam my mouth shut.
Hysteria, locked in, blows air bubbles in my
Churned-up cells.

The positive experience.
A few days later another young girl, about the same age.
She was at school, bought in by the class teacher.
She had taken a small overdose.
I was completely different with her.
'I was able to talk with her, let her know my concern was genuine.'
Chris inquires 'So what made it different?'
'It was a day shift 9 or 10 in the morning.
The department was quiet.
I had time.
And I wasn't tired.
She had taken the OD because her mum wouldn't let her visit her boyfriend the night before.
She was desperate about not seeing him.
I was the parent.
This was ok because she was frightened – she needed comforting.'
Chris informs 'The parent-child pattern of communication within Transactional Analysis can be therapeutic when the practitioner is mindful of adopting that pattern rather than simply reacting to the situation because it evokes a maternal response.'
I answer 'Yes, my response was reactive – I see your point that emotional reaction reflects the way I had absorbed the girl's suffering as a mother does for her child.
Does this distort my decisions and actions?'
What accounts for the difference in my response to these two young girls?
The first girl was outside my emotional limits the second girl within them.
I felt guilty.
Chris offers a positive spin 'Perhaps your first experience was also positive because you learnt from it?'
Now that's a better way to look at it.

CHAIR 7

My mother asked where I was going,
I told her, was told, 'no.'
'But'
'No'
'But'
'No'
Captive in the cell of my bedroom
Unable to go to my boyfriend
But I needed to talk to him

My thoughts, loud, crowded, hurt,
In my drawer I had something
To help with the pain
More will be better to numb

I swallow
My words
Feel poison in me
Go weak, world tweeked gray
My sluggish feet carry me
To school
Teacher sees what isn't in my eyes
Sends me to the big house
Where people in coats look into me

No scurrying
Not like on TV
All in slow mo
Except for my brain,
Up on two wheels
Careening around corners
And the nurse listens to me
Perhaps she remember what it's like
When life gets too hard
Ball and chain around my ankles
Tripping me up

I am frightened
Have never felt this before
Wish I could puke
Empty my gut of all that has choked out
My innocence

Between sessions I read

Pp 16>

> 'Poor information and communication systems, lack of knowledge about suicide; negative attitudes towards people who self-harm does not help the rising number of patients presenting with DSH ... A&E staff must become more involved with education/training where negative attitudes are challenged' [17, p. 11].

Pp 17> Session 8

Another deeply distressed girl who had OD, also around fifteen year of age, verging on hysteria, difficult to deal with ...
I felt her suffering.
I responded with care without judgment, more mindful, more poised.
The difference was palpable.
Variables were different.
It was during the day, quiet early in the shift, the workload was light and I could concentrate on her care.
Dwelling with her, I remember the other teenager, remembering the lessons.
I convened a debate with my A&E colleagues – they are interested in my study.
Chris approvingly 'That's good'.
They are divided on their own feelings about DSH patients.
Some feel they firmly understood and treated the patient group in exactly the same way they would any other.

Yeah, but I doubt that is true knowing them.

It's not easy to face up to being uncaring.

Some found themselves, perhaps like myself, somewhere in the middle, lacking real knowledge of DSH and experiencing difficulty with caring for such patients.

Not surprisingly, some felt that DSH patients were selfish and time wasters who manipulate both nurses and the medical system.

I read

Pp 18>

> 'Nurses and doctors do not support the notion that suicidal behaviour reflects mental illness' One staff nurse who took part in the research stated – 'Sometimes I think they are time wasters – occasionally, and quite selfish – if you have a good reason to self harm then that's that ... but if not then I think it's quite selfish' [18, p. 6/8].

One colleague stated that she is 'resigned' to nursing DSH patients.

I ask her to explain ... she says that the only DSH patients we meet are those in crisis, that we never see patients who recover.

Chris inquires 'What does recover mean?'

I wish I knew. The debate with my colleagues enabled our thoughts and feelings to surface and, whilst I was not able to change their opinion there and then, perhaps a seed was sown, a seed that may surface later, at a time that is right for the individual to address their own contradictions.

Chris prods 'You've become an agitator'.

I answer 'Yes, just like you!'

The meaning of my practice shifts with each new experience and insight.

Most significantly I no longer fear involvement with DSH patients.

Like I've broken through the fear barrier.

From the outset of this self-inquiry, I was concerned that any changes I made to my practice in relation to my care of DSH patients would leave me vulnerable.

By this I mean that emotions have significance and that respect for knowledge and wisdom is gained if the individual allows their emotions to direct their thoughts and attention.

As a result of my inquiry, a host of factors including cultural and religious beliefs have emerged that influence my practice with DSH patients.

Chris encouraging 'Say more?'

I sense how being raised in a predominately Christian society with strong cultural beliefs about self-harm and suicide has impacted on me.

I was reading that as recently as 1961 suicide and attempted suicide fell into the same category as murder and there were a number of prosecutions.

Decriminalisation in 1966 did not lead to any great change to the prevailing Christian ethic even as the world became more secular.

Pp 19>

I read 'In the Judeo-Christian cultures there has always been a belief that suicide is reprehensible and ethically wrong' [9, p. 1112].

Reading the Metro recently I sense that attitudes have not changed

Pp 20> newspaper clipping

I can see the way my past relationships with DSH patients have always been tinged with hostility.

Is that Christian?

Yes I know it's risky bringing God into the picture.

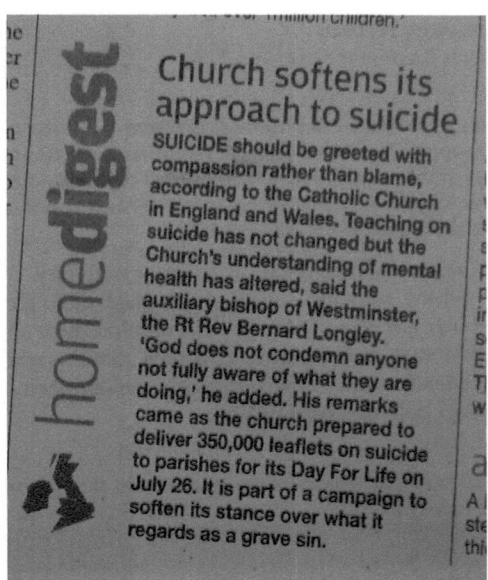

Church softens its approach to suicide

SUICIDE should be greeted with compassion rather than blame, according to the Catholic Church in England and Wales. Teaching on suicide has not changed but the Church's understanding of mental health has altered, said the auxiliary bishop of Westminster, the Rt Rev Bernard Longley. 'God does not condemn anyone not fully aware of what they are doing,' he added. His remarks came as the church prepared to deliver 350,000 leaflets on suicide to parishes for its Day For Life on July 26. It is part of a campaign to soften its stance over what it regards as a grave sin.

Chris challenged me earlier to identify the nurses' role in A&E. Is it holistic or merely patch work?

The word holistic is difficult – I mean about the whole person.

But I know better that my response to the DSH patient does makes a difference.

That compassion and non-judgmental acceptance works better than indifference or worse, rejection and thinly veiled contempt.

Only when nurses, like myself, resolve contradiction, can they realise their visions of practice as a lived reality and lead more satisfactory lives.

In acknowledging and confronting my prejudice I discover myself as a person and have found that this, in itself, naturally leads to, not just tuning into others and their needs, but also myself.

It feels astonishing to realise such self-neglect.

And yet I sense that nurse education gives little emphasis to developing and sustaining effective therapeutic relationships, especially with patients experiencing DSH.

Chris hits the nail on the head 'All experience is positive if we can learn from it'.

Sounds like a cliché?

My empowerment to act came from within because I could no longer live with the contradiction, once my protective veneer had been torn off within supervision.

I had a choice: to retreat or push forward.

But in reality, I had no choice because where could I have retreated too?

Pp 21> Session 9

My arms around a woman in great distress, crying a steady stream of tears.

Suddenly, I realised I genuinely cared.

No masks it was the real me!

We talked as I carried out clinical observations.

I was so in-tune with this woman I instinctively knew what she wanted from me.

I sat next to her and her tears began.

She physically moved towards me.

I believe she sensed my empathy and the genuineness of my caring response.

As I encircled her in my arms, I felt emotional.

I felt sadness for her, but realised the truth of Ramos's words [16] –

'Nurses described an emotional identification which was real, not devastating to the nurse, but a motivator'.

Such a relationship as the very cornerstone of nursing care.

I wanted to hold this woman because she needed me to hold her.

I felt very comfortable doing so.

A burden had lifted from my shoulders.

It was almost spiritual.

CHAIR 8

I mean to be strong
With this nurse though,
No need.
I see in her eyes
Some understanding of the pain
I must have endured
To go so far this far
I feel she cares wants to help
And the knowledge of that
That I am not invisible
That maybe just maybe
I matter
Have worth
Undoes me
And the tears come
The years of tears
The pain that's been growing festering
Rising to boil
And now
Valve on pressure cooker adjusted
So I can safely spend
Some of this gunk inside of me

And I cry and I cry and I cry
And the nurse's arms are around me
And I can feel she wants to cry too
And sharing it
It's not so heavy
Sharing it
The tears fly out faster
And I can feel the beginnings of places, spaces inside me
Where maybe the light can come in

For so long
Hopeless
So long
I thought that's all there was

I have always been depressed
I am depressed
I always will be depressed
So I thought so I knew

And then her arms
Nudging the pain out of me
And in the space
Maybe
Maybe I can feel something other than
The grip of inevitable death

I sense her heart beating
In time with my own

It has been a relatively short journey.
The terrain has been tough yet productive.
I've discovered myself.
This 'new self' is still to be tested for its robustness in face of more difficult interactions.
I know that my attitude and those of my colleagues is at the core of person-centred practice.
Logtsrup's words inspire me [19, p. 18]

Pp 22>

> By our attitude to one another we help to shape one another's world.
>
> By our very attitude to the other person, we help to determine the scope and hue of his or her world.
>
> We make it large or small, bright or drab, rich or dull, threatening or secure.
>
> We help to shape his or her world not by theories and views but by our very attitude towards him or her.
>
> Herein lies the unarticulated and one might say anonymous demand that we care for the life which trust has placed in or hands.

The End

Ensuing Dialogue

For a moment there is silence then someone says 'The whole performance was emotional but those final words brought tears to my eyes. Indeed my eyes have been opened. We get so embroiled in doing things we can so easily lose sight of our purpose as nurses'.

A nurse immediately stands up and says 'I'm a third year nursing student. I have learnt more about caring for self-harm patients in the past 30 minutes than I have in the whole of my nurse training. Thank you'.

Her comment is a show stopper and hard to follow as if the audience is stunned.

In the pause that follows I ask the students who read the empathic poems how they felt. Two of the students note their emotional response. One said she had self-harmed in the past and that the performance was actually therapeutic for her, empathically putting herself in the young girl's shoes. She felt that it was now ok for her to say she had self-harmed whereas previously she felt stigmatised.

Someone says 'I think Jane was immensely brave to tackle this topic for her dissertation, almost a confession. It reinforced in my mind the power of reflection as a learning process about becoming a better person, as Johns says in his books about cleaning smudges of the mirror to see oneself truly'.

An audience person says 'Yes. I also felt the performance was deeply moving as if Jane's confession came alive! I don't work in A & E but I sense how its environment is not sympathetic. As a teacher the performance was very powerful. It has set my mind racing about how I could use it'.

Another audience person 'Yes, I agree with the last person. The idea of using empathic poems was extremely powerful. It showed such insight. I did wonder if the self-harm people would have said something similar?'

I respond 'It would have been difficult to trace them to ask. However, I felt it was important to give them an independent voice'.

The person responds: 'I can feel that. It does add perspective. You do wonder what self-harm patients are really thinking. Did they really want to kill themselves or just seeking attention? A gesture in the moment?'

Another audience person notes 'Picking up what the last person said, I work for a mental health charity. I will be in contact with you about the possibility of performing Jane's rap to another audience. Thank you. I really appreciated the rap'.

Another voice chips in 'What strikes me is the way Jane could share her experience with colleagues to make them think about their own attitudes. It showed me how individual reflection can spread within a team. I've wondered about the limitation of individual reflection to change things as if people are essentially cocooned within their own practice. I can see a bigger picture now'.

I direct his response to the audience 'Is that others' experience?'

In the pause that followed I said 'Jane's experience reveals how guided reflection nurtures commitment and responsibility towards ensuring a better attitude and response to self-harm patients. The contradiction between her person-centred values and actual practice was stark and uncomfortable'.

A man responds 'I am a senior manager. I was intrigued to come along to the performance today. It's true we talk the rhetoric of person-centred practice but do little to ensure it. The performance is so much food for thought'.

'And action?' I add.

He smiled.

References

1. Mattigley, C. (1988) *Healing Dramas and Clinical Plots: The Narrative Structure of Experience.* Cambridge University Press, Cambridge.

2. Johns, C. (2009) Reflection on my mother dying: a story of caring shame. *Journal of Holistic Nursing* 27, 136–140.

3. Gray, R., Ivanoffski, V., Sinding, C. (2002) Making a mess and spreading it around: articulation of an approach to research based theatre. In A. Bochner, C. Ellis [Eds.] *Ethnographically Speaking; Autoethnography, Literature and Aesthetics.* AltaMira Press, Walnut Creek.

4. Loori, J. D. (2007) *The Zen of Creativity.* A Peekamoose Book, Ballantine Books, New York, NY.

5. Park-Fuller, L. (2003) Audiencing the audience: playback theatre, performative writing and social activism. *Text and Performance Quaterly* 23, 288–319.

6. Maddison, D. S. (1988) Performance, personal narratives and the politics of possibility. In S. Dailey [Ed.] *The Future of Performance Studies: Visions and Revisions.* National Communication Association, Annandale, 276–286.

7. Groom, J., Johns, C. (2010) Shifting attitude with deliberate self-harm patients in Accident & Emergency (A&E). In C. Johns [Ed.] *Guided Reflection; A Narrative Approach to Advancing Professional Practice* (second edition). Wiley-Blackwell, Hoboken, 215–235.

8. Anderson, M. (1999) Waiting for harm: deliberate self-harm and suicide in young people – a review of the literature. *Journal of Psychiatric and Mental Health Nursing* 37, 1–10.

9. McLaughlin, C. (1994) Casualty nurses attitudes to attempted suicide. *Journal of Advanced Nursing* 20, 1111–1118.

10. Lynn, F. (1998) The pain of rejection. *Nursing Times* 94, 27.

11. Corley, M., Goren, S. (1998) The dark side of nursing: impact of stigmatizing responses on patients. *Scholarly Inquiry for Nursing Practice* 12, 99–121.

12. Carveth, J. (1995) Perceived patient deviance and avoidance by nurses. *Nursing Research* 44, 173–178.

13. Eldrid, J. (1988) *Caring for the Suicidal.* Constable, London.

14. Kelly, P., May, D. (1982) Good and bad patients: a review of the literature and a theoretical critique. *Journal of Advanced Nursing* 7, 147–156.

15. Trexlar, T. (1996) Reformulation of deviance and labeling theory for nursing. *Image: Journal of Nursing Scholarship* 28, 131–136.

16. Ramos, M. (1992) The nurse-patient relationship: theme and variations. *Journal of Advanced Nursing* 17, 496–506.

17. Repper, J. (1999) A review of literature on the prevention of suicide through interventions in Accident and emergency departments. *Journal of Clinical Nursing* 8, 3–12.

18. Anderson, M., Standen, P., Nazir, S., Noon, J. (1999) Nurses' and doctors' attitudes towards suicidal behaviour in young people. *International Journal of Nursing Studies* 37, 1–10.

19. Logstrup, K. (1997) *The Ethical Demand.* University of Notre Dame Press, Notre Dame.

Notes

i.   As evidenced in the performance of 'My mother's death' [2]. I was accompanied by pianists who extemporised in dialogue with the words. (My thanks to Patrick Dean). At times. I would pause in the reading to let the pianist respond. It created a complimentary narrative that enhanced dramatically the performance by creating a powerful sense of mood.

ii. The performance was an accepted paper entitled 'Reflection as dialogue' presented at the Carfax Reflective practice conference held at University College Worcester in July 2000.

iii. If readers are inspired by Jane's Rap and would like to commission a performance or indeed perform it themselves please contact myself through Wiley.

CHAPTER 26

'Wrap-up'

Wrap-up is the last cue of the Model for Structured Reflection. It wraps up how the whole book has unfurled to reveal the processes and insights of guiding practitioners towards becoming reflective practitioners and realising their visions of practice.

Reflection is like opening your eyes to see self, as if for the first time. It can feel startling and disturbing when you have been going around blind like 'nurse fantastic' in Chapter 6 exercising her robotic unreflective approach to practice. Yet, you must ask, Why does the nurse respond like that? Does it reflect the clinical culture of high technology where nurses become technicians, as if their uniforms are laboratory white coats, and persons merely bodies to determine morbidity? If so, it is a far cry from a vision of person-centred practice. Perhaps it is the need to protect one's vulnerability from the other's suffering as if one might become infected and suffer. Better to wear a metaphoric mask to keep a distance. Asking 'who is this person' opens a potential can of worms. Reflective practice does just that. It asks 'who is this practitioner'? It invites the practitioner to 'open your eyes'. You may, of course, prefer to keep them closed.

The stories practitioners share through guided reflection reveals and lifts the significance and value of their practice. It transforms the mundane into the profound.

The writing and sharing of experience bring buried things to light, significant things that may have, on the surface, seem insignificant.

Becoming a reflective practitioner is like flying a plane and emerging through the storm into clear blue sky where the practitioner can see everything clearly for what it is. It invokes a deep sense of calm and grace. It is as if the mind is now hard wired for reflection whereby reflection is lived, has become a natural way to see and respond to the world. I can best describe this as an 'era of enlightenment', adding a dimension to Kieffer's (1) framework for participatory competence (Figure 5.4). The need for guidance falls away, yet maintaining a reflective journal is important to sustain oneself, reminding the practitioner to pay attention and continue to learn through experience, and, as a bonus, maintain a professional journal for re-registration.

I kept a continuous journal for four years (2, 3) in my role as a bank nurse and holistic therapist working in a hospice. Reading these journals again, reinforces in my mind the power of journaling as revealed in a short excerpt from my journal (3, p. 162).

Callum sits in the corner of his room. I have been informed that 'He has been difficult to get on top of, restless, agitated'.

I kneel before him and say 'Hi Callum, I'm Chris'.

He looks blank and then after about 30 seconds speaks 'I can come tomorrow with my with son and measure up if you let me know what needs to be done'.

At first, I can make no sense of his words and then I understand. He was a carpenter. Is this the way his agitation works itself out? Yet the word 'agitation' immediately labels him – I must be sensitive to who he is, not simply an 'agitated' person that risks framing my reference for seeing him.

Silence. Patiently I wait …. and then he says 'I can't stop here. I've been here for four days and must get home'.

I ask him who is at home. He stands and shows me the photograph on the window ledge. In it, he stands with his wife Rachel and their five grandchildren. The youngest, held by Rachel, is just a few months old. I say 'the little girl, she looks about four, is cute'.

He says 'She's the apple of my eye'.

Such poignancy, such connection. Dwelling with him in silence had cut through the agitation to reveal his deep despair that, from time to time, spins him into apparent 'confusion' as if he returns to a part of his life when, as a competent carpenter, he was the master of his life – in stark contrast with the helplessness he now feels.

Julie, a care assistant, enters the room and asks Callum about lunch. At first, he says he has no appetite. I imagine his stomach full of sorrow. But she persists 'Fish and chips?'

She shows him and he changes his mind. His talk flips back into him and his son coming to work here. Julie gently reminds him that he is at the hospice, he apologises that he didn't know what he was saying. It seems his despair is on the cusp.

We leave him to eat. Kirsty, a staff nurse, fills me in with Callum's history. He recently retired as a carpenter and was hoping to move to Spain. His cancer is very advanced, mesothelioma diagnosed about three years ago. He knows he is dying. He has worked hard, and now his dreams are crushed. Kirsty tells me how he followed her about one day, and again I could sense his regression, that Kirsty became a safe place to shelter from the storm, a kind of surrogate mother. The question now facing the team is, How best to help him? Perhaps being at home surrounded by his family would be best? Kirsty is uncertain because she doubts the ability of Rachel to cope. Clearly emigrating to Spain is not an option.

Rachel and her sister arrive. She is just like the photograph. On the surface she is contained, easy going. As I sit with them, she reveals her distress and exhaustion. She is full of stuff she needs to let out. I can *feel* Kirsty's words.

Rachel says 'He wants me here 24 hours'.

I can see the way he has attached himself to Kirsty in Rachel's absence. Like a frightened boy alone and drowning in the sea of despair he needs to be comforted. I feel anxious because we talk over him as if he wasn't there. He says nothing.

Wanting to be helpful, I suggest to Callum a foot massage might be relaxing? He accepts.

His feet surprise me. They are soft for a builder. He further surprises me by relaxing quickly. Within a few minutes, a muffled snore permeates the room. I gaze at Rachel and feel her smile lift my energy. I too smile.

I move into reflexology, working along the spine and balancing the chakras. I work the head, lungs and diaphragm. After 30 minutes, he has not stirred. He is asleep. I beckon Rachel and her son Martin who has arrived. They have been drinking tea. Rachel visibly relaxes seeing Callum so still. She says 'It's like magic'. I take her hand and say, 'It must seem like that'.

We pause, and still holding her hand I say 'your hands are dry'. She says 'they are always like that'. I say 'let me massage them for you'. He subdued smile radiates through the gloom. Holding her hand is an invitation to intimacy, a gateway to opening a healing space. Like a prop to ease the burden of her suffering. Like an olive branch of peace.

I mix patchouli, frankincense and juniper berry essential oils into the reflexology cream. She likes the smell, she relaxes into the massage and through my hands I feel her anxiety melt and stillness radiate through her body. Afterwards I gift her some massage cream to nourish her dry hands and, perhaps more significantly to nourish her spirit. Applying the cream with its aroma will evoke the healing she experienced with the hand massage.

Later, in the sun-drenched courtyard, I sit and reflect on Callum and Rachel. Lives torn apart. The soft sound of the water fountain is very calming. I write my notes and read his history. The notes spell out his physical deterioration and worsening mental anguish. He resisted admission because it meant accepting how poorly he was and hospice meant death. Murray Cox helps me puts things into perspective (4, p. 11)

> 'Sometimes the patient presents with finely chiselled, clearly delineated symptoms. At other times he conveys a baffling sense of swirling, inchoate, undifferentiated affective surge, he uses many words to try and describe this sense of turbulence, but chaos often seems to get nearest the mark'.

Callum's cry across the wasteland 'I am chaos!'

Do I hear him well enough? I am a surf rider who tunes into the rhythm of his chaotic waves to ride its length. Callum's is a large wave to surf!

As Murray Cox writes (4, p. 11)

> 'The surf rider has a persistent sense of being on the brink of something more, always wondering where the next wave will carry him further still. He is poised at the unfolding invitational edge of experience that flows out of previous experience'.

Maya, a staff nurse, seeks my advice. She is uncertain about using midazolam with Callum. I give my opinion that midazolam would be a blanket to suffocate him, that his deep despair needs to surface rather than be dampened down. I say 'I don't know what's best. Touch would be my way of being with him, holding and comforting him whilst also easing Rachel's suffering'.

A brief pause and then I add 'Perhaps a small dose might take the edge of his fear?'

My words surprise me given my resistance to sedation. Maya remembers an earlier conversation with me when I had challenged her attitude to midazolam. Now she is more mindful of using midazolam too quickly as a way of easing her anxiety to fix Callum's agitation. We acknowledge it is hard to watch someone in emotional turmoil. It is also difficult to resist the family's plea to do something to calm him. At such times these conversations are vital.

Thirty minutes later, Callum remains relaxed. I kneel by his side and call him. He stirs and opens one eye and then closes it. Rachel tells me how he was meticulous about his appearance. Designer suits with the tags still on them and now this. It is hard for Rachel to see her proud man reduced to rubble.

Dr Brown has heard how effective my touch was in calming Callum. He asks my advice in managing Callum's agitation. I caution against going over board with midazolam and suggest we ask the staff to give touch. Dr Brown agrees. He too is doubtful about using neuroleptic drugs.

I am surprised to be consulted because he has never asked my views before. I have always felt invisible to him: that the use of complementary therapies is not within his medical gaze. As a consequence, I work in the margins of mainstream hospice care and felt that complementary therapy is viewed with no more than a benign tolerance to help people relax.

(continued)

Such is the nature of my hospice practice. My journal words bring my practice alive in ways the reader can relate to, feel engaged with, engendering personal reflection and imagination in ways that theory or conventional texts fail to open up the mystery of human existence.

Yet, despite my claim, readers may ask in a world still dominated by evidence-based practice, 'What evidence is there that learning through reflection is efficacious?' Well, the proof is in the pudding, not from statistical surveys or controlled trials but from the practitioner's own words. The narratives in the book are not mere anecdote. They have been systematic and well-crafted self-inquiry. They offer compelling and convincing evidence of the power of reflection to transform practice.

In Chapter 14, I suggested that empirical studies of the efficacy of reflective practice in relation to outcomes were limited. To take one example by Coleman and Willis's paper (5) (as cited in Chapter 19) entitled – 'Reflective writing; the student nurse's perspective on reflective writing and poetry writing'. On face value the paper supported the value of poetry as a medium for reflection based on reports from 20 students in focus groups.

They state their results (5, p. 906) –

'Students found the process of reflective writing daunting but valued it over time. Current educational methods, such as assessing reflective accounts, often lead to the "narrative" being watered down and the student feeling judged. Despite this, reflection made students feel responsible for their own learning and research on the topic. Some students felt the use of models of reflection constricting, whilst poetry freed up their expression allowing them to demonstrate the compassion for their patient under their care.

There is a need for students to have a safe and supportive forum in which to express and have their experiences acknowledged without the fear of being judged'.

I agree with their conclusions. I have made similar observations as evidenced throughout the book. However, anybody judging the efficacy of any study of reflective practice would need to heed the variables involved:

1. The organisation role of the guide in relation to the practitioner.
2. The guide's expertise in guiding the practitioner.

3. The guide's values in relation to the practitioner's values.
4. The extent the guide knew the people involved in the practitioner's experiences.
5. The practitioner's knowledge and experience of learning through reflection.
6. The time span and continuity of the reflective experience.
7. The use of a model of reflection and journaling.
8. How learning was judged in terms of both process and outcomes.
9. Whether learning took place as an individual or in groups.
10. Whether participation by practitioners was voluntary or mandatory.
11. The particular relationship between guide and practitioner.

The last point is itself vast, raising such variables as personal connection, the balance of challenge and support, and the way sessions are wrapped up – indeed all the steps of the 10-step process model of guided reflection (Figure 9.1). They are all significant in interpreting the efficacy of guided reflection from empirical studies beyond abstract generalisations. These variables can all be discerned within the narrative.

Paradigms of Knowing

Wilber [6] offers an integral model to different approaches to knowledge split into four quadrants based on whether the researcher is interior to the research (left hand path) or exterior to the research (right hand path), and whether the researcher is an individual or a collective. Reflexive narrative research is self-inquiry, which is individual and subjective in contrast with empirical research that stands objectively outside the research topic.

Wilber refers to rules on injunction whereby truth is ascertained. Self-inquiry research is governed by 'I' – reflecting its subjective nature. 'I' am researching myself along a journey of being and becoming who 'I' seek to be. 'I' do not stand outside myself as if observing some object although my subjectivity is tempered by guidance. Whereas empirical research seeks to draw statistical proof that its focus of research exists as a fact leading to generalisations that claim to exist for all such situations. The proof of 'I' is revealed in narrative form. That is its claim to truth. 'I' might state 'this is my truth'. The reader will discern the authenticity of that claim in relation to their own experiences and draw their own truth.

These paradigms are very different. However, self-inquiry critically draws on objective empirical knowledge as information, thus integrating the paradigms. Yet the 'I' is the master and the 'it' the servant. All empirical knowledge needs to be interpreted to fit the particular human situation.

Wilber [6, p. 23] notes –

'The entire right hand imperialism, which in many ways has been the hallmark of Western modernity, is known generally as *scientism*, which, as I would define it, is the belief that the entire world can be fully explained in "it-language". It is the assumption that all subjective and intersubjective spaces can be reduced, without remainder, to the behavior of objective processes, that human and nonhuman interiors alike can be thoroughly accounted for as holistic systems of dynamically interwoven its'.

Scientism equates with evidence-based practice and remains the hallmark of what counts as knowledge. As such, narrative proof is paradigmatically resisted as acceptable evidence. As Sweet notes [7]

'One day, it will be as unusual to find an educational strategy, instructional practice, or program that has not been validated by scientific evidence as it is to find a doctor who uses leeches to cure a fever'.

Evidence-based practice has its place. However, people are not 'its', and what is determined objectively cannot be simply applied to the individual without reducing the person to the status of an object to be manipulated.

Only the reflective perspective of reflexive narrative can illuminate the complex and indeterminate nature of becoming towards realising person-centred practice through guided reflection given the uniqueness of both process and outcome. Such nature can never be reduced to 'its' without gross distortion of its reality.

Any practitioner serious about realising person-centred practice would choose guided self-inquiry towards realising it and contributing to its understanding.

Four Student Reflections on Guided Reflection

To substantiate 'the proof is in the pudding', I offer four students' reflections on their experience of guided reflection, distilled from many similar written observations in reflexive narrative assignments and dissertations.

One student writes of the liberating sensation of reflective practice in her assignment

> 'Reflection is transforming my practice in so many meaningful and profound ways. I have never felt so free to care and to be true to what I consider to be ideal practice. Reflection has enabled me to contextually refocus on the individual. My interactive skills are being sharpened and I am rediscovering the therapeutic value of establishing a close relationships with clients. Until now I have never been able to find an approach to nursing which recognizes the true potential of this unique relationship. My first few reflections were triggered by a feeling that I had failed to achieve my goals in some way. Guided reflection has enabled me to make use of the creative energy of conflict. I have been challenged to stoke up a far more challenging style of practice. I have become empowered to provoke and maintain the contradictions I feel between my goals of desirable practice and actual practice. Just as there are no limits to my expanding consciousness'.

Susan[i] [8] notes

> 'However', I quickly became alive to the possibilities that this course would offer me in terms of self-perception and development. I was, in a sense, forced to come face to face with myself – an experience that on occasions I found disturbing – yet it led to the discovery of a new way of far more satisfying learning and a set of new horizons and vistas to explore. On a personal note, the process has proved literally life changing. I am happier, more content with self and have developed a confidence and self-regard that has not only benefited me professionally but in my personal life also. This seems to be a highly significant outcome since Bennis and Nanus [9] describe a positive self-regard as the most essential personal trait of successful leaders. Self-esteem signifies a deep down, inside the self-feeling of personal worth which generates from real capacity, competence and adequacy of role performance [10].
>
> My commitment to transformational leadership and my practice of the art still seem to be anathema to the prevailing transactional culture in the NHS. Is the NHS and my organisation truly ready then for leaders like myself who adopt a transformative stance when this may mean, as it frequently does, that the leader is in conflict with the undeniably pervasive transactional nature of the health service as it exists today? The answer to this is probably 'not yet' but I believe that the time will come and feel rather like a missionary in the field in my own workplace filled with a zeal to spread the word. I share the view of William Blake, the imaginative and mystic visionary who expressed a unique and vital view when he wrote [11, p. 293].
>
> 'I must create a system or be enslaved by another Man's.
>
> I will not reason and compare: my business is to create'.

Mary is the CEO of a child bereavement service. She writes[ii] [12, p. 169–171]

'The leadership programme has transformed me from being a transactional manager into a transformational leader. Although, as a manager I believed I led with a transformational flavour, you had to get deep down and peep through the keyhole to see it. I have learnt along my journey that leadership is much more than being taught; it is learning, and that the leader keeps learning [13] and continuously facilitates learning around those with whom she works. Learning has become natural for me as I have become more mindful of myself as a leader. It is a simple equation.

My journey from a transactional manager to transformational leader has been a journey from darkness into light. It has not been easy. I have struggled with many difficult feelings and extreme emotions that I have never experienced before. I had an ongoing internal battle that raged as I grappled at leadership theories and the reality of how I was going to manage the service – weaving management within my leadership in congruent ways. "The Service" was my baby! I had nurtured it from infancy into this huge and increasingly complex organisation. But as I grew along the journey and embraced the wider culture of the Primary Care Trust, and told to conform to its transactional culture, the frustration I felt was immense. I have struggled with the tension of my current reality and my vision of where and who I would like to be. Now, looking back I can see my reflexive journey with astonishing clarity. I truly feel liberated and transformed and recognise that the service too has been transformed for the better. I honestly feel that if I had not completed this course, I would no longer be manager of "The Service". Before embarking on the programme, the joy had gone out of my life and I was just going through the motions. This would eventually have been too much and I would have abandoned my vision in favour for sanity. There is always a transactional price to pay for not conforming! That would have been such a waste and left me leaving a failure and regretful. Wheatley [14] suggests that if I believe that, as a leader, I must have my hands into everything, controlling every decision, every person and every moment, then I cannot hope for anything except what I already have – a treadmill of frantic effort that would ultimately result in destroying myself and the collective vitality with those who I work with. It was certainly going that way. The bigger "The Service" became the more frantic I became. It was so insidious I didn't see it creeping up. "The Service" has blossomed into a thriving innovative service. I have been able to let go of my stranglehold and empower others to take responsibility and thrive. I know I will always surface challenges to the way I lead as others' actions make me anxious from time to time. Yet being mindful I can see myself more clearly. Smile instead of frown and see the anxious moment as a learning moment. Yet such lessons have been difficult to learn wrapped up in the moment. Coming to the community of inquiry, I can tell the story and see it and slowly I began to resolve the tension within practice. I have opened my existing windows wider and opened windows I didn't know existed to see an amazing landscape full of possibilities. I now live leadership. It is transparent.

Glouberman [15] suggests we live in a culture where we are valued more for what we achieve in the eyes of others than what we achieve in our own eyes. I feel good when people acknowledge what has been achieved. It has not been easy to let go of control and have others received acclaim for their work. But giving power away has given me the freedom to explore other possibilities that I could only have ever dreamed about and would never have had the courage to take these dreams forward. In letting go of control I have learnt that things evolve and pattern around vision and intent. I now see a future full of exciting possibilities! I relate very much to Glouberman's [15] idea of spending much of my previous life as a manager as a rat on an exercise wheel in a cage, trying to keep up with the inner and outer expectations that dominated my life. Every now and then I kicked the exercise wheel or rattled the bars of the cage but doing this just delayed me: eventually I would go back to the wheel, running faster to make up or lost time. Whatever I did, whether it was something I really wanted to do or something I didn't, the inner result was just the same: even my most creative desires were transformed into expectations that ended up oppressing me. I was constantly trying to do too much! This is not the end of my journey; my journey is now a life long commitment that I under take in my quest to be a true leader. It has given new meaning to my life, my role as manager and the service as a whole. Such was the vitality of the community of learning that we plan to continue to meet. We have formed a strong bond that can never be broken'.

Mary's testament is of particular significance because of her CEO status. As a consequence of her leadership learning experience, she implemented guided reflection throughout the organisation.

Priest[iii] and Johns [16, p. 213] write

'For me the journey has been like standing on the shore where the ground is firm and familiar, looking out into the ocean that glimmers in the sun. But beneath the waves its true depth is hidden from view. At first you struggle against the tide, currents and waves, but upon returning to the water you have learnt a little bit more about the ocean. The more I return to the chopping waves the more graceful I move within its waters, until I swim in liquid light where I can see the shells and pearls and poisonous fish. Reflection is a skill in itself and when you finally get used to it, it usually shows that you are the root of most of your problems'.

The words of these practitioners are both compelling and humbling to read. They stand in testament to the transformational power and grace of guided reflection over a period of time. They reflect the ontological nature of self-inquiry, how we can come to know ourselves through becoming a reflective practitioner as the gateway towards realising our visions of self and practice. Journeys of self-inquiry can be disturbing. Hence the invaluable support by guides and peers.

Christopher Johns

References

1. Kieffer, C. (1984) Citizen empowerment: a developmental perspective. *Prevention in Human Sciences* 84, 9–36.

2. Johns, C. (2004) *Being Mindful, Easing Suffering.* Jessica Kingsley Publishers, London.

3. Johns, C. (2006) *Engaging Reflection in Practice.* Blackwell Publishing, Oxford.

4. Cox, M. (1988) *Structuring the Therapeutic Process: Compromise with Chaos* (revised edition). Jessica Kingsley Publishers, London.

5. Coleman, D., Willis, D. S. (2015) Reflective writing; the student nurse's perspective on reflective writing and poetry writing. *Nurse Education Today* 35(7), 906–911.

6. Wilber, K. (1997) *The Eye of Spirit: An Integral Vision for a World Gone Slightly Mad.* Shambhala, Boston.

7. Sweet, R. W., Jr. (2004) The big picture: where we are nationally on the reading front and how we got here. In P. McCardle, V. Chhabra [Eds.] *The Voice of Evidence in Reading Research.* Paul H. Brookes Publishing Co, Baltimore, 13–44.

8. Brooks, S. (2004) *Becoming a transformational leader.* Unpublished Masters in Leadership dissertation. Bedford, University of Bedfordshire.

9. Bennis, W., Nanus, B. (1985) *Leaders: Strategies for Taking Charge.* Harper Row, New York.

10. Waitley, D. (1996) *Psychology of Success: Developing Your Self-Esteem.* Irwin Professional Publishers, Burr Ridge, IL.

11. Blake, W. (1997) *Jerusalem: The Emanation of the Giant Albion: The Illuminated Books Volume 1.* M. D. Paley, D. Bindman [Eds.] Princeton University Press, New Jersey.

12. Johns, C. (2016) *Mindful Leadership: A Guide for the Healthcare Professions.* Palgrave, London.

13. Vail, P. (1996) *Learning as a Way of Being: Strategies for Survival in a World of Permanent White Water.* Jossey-Bass, San Francisco.

14. Wheatley, M. J. (1999) *Leadership and the New Science.* Berrett-Koehler Publisher, San Francisco.

15. Glouberman, D. (2003) *The Joy of Burnout.* Hodder & Staughton, London.

16. Priest, J.-M., Johns, C. (2010) More than eggs for breakfast. In C. Johns [Ed.] *Guided Reflection: A Narrative Approach to Advancing Professional Practice* (second edition). Wiley-Blackwell, Oxford, 195–214.

Notes

i. Susan was a student on the MSc Leadership in Healthcare.

ii. Mary was also a leadership student.

iii. John-Marc Priest was also a leadership student.

APPENDIX

The classroom critical incident questionnaire (Brookfield [1, p. 115])

The guide invites the student to submit these anonymously. He analyses the responses and gives feedback next session and invites dialogue. Brookfield recognises the benefits of this approach to build trust, alert the group to problems before a disaster occurs and to give the guide feedback about ways he might develop his facilitation.

- At what moment in the class this week did you feel most engaged with what was happening?
- At what moment in the class this week did you feel most distanced from what was happening?
- What action that anyone [teacher or student] took in class did you find most affirming or helpful?
- What action that anyone (teacher or student) took in class this week did you find the most puzzling?
- What about the class surprised you the most? (This could be something about your own reactions to what went on, or something that someone did, or anything else that occurs to you.)

Reference

1. Brookfield, S. (1996) *Becoming A Critically Reflective Teacher*. Jossey-Bass, San Francisco.

INDEX